# Health Education: Theory, Research and Practice

# Health Education: Theory, Research and Practice

Edited by Percy Shields

hayle medical

New York

Hayle Medical,
750 Third Avenue, 9th Floor,
New York, NY 10017, USA

Visit us on the World Wide Web at:
www.haylemedical.com



ISBN: 978-1-63241-434-2

The publisher's policy is to use permanent paper from mills that operate a sustainable forestry policy. Furthermore, the publisher ensures that the text paper and cover boards used have met acceptable environmental accreditation standards.



Printed in the United States of America.

**Cataloging-in-Publication Data**

Health education : theory, research and practice / edited by Percy Shields.
p. cm.
Includes bibliographical references and index.
ISBN 978-1-63241-434-2
1. Health education. 2. Health literacy. 3. Public health. 4. Medical care. I. Shields, Percy.
RA440 .H43 2017
613--dc23

# Table of Contents

# Preface

Every book is a source of knowledge and this one is no exception. The idea that led to the conceptualization of this book was the fact that the world is advancing rapidly; which makes it crucial to document the progress in every field. I am aware that a lot of data is already available, yet, there is a lot more to learn. Hence, I accepted the responsibility of editing this book and contributing my knowledge to the community.

Health education is defined as the area of health concerned with education. Environmental, emotional, physical and social health are some of the key areas of health education. Increased awareness is facilitated by both surveying as well as policy-making. This book outlines the processes and applications of health education in detail. The topics included herein are of utmost significance and bound to provide incredible insights to readers. This book is vital for students and researchers in the field of hospital management, public health and pharmaceutical sciences.

While editing this book, I had multiple visions for it. Then I finally narrowed down to make every chapter a sole standing text explaining a particular topic, so that they can be used independently. However, the umbrella subject sinews them into a common theme. This makes the book a unique platform of knowledge.

I would like to give the major credit of this book to the experts from every corner of the world, who took the time to share their expertise with us. Also, I owe the completion of this book to the never-ending support of my family, who supported me throughout the project.

**Editor**

1

# A National Survey of Skin Infections, Care Behaviors and MRSA Knowledge in the United States

**Jocelyn R. Wilder[1]*, Duane T. Wegener[2], Michael Z. David[1], Charles Macal[1,3], Robert Daum[1], Diane S. Lauderdale[1]**

1 The Department of Health Studies, The University of Chicago, Chicago, Illinois, United States of America, 2 The Department of Psychology, The Ohio State University, Columbus, Ohio, United States of America, 3 Decision and Information Sciences Division, Argonne National Laboratory, Argonne, Illinois, United States of America

## Abstract

A nationally representative sample of approximately 2000 individuals was surveyed to assess SSTI infections over their lifetime and then prospectively over six-months. Knowledge of MRSA, future likelihood to self-treat a SSTI and self-care behaviors was also queried. Chi square tests, linear and multinomial regression were used for analysis. About 50% of those with a reported history of a SSTI typical of MRSA had sought medical treatment. MRSA knowledge was low: 28% of respondents could describe MRSA. Use of protective self-care behaviors that may reduce transmission, such as covering a lesion, differed with knowledge of MRSA and socio-demographics. Those reporting a history of a MRSA-like SSTI were more likely to respond that they would self-treat than those without such a history (OR 2.05 95% CI 1.40, 3.01; $p<0.001$). Since half of respondents reported not seeking care for past lesions, incidence determined from clinical encounters would greatly underestimate true incidence. MRSA knowledge was not associated with seeking medical care, but was associated with self-care practices that may decrease transmission.

**Editor:** Gerardo Chowell, Arizona State University, United States of America

**Funding:** The survey was supported by Time-Sharing Experiments for the Social Sciences program (TESS; National Science Foundation Grant 0818839; J. Freese and P. S. Visser, principal investigators). Analysis was supported by the National Institute of General Medical Sciences (NIGMS) U01 Gm087729 MIDAS. The funders had no role in study design, data collection and analysis, decision to publish, or preparation of the manuscript.

**Competing Interests:** The authors have declared that no competing interests exist.

* Email: jwilder@uchicago.edu

## Introduction

The number of outpatient visits for medical care in the United States for a skin or soft tissue infection (SSTI) is estimated to have risen from 8.6 million in 1997 to 14.2 million in 2005, a 65% increase [1,2]. The increase is likely related to the appearance of new strains of methicillin-resistant *Staphylococcus aureus* (MRSA) spreading among healthy people in the United States. These new strains, recognized in the late 1990s, as Community-Associated MRSA (CA-MRSA), are distinct from older strains of MRSA which were usually confined to healthcare settings and typically infecting patients with previous health care exposures. While SSTIs may be caused by various conditions the majority of CA-MRSA infections are SSTIs that present as either abscesses or cellulitis. CA-MRSA strains likely account for a majority of SSTIs among ambulatory patients in recent years [3–7].

Data on the incidence of SSTIs in the United States are not systematically collected. Even if collected, such data would not represent the true incidence of SSTIs in the general population because we think it is likely that not all SSTIs are brought to medical attention. The changing incidence in SSTIs observed in clinical settings might reflect trends in the overall incidence in the population, but it is also possible that a change in the incidence of clinically attended SSTIs reflects a change in the proportion of individuals with SSTIs who seek medical care. Media attention to CA-MRSA has likely raised popular awareness of the risks of progression of MRSA SSTIs to invasive infections. For example, there was significant media attention and public interest focused on CA-MRSA after a high profile medical publication estimated that in the United States more individuals had died from MRSA than AIDS in 2005 [8–10]. Therefore, it is not certain from current data how prevalent MRSA infections (or SSTIs in general) are in the population, what proportion of such infections present in clinical settings, or whether trends in clinically attended skin infections may be due in part to heightened awareness of MRSA.

We designed a survey to assess how frequently adults in a nationally representative sample reported having ever had a lesion similar to one described in a vignette that was typical of a CA-MRSA SSTI. After six months, respondents were resurveyed and asked about occurrence of described lesion in the six months between the survey waves. For those who reported having a lesion, we asked whether they had sought medical care. The purpose of this study was threefold: (1) to estimate the lifetime prevalence and six-month occurrence of an SSTI similar to a CA-MRSA skin infection; (2) to estimate the proportion of such skin infections brought to medical attention; and (3) to assess whether a past sore and/or knowledge of MRSA influences care-seeking and treatment behaviors, both actual and intended.

## Methods

The survey was supported by the Time-Sharing Experiments for the Social Sciences (TESS) program with funding from the National Science Foundation. Analysis was support by the

National Institute of General Medical Sciences (NIGMS). The survey (File S1) was conducted by Knowledge Network and distributed to their KnowledgePanel. KnowledgePanel is a probability-based Internet panel with a sampling frame of approximately 50,000 individuals (ages 18 and older) who are sampled from the United States Postal Service's Computerized Delivery Sequence file, which comprises approximately 97percent of the physical addresses in all 50 states. Further details for Knowledge Network's Panel design are available at www.knowledgenetworks.com/knpanel/docs/knowledgepanel(R)-design-summary-description.pdf Basic demographic data are collected from all participants when they join the panel. In this study, African American and Hispanic households were oversampled in order to ensure a sufficient sample size to assess differences across major racial/ethnic groups. The data received from Knowledge Network was de-identified. The University of Chicago and The University of Ohio IRBs approved the research.

The initial survey was completed by 1980 adults in August 2011. Six months later, 1379 of the participants in the initial sample completed the follow-up survey.

The descriptions of the lesions represented in the vignettes are typical of abscesses caused by MRSA. The description represents a moderately severe infection and was used to elicit care seeking for a level of severity that a physician would recommend clinical care. At baseline, participants were randomly assigned to receive one of two vignettes that varied in one respect. In one version the SSTI was described as draining pus (Figure 1); it was thought that presence of a draining lesion may influence one's care seeking and self-care behaviors, and in the other vignette, pus was mentioned but the sore was not described as draining (Figure 2). Note that a draining SSTI would have passed through a non-draining phase first, whereas not all non-draining SSTIs progress to a draining phase.

After the description, respondents were asked if they had ever had an SSTI similar to that described and whether they had sought medical care. All respondents were then asked how likely they would be to self-treat such an infection if they experienced it now, using a 9 point rating scale ranging from 1 (not at all likely to self-treat) to 9 (very likely to self-treat). For analysis, self-treatment was collapsed into three levels: 1 (not at all likely to self-treat) through 3 were categorized as likely to seek care, 4 through 6 were categorized as equally likely to seek care or self-treat and 7 through 9 (very likely to self-treat) were categorized as likely to self-treat.

Respondents were asked whether they would use each of three self-care behaviors that may alter the likelihood of MRSA transmission to others: "covering the sore" and "avoid sharing personal items like towels with household members," both of which should decrease risk of transmission, and "try to squeeze out the pus" which may spread bacteria and increase risk of transmission. Respondents were then asked whether they had heard of MRSA and whether they knew what MRSA was. If a respondent indicated that they knew what MRSA was, a free-text box was provided for them to define MRSA. We used the responses to these questions to assign individuals to three mutually exclusive groups: those who had not heard of MRSA ("unaware"), those who had heard of it but did not know what it was ("aware") and those who could define MRSA ("knowledge"). Those in the aware and knowledge groups were asked about the likelihood of the SSTI described earlier being caused by MRSA, using a 9 point rating scale from 1 (not at all likely to be MRSA) to 9 (very likely to be MRSA). They were also asked how many people they knew who had had a MRSA infection.

There was an experiment also embedded in the survey. A random half of the respondents received an informational message based on CDC's MRSA website information. The following questions were asked of those receiving and not receiving the informational message: (1) How likely would you be to seek medical care if you had a sore similar to the one described, with responses ranging from 1 (not at all likely) to 9 (very likely). (2) If left untreated, the consequences of the described sore are: 1 (not serious) to 9 (very serious). (3) How likely is the described sore to be MRSA: 1 (not at all likely) to 9 (very likely). Six months after the initial survey all respondents (both those who had received the MRSA information and those who had not) received a follow-up survey with the same sore description. They were asked if during the prior six months they had had a sore similar to the one described and whether they had sought medical care.

### Data Analysis

The proportions of those with a lifetime and six-month history of SSTIs similar to the description were determined for all respondents and stratified by demographics and other character-

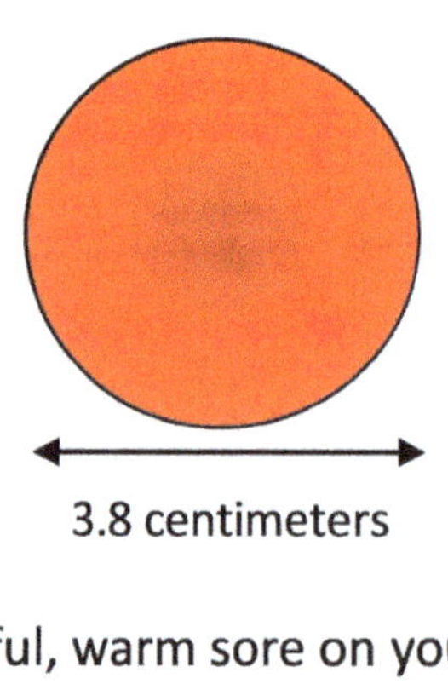


Imagine that you have a red, painful, warm sore on your skin that is about 1.5 inches across. The sore hurts more when you touch it and is starting to ooze thick pus (white liquid). You have had the sore for a few days, and it seems to be getting worse not better

**Figure 1. Description of Draining Sore Vignette.**

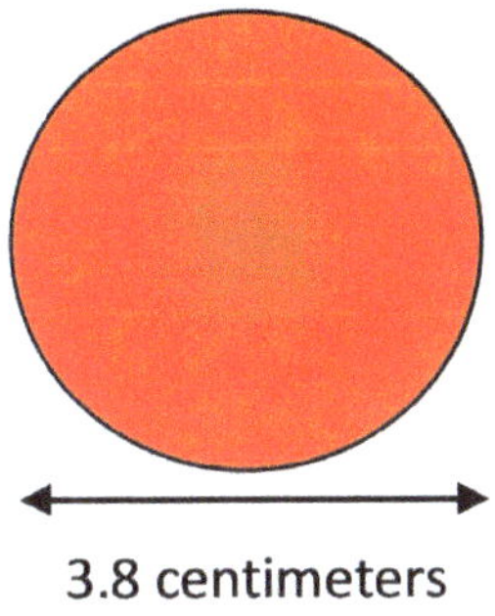


Imagine that you have a red, painful, warm sore on your skin that is about 1.5 inches across. The sore is firm to the touch, hurts more when you touch it, and feels like there might be pus under the skin. You have had the sore for a few days, and it seems to be getting worse not better.

**Figure 2. Description of Non-Draining Sore Vignette.**

istics. Variation in seeking medical care was examined by individual characteristics, including knowledge of MRSA. Variation in intention to self-treat and use of self-care behaviors were examined by lesion history, socio-demographics, and MRSA knowledge. Significance in differences between groups was assessed by chi-square tests for categorical and dichotomous variables and by linear regression for continuous variables. Age and income were tested for linear trend in proportions using linear regression. Covariates that were significantly associated with the dependent or exposure variables at $p<0.10$ were included in the multivariable models.

Logistic regression was used to identify factors related to having had a previous sore. A multinomial logistic regression model was used to determine whether history of a previous lesion was associated independently either with intention to seek medical care or with intention to self-treat, each compared to those who responded in the middle of the scale (noncommittal as to whether they would self-treat or not). The model is adjusted for characteristics associated with care-seeking. All analyses used sampling weights to adjust raw responses and generate estimates representative of the U.S. population. Data were analyzed in STATA 12, and all analyses use variances for weighted survey data.

## Results

Demographic characteristics of the initial sample of 1980 adult respondents and the 1376 that completed the six-month follow-up survey are presented in Table 1. Those that participated in the six-month follow-up had similar demographic characteristics to those who participated in the initial survey. Although the informational message that half of respondents received at the end of the initial survey had an immediate influence on perceptions of the severity of a SSTI, compared to those who did not receive the message, (mean 7.67 vs. 7.08, $F=18.09$, $p<0.001$) and on the likelihood that a sore such as that described was MRSA (mean 6.36 vs. 5.54, $F=58.24$, $p<0.001$), neither effects persisted over the 6-month period. Nor was there any difference in care seeking for those who had a sore in the six months between the surveys ($\chi2=0.03$, $p=0.87$). Therefore, we have combined all responses from the six-month follow up in this report.

### Lifetime Prevalence and Incidence of SSTIs Typical of CA-MRSA

Table 2 displays the lifetime prevalence and six month incidence of lesions. Thirteen percent of respondents reported having had a lesion similar to the one described prior to the survey, 53% of those with a previous lesion responded that they had not sought medical care. Respondents with lower household income were more likely to respond that they had a previous lesion ($p^{trend}<0.001$) than those with higher household incomes. In the follow-up survey, 6% of respondents reported having had an SSTI in the six months between the initial and the follow-up survey. Among those with an SSTI in this interval, 48 percent had not sought medical treatment. In the logistic regression displayed in Table 3, after adjusting for, gender, age, race/ethnicity, education, income and having a regular health care provider, significant factors associated with reporting a previous sore were having a household income below 60,000 ($p<0.05$) and having a regular care provider ($p=0.03$). Hispanic race was marginally significant ($p=0.05$). In the second wave, Hispanics were more likely to respond that they had had a lesion in the past six months than Whites ($p<0.001$).

### Associations with MRSA Knowledge

MRSA knowledge varied significantly by gender, race/ethnicity, age, household income and education (Table 4). The majority of respondents reported that they had heard of MRSA (53%); approximately half of those (28% of all respondents) could define MRSA. Since definitions were almost all plausible, we did not divide them into more or less correct ones. Correlates of awareness and knowledge were similar. Women, Whites, and those with higher education and greater income were all more likely to have both awareness and knowledge.

**Table 1.** Demographic Characteristics of Survey Respondents, Weighted to Reflect the National Population.

| | Initial survey | | Follow-up survey | |
|---|---|---|---|---|
| **Variables** | **Weighted % (N)** | **95% CI** | **Weighted % (N)** | **95% CI** |
| **All** | 100.0 (1980) | | 100.0 (1376) | |
| *SOCIODEMOGRAPHIC FACTORS* | | | | |
| **Gender** | | | | |
| Male | 48.3 (964) | 45.5, 51.2 | 49.8 (689) | 46.4, 53.2 |
| Female | 51.7 (1016) | 48.8, 54.5 | 50.2 (687) | 46.8, 53.6 |
| **Age, years** | | | | |
| 18–29 | 21.7 (355) | 19.9, 24.3 | 19.8 (216) | 17.0, 23.0 |
| 30–44 | 26.0 (508) | 23.6, 28.6 | 24.5 (333) | 21.7, 27.5 |
| 45–59 | 27.7 (602) | 25.3, 30.2 | 28.5 (436) | 25.7 31.6 |
| ≥60 | 24.6 (515) | 22.3, 27.1 | 27.2 (391) | 24.3, 30.2 |
| **Race/Ethnicity** | | | | |
| Non-Hispanic White | 67.9 (1077) | 65.4, 70.3 | 69.7 (789) | 66.7, 72.5 |
| Non-Hispanic Black | 11.5 (406) | 10,2, 12.9 | 10.4 (262) | 8.9, 12.0 |
| Hispanic | 13.9 (409) | 12.3, 15.7 | 13.4 (265) | 11.5, 15.5 |
| Non-Hispanic Other | 6.7 (88) | 5.2, 8.5 | 6.5 (60) | 4.9, 8.8 |
| **Education** | | | | |
| ≤High school | 43.7 (890) | 40.9, 46.5 | 42.4 (612) | 54.3, 60.9 |
| >High school | 56.3 (1090) | 53.3, 59.1 | 57.6 (764) | 39.1, 45.7 |
| **Household Income** | | | | |
| <20 k | 16.3 (329) | 14.4, 18.5 | 14.1 (199) | 11.9. 16.5 |
| 20 k-<40 k | 23.1 (429) | 20..7, 25.6 | 23.8 (289) | 21.0, 26.9 |
| 40 k-<60 k | 16.8 (358) | 14.7, 19.1 | 16.3 (232) | 14,0, 19.0 |
| ≥60 k | 894 (43.8) | 41.0, 46.6 | 45.8 (656) | 42.2, 49.2 |
| **Geography** | | | | |
| Non metropolitan area | 16.1 (286) | 14.1, 18.3 | 15.9 (197) | 13.5, 18.5 |
| Metropolitan area | 83.9 (1694) | 81.7, 85.9 | 84.1 (1179) | 81.5, 86.5 |
| **Children in Home** | | | | |
| No children | 67.3(1,286) | 64.6, 69.8 | 69.7 (935) | 66.6, 72.7 |
| Children | 32.7 (694) | 30.2, 35.4 | 30.3 (441) | 27.3, 33.4 |
| **Health care provider** | | | | |
| No regular provider | 20.4 (366) | 18.1, 22.9 | 21.2 (253) | 18.4, 24.3 |
| Regular provider | 79.6 (1589) | 77.1, 81.9 | 78.8 (1109) | 75.7, 81.6 |
| *MRSA-RELATED FACTORS FROM INITIAL SURVEY* | | | | |
| **Knowledge of MRSA** | | | | |
| MRSA unaware | 46.7 (921) | 43.9, 49.0 | 46.7 (643) | 43.3, 50.1 |
| MRSA aware | 24.9 (486) | 22.5, 27.4 | 25.7 (346) | 22.8, 28.7 |
| MRSA knowledge | 28.3 (28.3) | 25.9, 30.9 | 27.6 (393) | 24.7, 30.7 |
| **Knew someone who had MRSA** | | | | |
| Does not know | 59.9 (633) | 56.0, 63.6 | 57.6 (436) | 53.0, 62.1 |
| Knows someone | 40.1 (415) | 36.4, 44.0 | 42.4 (302) | 37.9, 47.0 |

TESS Survey 2011.

## Draining Vignette vs. Non-draining vignette

There was not a significant difference in care seeking among those with lesions that resembled the draining vignette compared to those with lesions that resembled the non-draining vignette. The likelihood of self-treatment for a hypothetical lesion was slightly lower among those who had a draining vignettes compared to those with a non-draining vignette (draining mean 4.4 vs. non-draining mean 4.7; $p = 0.04$) (Table 4). Additionally, those who received the draining vignette were significantly more likely to report that they would cover the lesion (67.4% vs. 57.7%, $p < 0.001$) and avoid sharing

**Table 2.** Lifetime Prevalence and Subsequent Six-month Occurrence of SSTIs similar to CA-MRSA by Selected Characteristics.

| | Lifetime Prevalence (%) | 95% CI | *p* value | 6 month Prevalence (%) | 95% CI | *p*-value |
|---|---|---|---|---|---|---|
| **All** | 13.5 | 11.7, 15.5 | | 6.2 | 4.8, 8.0 | |
| Sought Medical Care | 47.2 | 39.8, 54.7 | | 52.0 | 38.4, 64.7 | |
| Self-Care | 53.0 | 45.3, 60.3 | | 48.0 | 35.3, 61.6 | |
| *SOCIO-DEMOGRAPHIC FACTORS* | | | | | | |
| **Gender** | | | 0.95 | | | 0.65 |
| Male | 13.5 | 11.2, 16.5 | | 5.8 | 4.0, 8.3 | |
| Female | 13.4 | 11.0, 16.3 | | 6.5 | 4.5, 9.3 | |
| **Race/Ethnicity** | | | 0.07 | | | <0.001 |
| Non-Hispanic White | 11.8 | 9.7, 14.2 | | 4.1 | 2.7, 6.2 | |
| Non-Hispanic Black | 16.3 | 12.3, 21.3 | | 6.7 | 4.1, 10.7 | |
| Hispanic | 18.3 | 13.8, 23.7 | | 11.8 | 7.7, 17.6 | |
| Non-Hispanic Other | 16.3 | 8.8, 18.2 | | 14.8 | 6.5, 29.0 | |
| **Age, years** | | | 0.67 | | | 0.22 |
| 18–29 | 14.0 | 10.0, 19.3 | | 8.1 | 4.6, 13.9 | |
| 30–44 | 14.9 | 11.4, 19.2 | | 7.7 | 4.9, 12.0 | |
| 45–59 | 13.4 | 10.4, 17.1 | | 4.5 | 2.9, 6.9 | |
| ≥60 | 11.6 | 8.6, 15.5 | | 4.7 | 2.7, 8.2 | |
| **Education** | | | 0.73 | | | 0.99 |
| ≤High school | 13.9 | 11.2, 17.0 | | 6.2 | 4.1, 9.3 | |
| >High school | 13.2 | 10.9, 15.9 | | 6.2 | 4.5, 8.5 | |
| **Income** | | | $p^{trend}<0.01$ | | | $p^{trend}=0.06$ |
| <20 k | 17.3 | 12.9, 22.8 | | 10.7 | 6.5, 17.3 | |
| 20 K-<40 k | 14.8 | 11.0, 19.7 | | 7.0 | 4.2, 11.3 | |
| 40 k-<60 k | 16.9 | 12.3, 22.8 | | 4.0 | 1.8, 8.9 | |
| ≥60 k | 10.0 | 7.9, 12.8 | | 5.0 | 3.2, 7.5 | |
| **Geography** | | | 0.90 | | | 0.41 |
| Non metropolitan area | 2.2 | 1.5, 3.3 | | 1.7 | | |
| Metropolitan area | 11.5 | 9.6, 13.1 | | 11.2 | | |

TESS Survey 2011.

personal items (67.2% vs. 55.1%, $p<0.001$) than those who received the non-draining vignette.

## Determinants of Self-Care Behaviors and Intention to Self-Treat

Reported intention to use at least one the three specific self-care behaviors that may affect MRSA transmission varied by socio-demographic characteristics. However, the only significant demographic predictor of avoiding sharing personal items was having children in the home ($p = 0.02$) (Table 5). MRSA knowledge was significantly related to all three self-care behaviors; those who reported knowledge of MRSA were more likely to report intentions to use behaviors associated with lower transmission risk: covering a lesion ($p<0.01$) and avoiding sharing personal items ($p<0.001$).

In univariate analyses, the likelihood of self-treatment was higher for respondents who were younger in age ($p^{trend} = 0.01$), did not have a regular health care provider ($p = 0.001$) or had a history of an SSTI ($p = 0.001$). The intention to self-treat decreased as household income increased ($p^{trend}<0.001$). Among those with awareness or knowledge of MRSA, the likelihood of self-treating was lower among those who believed the lesion was caused by MRSA ($p<0.001$).

A stepwise multinomial logistic model indicates, after adjusting for, gender, age, race, ethnicity, education, income and having a regular health care provider, that those with a previous lesion were twice as likely to self-treat (RR = 2.09 95% CI 1.41, 3.01; $p<$ 0.004) and half as likely to seek care (RR = 0.53, 95% CI 0.34, 0.82; $p = 0.004$), compared to those who were noncommittal as to whether they would seek care or self-treat (Table 6). Women were less likely to self-treat (RR = 1.37; 95%CI 1.04, 1.80, $p = 0.02$). Increasing age strongly predicted increased care-seeking. Having a lower income was associated with a higher intent to self treat (RR = 1.72; 95%CI 1.07, 2.76 $p = 0.03$). Those with a regular physician were less likely to self-treat (RR 0.64; 95%CI 0.44, 0.95, $p = 0.03$).

## Discussion

This nationally representative survey suggests that estimating the occurrence of SSTIs typical of CA-MRSA just from those presenting with lesions at ambulatory care settings would underestimate the true occurrence of SSTIs in the population

**Table 3.** Logistic Regression Analysis for Factors associated with having a previous sore.

| Variables | Unadjusted OR (95% CI) | p-values | Adjusted OR (95% CI) | p-value |
|---|---|---|---|---|
| **Gender** | | | | |
| Male | 1.00 | | 1.00 | |
| Female | 0.99 (0.12, 0.20) | 0.96 | 0.94 (0.98, 1.31) | 0.73 |
| **Age (per year)** | 1.00 (0.99, 1.01) | 0.38 | 0.99 (0.98, 1.01 | 0.26 |
| **Race** | | | | |
| White | 1.00 (Ref) | | 1.00 (Ref) | |
| Black | 1.47 (0.99, 2.18) | 0.05 | 1.30 (0.83, 1.97) | 0.26 |
| Hispanic | 1.67 (1.13, 2.49) | 0.01 | 1.53 (0.99, 2.36) | 0.05 |
| Other | 1.46 (0.70, 3.05) | 0.31 | 1.46 (0.69, 3.07) | 0.33 |
| **Education** | | | | |
| <High School | 1.00 (Ref) | | 1.00 (Ref) | |
| High School graduate plus | 0.94 (0.68, 1.31) | 0.83 | 1.17 (0.80, 1.71) | 0.41 |
| **Income** | | | | |
| <20 k | 1.87 (1.21, 2.91) | 0.01 | 1.96 (1.18, 3.26) | 0.01 |
| 20 k-<40 k | 1.56 (1.00, 2.41) | 0.05 | 1.66 (1.03, 2.62 | 0.04 |
| 40 k-<60 k | 1.83 (1.15, 2.89) | 0.01 | 1.92 (1.20, 3.06) | 0.01 |
| ≥60 k | 1.00 (Ref) | | 1.00 (Ref) | |
| **Health Care Provider** | | | | |
| No Regular Health Care Provider | 1.00 (Ref) | | 1.00 (Ref) | |
| Regular Health Care Provider | 1.38 (0.88, 2.18) | 0.16 | 1.72 (1.05, 2.81) | 0.03 |

and probably misrepresent the descriptive epidemiology of SSTIs. We found that about half of individuals reporting a lifetime history of an SSTI similar to a moderately severe CA-MRSA infection had not sought medical care. Similarly, about half of individuals with such a lesion in the subsequent six-month period also reported that they had not sought medical care. MRSA knowledge was not related to care-seeking. Therefore there is no evidence here to suggest that the reported increase in the numbers of SSTIs, based on clinical encounter data is an artifact of increased awareness of the seriousness of MRSA in the United States [8].

We believe these data represent the first nationwide estimates of the occurrence of SSTIs typical of CA-MRSA lesions in the United States among adults, as well as care-seeking behaviors related to these SSTIs. While our findings cannot be used to precisely adjust the numbers seen in the clinical setting to determine true population incidence, they do suggest that roughly twice the number of infections that present in clinical settings are occurring in the population. To date there are no studies that try to elucidate the proportion of SSTIs that are not brought to the attention of a health care provider.

Our findings of lifetime history and six-month incidence are not consistent with each other: lifetime history reported in the first survey (13%) was double the subsequent six-month occurrence (6%), although one would expect it to be much larger. There are a number of possible explanations. The first may be recall bias: respondents may have underreported SSTIs in the first survey because these may not be memorable health events. The other possibility is that a secular increase in the incidence of CA-MRSA SSTIs in part explains this striking contrast. That is, if a large majority of these infections have occurred relatively recently, then lifetime history might more closely reflect recent history. The first survey may have heightened awareness of SSTIs and contributed to more complete recall six months later (or perhaps even over-identification of lesions during the six-month period). It could also be that the lesions recur reasonably often for the same people and that a relatively large proportion of those who have had such lesions in recent years had a recurrence during the six month period [11]. In other words, because the incidence of such infections is not purely random, one would not interpret the proportion of infections during the six months to suggest that a different 6 percent of the population would get such infections during each six-month period. In any case, the six-month data suggest very high rates of SSTIs similar to CA-MRSA infections in the general U.S. population. Extrapolating from the six-month data and assuming 0–100 percent recurrence in the next six months, somewhere between 6 percent and 12 percent of the U.S. population would have an SSTI similar to those described in our vignettes annually. If the non-responders to the second survey wave were all assumed to have not had an infection, then the estimate would be 4 percent to 8 percent.

The adjusted multinomial regression suggests that intention to self-treat was approximately twice as high among those with experience of a previous lesion. Why previous lesions actually decrease the likelihood of seeking professional care is unclear, although those whose sores resolved without complications may feel there is no gain to professional care. In addition, those without a regular doctor were significantly more likely to self-treat, and it is estimated that about one in five in the United States do not have a usual source of care [12]. Thus reported socioeconomic disparities in MRSA incidence likely underestimate true disparities.

**Table 4.** Demographic Characteristics by Knowledge of MRSA.

| Variables | MRSA UNAWARE (N = 921) | | MRSA AWARENESS[a] (N = 486) | | MRSA KNOWLEDGE[b] (N = 565) | | |
|---|---|---|---|---|---|---|---|
| | Weighted distribution (%) | 95% CI | Weighted distribution (%) | 95% CI | Weighted distribution (%) | 95% CI | *p*-value |
| **All** | 46.7 | 43.9, 49.6 | 24.7 | 22.5, 27.4 | 28.6 | 25.9, 30.9 | |
| ***SOCIO-DEMOGRAPHIC FACTORS*** | | | | | | | |
| **Gender** | | | | | | | <0.003 |
| Male | 50.1 | 46.1, 54.2 | 26.1 | 22.7, 29.9 | 23.8 | 20.5, 27.4 | |
| Female | 43.6 | 39.8, 47.6 | 23.8 | 20.5, 27.3 | 32.6 | 29.1, 36.4 | |
| **Race/Ethnicity** | | | | | | | <0.001 |
| Non-Hispanic White | 40.5 | 37.0, 44.1 | 26.6 | 23.5, 29.9 | 32.9 | 29.7, 36.4 | |
| Non-Hispanic Black | 51.5 | 45.3, 57.5 | 26.6 | 21.5, 32.5 | 21.9 | 17.4, 27.2 | |
| Hispanic | 67.6 | 61.6, 73.1 | 18.1 | 14.0, 23.0 | 14.3 | 10.4, 19.4 | |
| Non-Hispanic Other | 58.7 | 46.1, 70.2 | 19.4 | 11.4, 31.1 | 21.9 | 13.6, 33.3 | |
| **Age, years** | | | | | | | 0.007 |
| 18–29 | 48.0 | 40.4, 54.8 | 28.1 | 22.3, 34.6 | 23.9 | 18.4, 30.4 | |
| 30–44 | 54.0 | 48.5, 59.3 | 19.1 | 15.2, 23.7 | 27.0 | 22.6, 31.9 | |
| 45–59 | 41.6 | 36.6, 46.7 | 24.9 | 20.7, 29.5 | 33.6 | 28.9, 38.5 | |
| ≥60 | 43.8 | 38.4, 49.4 | 28.3 | 23.7, 33.5 | 27.9 | 23.3, 33.0 | |
| **Education** | | | | | | | <.001 |
| ≤High school | 52.5 | 48.3, 56.7 | 26.8 | 23.2, 30.7 | 20.7 | 17.4, 24.3 | |
| >High school | 42.3 | 38.5, 46.2 | 23.5 | 20.4, 26.9 | 34.3 | 30.8, 37.9 | |
| **Household Income** | | | | | | | <.0001 |
| <20 k | 53.4 | 46.6, 60.1 | 27.2 | 21.7, 33.6 | 19.4 | 14.5–25.5 | |
| 20 k-<40 k | 53.6 | 47.6, 59.6 | 26.1 | 21.1, 31.8 | 20.3 | 15.8–25.6 | |
| 40 k-<60 k | 47.3 | 40.3, 54.4 | 24.4 | 18.8, 31.1 | 28.3 | 22.6–34.9 | |
| ≥60 k | 40.5 | 36.4, 44.7 | 23.6 | 20.2, 27.4 | 35.9 | 32.0–40.1 | |
| **Geography** | | | | | | | 0.06 |
| Non-Metropolitan Area | 40.4 | 33.5, 47.6 | 31.2 | 24.9, 38.2 | 28.4 | 22.4, 35.4 | |
| Metropolitan Area | 48.0 | 44.9, 51.1 | 23.7 | 21.2, 26.4 | 28.3 | 26.7, 31.2 | |
| **Children in Home** | | | | | | | 0.23 |
| No children | 48.1 | 44.6, 51.6 | 25.0 | 22.1, 28.2 | 26.9 | 24.0, 30.0 | |
| Children | 44.0 | 39.3, 48.8 | 24.6 | 20.7, 29.1 | 31.4 | 27.0, 36.1 | |
| **Regular Health Care provider** | | | | | | | $p = 0.003$ |
| No regular provider | 54.5 | 47.8, 61.0 | 26.1 | 20.7, 32.4 | 19.4 | 14.7, 25.3 | |
| Regular provider | 44.7 | 41.6, 47.8 | 24.7 | 22.1, 27.6 | 30.6 | 27.8, 33.6 | |

TESS Survey 2011.
[a]MRSA Awareness is having heard of MRSA but unable to define MRSA.
[b]MRSA Knowledge is the ability to define MRSA.

**Table 5.** Weighted Percentages of Affirmative Reponses to Intention to Self-Treat a MRSA-like Sore and Use of Specific Self Care Behaviors.

| | Likely to Self-Treat (Weighted Means of 9-point scale) | Cover Sore (Weighted %) | Avoid sharing personal items (Weighted %) | Squeeze pus from Sore (Weighted %) |
|---|---|---|---|---|
| **All** | 4.59 | 62.53 | 61.11 | 55.01 |
| *SOCIO-DEMOGRAPHIC FACTORS* | | | | |
| **Gender** | | | | |
| Female | 4.46 | 63.86 | 63.16 | 48.01 |
| Male | 4.73 | 61.12 | 58.93 | 62.50 |
| | F = 3.66, t = −1.91, $p = 0.05$ | $p = 0.32$ | $p = 0.14$ | $p < 0.001$ |
| **Race** | | | | |
| Non-Hispanic White | 4.54 | 67.17 | 61.00 | 54.09 |
| Non-Hispanic Black | 4.39 | 54.91 | 61.83 | 53.28 |
| Hispanic | 4.76 | 41.68 | 57.34 | 61.05 |
| Non-Hispanic Other | 5.03 | 71.93 | 68.83 | 54.79 |
| | F = .93, t = 1.66, $p = .33$ | $p < 0.001$ | $p = 0.31$ | $p = 0.35$ |
| **Age** | | | | |
| 18–29 yrs. | 4.84 | 63.65 | 57.54 | 62.95 |
| 30–44 yrs. | 4.69 | 60.14 | 62.44 | 58.79 |
| 45–59 yrs. | 4.70 | 63.80 | 62.17 | 55.55 |
| ≥60 yrs. | 4.15 | 62.67 | 61.67 | 43.43 |
| | F = 8.69, t = −2.95, $p^{trend} = 0.01$ | $p^{trend}$ 0 = .91 | $p^{trend} = 0.40$ | $p^{trend} < 0.001$ |
| **Education** | | | | |
| ≤High School | 4.69 | 58.2 | 59.8 | 56.9 |
| >High School | 4.52 | 65.9 | 62.1 | 52.2 |
| | F = 5.67, t = −2.38, $p = 0.07$ | $p = 0.005$ | $p = 0.41$ | $p = 0.13$ |
| **Health care provider** | | | | |
| No regular physician | 5.06 | 65.49 | 58.59 | 60.37 |
| Regular Physician | 4.47 | 61.82 | 61.89 | 53.96 |
| | F = 11.79, $p < 0.001$ | $p = 0.30$ | $p = 0.37$ | $p = 0.09$ |
| **Income** | | | | |
| <20 k | 4.84 | 49.12 | 58.98 | 52.95 |
| 20 k-<40 k | 4.79 | 63.20 | 63.02 | 53.25 |
| 40 k-<60 k | 4.88 | 64.90 | 58.16 | 52.13 |
| ≥60 k | 4.29 | 66.28 | 62.04 | 55.01 |
| | F = 10.43, $p^{trend} < 0.001$ | $p^{trend} < 0.001$ | $p^{trend} < 0.68$ | $p^{trend} < 0.15$ |
| **Geography** | | | | |
| Non Metropolitan Area | 4.82 | 68.14 | 62.43 | 51.44 |
| Metropolitan Area | 4..54 | 61.49 | 60.86 | 55.70 |
| | F = 2.15, $p = 0.09$ | $p = 0.07$ | $p = 0.68$ | $p = 0.28$ |
| **Children in Home** | | | | |
| No children in Home | 4.52 | 62.74 | 58.84 | 54.16 |
| Children in Home | 4.73 | 62.11 | 65.79 | 56.78 |
| | F = 2.11, $p = 0.15$ | $p = 0.83$ | $p = 0.02$ | $p = 0.39$ |
| *MRSA-RELATED FACTORS* | | | | |
| **MRSA knowledge** | | | | |
| MRSA Unaware | 4.58 | 58.43 | 57.52 | 56.35 |
| MRSA Aware | 4.75 | 63.70 | 58.44 | 58.23 |
| MRSA Knowledge | 4.42 | 68.62 | 70.17 | 50.22 |
| | F = 1.89, $p = 0.15$ | $p < 0.01$ | $p < 0.001$ | $p = 0.08$ |
| **Received draining vignette** | | | | |

**Table 5.** Cont.

| | Likely to Self-Treat (Weighted Means of 9-point scale) | Cover Sore (Weighted %) | Avoid sharing personal items (Weighted %) | Squeeze pus from Sore (Weighted %) |
|---|---|---|---|---|
| Non-Draining | 4.73 | 57.71 | 55.05 | 55.96 |
| Draining | 4.44 | 67.35 | 67.16 | 54.07 |
| | F = 4.18, *p* = 0.04 | *p* < 0.001 | *p* < 0.001 | *p* = 0.51 |
| **Lifetime Prevalence of sore** | | | | |
| No previous lesion | 4.40 | 63.93 | 61.61 | 54.06 |
| Previous lesion | 5.80 | 55.31 | 59.72 | 62.40 |
| | F = 54.78, *p* < *0.001* | *p* = 0.03 | *p* = 0.63 | *p* = 0.04 |
| **Knew someone who had MRSA[a]** | | | | |
| No | 4.74 | 64.19 | 63.61 | 58.24 |
| Yes | 4.39 | 69.13 | 65.90 | 48.01 |
| | F = 3.49, *p* = 0.06 | *p* = 0.19 | *p* = 0.56 | *p* = 0.01 |
| **Likelihood of Sore being MRSA** | | | | |
| Sore is not MRSA[b] | 5.42 | 59.8 | 60.3 | 57.9 |
| Sore is MRSA[c] | 4.22 | 69.2 | 64.0 | 50.3 |
| | F = 16.72, *p* < 0.001 | P0 = .04 | p = 0.46 | p = 0.13 |

[a]Among those who were aware of MRSA and those who could define MRSA.
[b]Those who responded 1(very unlikely) through 3 to the likelihood of the sore being MRSA.
[c]Those who responded 7 through 9 (very likely) to the likelihood of the sore being MRSA.

**Table 6.** Multinomial Regression Analysis of Intention to Self-treat.

| Variables | Intention to Self-treat | | | | |
|---|---|---|---|---|---|
| | More likely to seek care | *p*-values | Equally likely to seek care or self-treat | More likely to self-treat | *p*-values |
| | RR (95% CI) | | | RR (95% CI) | |
| **Lesion History** | | | | | |
| No previous lesion | 1.00 (Ref) | | 1.00 | 1.00 (Ref) | |
| Previous lesion | 0.53 (0.34, 0.82) | 0.004 | 1.00 | 2.09 (1.40, 3.07) | <0.001 |
| **Female** | 1.37 (1.04, 1.80) | 0.02 | 1.00 | 1.14 (0.84, 1.53)c | 0.42 |
| **Age (per year)** | 1.02 (1.01, 1.92) | <0.001 | 1.00 | 1.01 (1.00, 1.02) | 0.005 |
| **Race/Ethnicity** | | | | | |
| White | 1.00 (Ref) | | 1.00 | 1.00 (Ref) | |
| Black | 1.35 (0.95, 1.92) | 0.10 | 1.00 | 1.02 (0.68, 1.55) | 0.92 |
| Hispanic | 0.99 (0.68, 1.45) | 0.98 | 1.00 | 0.81 (0.53, 1.22) | 0.41 |
| Other | 0.83 (0.41, 1.67) | 0.60 | 1.00 | 1.10 (0.58, 2.07) | 0.78 |
| **Education** | | | | | |
| <High School | 1.00 (Ref) | | 1.00 | 1.00 (Ref) | |
| High School graduate plus | 0.97 (0.72, 1.29) | 0.83 | 1.00 | 0.80 (0.57, 1.12) | 0.19 |
| **Income** | | | | | |
| <20 k | 0.94 (0.61, 1.45) | 0.81 | 1.00 | 1.89 (1.21, 2.95) | 0.03 |
| 20 k-<40 k | 0.77 (0.53, 1.09) | 0.15 | 1.00 | 1.10 (0.72, 1.67)c | 0.67 |
| 40 k-<60 k | 0.70 (0.47, 1.03) | 0.07 | 1.00 | 1.10 (0.70, 1.77)c | 0.69 |
| ≥60 k | 1.00 (Ref) | | 1.00 | 1.00 (Ref) | |
| **Health Care Provider** | | | | | |
| No Regular Health Care Provider | 1.00 (Ref) | | 1.00 | 1.00 (Ref) | |
| Regular Health Care Provider | 1.15 (0.77, 1.70) | 0.50 | 1.00 | 0.64 (0.44, 0.95) | 0.03 |

Increased MRSA knowledge did not increase the likelihood of seeking care, although there was a trend towards significance for knowing someone who had had a MRSA infection being more likely to seek care (among respondents who were aware of MRSA). However, MRSA knowledge was strongly associated with the use of self-care behaviors likely to reduce MRSA transmission (covering an SSTI, not squeezing pus from an SSTI and avoiding sharing personal items with household members) suggesting there is a role for public health information to affect transmission of CA-MRSA.

This study has limitations that should be acknowledged. Respondents' reported SSTIs may have been caused by conditions other than MRSA. However our estimate that about 50% of those with similar SSTIs sought care should apply to all etiologies of similarly severe sores. We only assessed prior history of SSTIs typical of CA-MRSA infection by self-report, and we do not know if the respondents' previous SSTIs were due to CA-MRSA. While the description was of a moderately severe SSTI typical of MRSA; milder SSTIs may also be caused by MRSA and would not have been captured in our survey. Furthermore, the self-report of lesions may be affected by recall bias, respondents with comorbidities or other symptoms may be more likely to recall previous lesions which may also be related to care-seeking. Because of the relatively low incidence of infection, we are primarily examining specific self-care behaviors for a hypothetical SSTI and cannot necessarily assume that these behaviors would be the same in the event that a respondent was faced with an actual SSTI. Although the internet panel is based on United States Postal Service's Computerized Delivery Sequence file, there may be differences among those who agree to take part in the panel; however recruitment of participants is done across a large population and may capture a greater proportion of the population compared to telephone sampling. Our survey over-samples African American and Hispanic individuals, allowing estimates of group rates. Furthermore, while SSTIs have various etiologies, the study highlights that approximately half of those with SSTIs do not seek care. We are unaware of any other data about the occurrence of SSTIs among a nationally representative sample in the United States.

## Conclusions

Our data suggest the magnitude of SSTI incidence in the population is greater than estimates based on patients who have sought medical care. We found that roughly 50% of people with a moderately severe SSTI said that they had or would care for such a lesion themselves and not seek medical care. A large proportion of the population is unaware of MRSA and only about a quarter of adults in the U.S. could define MRSA. Intention to self-treat was not influenced by knowledge of MRSA, and thus increasing knowledge of MRSA is unlikely to explain much of the apparent increase in incidence in the United States. While knowing what MRSA is does not seem to be associated with seeking care, it is associated with self-care behaviors that may reduce the transmission of MRSA, and thus public health informational campaigns could reduce transmission.

## Author Contributions

Conceived and designed the experiments: DW MD RD CM DL JRW. Analyzed the data: JRW. Wrote the paper: JRW. Reviewed and revised for important intellectual content: MD DW DL.

## References


1. Edelsberg J, Taneja C, Zervos M, Haque N, Moore C, et al. (2009) Trends in U.S. hospital admissions for skin and soft tissue infections. Emerging Infectious Diseases 15: 1516–1528.
2. Hersh AL, Chambers HF, Maselli JH, & Gonzales R. (2008) National trends in ambulatory visits and antibiotic prescribing for skin and soft-tissue infections. Archives of Internal Medicine 168:1585–1591.
3. Chen AE, Goldstein M, Carroll K, Song X, Perl TM, et al. (2006) Evolving epidemiology of pediatric *Staphylococcus aureus* cutaneous infections in a Baltimore hospital. Pediatric Emergency Care 22:717–723.
4. Kaplan SL, Hulten KG, Gonzalez BE, Hammerman WA, Lamberth L, et al. (2005) Three-year surveillance of community-acquired *Staphylococcus aureus* infections in children. Clinical Infectious Diseases 40: 1785–1795.
5. Moran GJ, Krishnadasan A, Gorwitz RJ, Fosheim GE, McDougal LK, et al. (2006) Methicillin-resistant *S. aureus* infections among patients in the emergency department. The New England Journal of Medicine 355: 666–674.
6. Purcell K, Fergie J (2005) Epidemic of community-acquired methicillin-resistant *Staphylococcus Aureus* infections: a 14-year study at Driscoll Children's Hospital. Archives of Pediatrics & Adolescent Medicine 159: 980–985.
7. Talan DA, Krishnadasan A, Gorwitz RJ, Fosheim GE, Limbago B, et al. (2011) Comparison of *Staphylococcus Aureus* from skin and soft-tissue infections in US emergency department patients, 2004 and 2008. Clinical Infectious Diseases 53: 144–149.
8. Klevens RM, Morrison MA, Nadle J, Petit S, Gershman K, et al. (2007) Invasive methicillin-resistant *Staphylococcus Aureus* infections in the United States. The Journal of the American Medical Association 298: 1763–1771.
9. Hahn W, Morley CP, Morrow C, Epling JW (2009) The effect of media attention on concern for and medical management of methicillin-resistant *Staphylococcus Aureus*: a multimethod study. Journal of Public Health Management and Practice 15: 150–159.
10. Dukic VM, David MZ, Lauderdale DS (2011) Internet queries and methicillin-resistant *Staphylococcus aureus* surveillance. Emerging Infectious Diseases 17: 1068–1070.
11. Cenizal M, Skiest D, Luber S (2007) Prospective randomized trial of empiric therapy with Trimethoprim-Sulfamethoxazole or Doxycycline for outpatient skin and soft tissue infections in an area of high prevalence of Methicillin-resistant *Staphylococcus aureus*. Antimicrobial Agents and Chemotherapy 51, 2628–2360.
12. Kirby JB (20 December 2010) Main reason for not having a usual source of care by race, ethnicity, income, and insurance status, 2007. Agency for Healthcare Research and Quality, Rockville, MD. Available: http://meps.ahrq.gov/mepsweb/data_files/publications/st308/stat308.pdf. Accessed 17 July 2014.

2

# Compliance of Disease Awareness Campaigns in Printed Dutch Media with National and International Regulatory Guidelines

**Teresa Leonardo Alves[1], Auramarina F. Martins de Freitas[1], Martine E. C. van Eijk[2], Aukje K. Mantel-Teeuwisse[1]***

1 World Health Organization Collaborating Centre for Pharmaceutical Policy and Regulation, Utrecht Institute for Pharmaceutical Sciences (UIPS), Utrecht University, Utrecht, The Netherlands, 2 Independent Consultant, Utrecht, The Netherlands

## Abstract

***Background:*** The European legislation prohibits prescription-only medicines' advertising but allows pharmaceutical companies to provide information to the public on health and diseases, provided there is no direct or indirect reference to a pharmaceutical product. Various forms of promotion have become increasingly common in Europe including "disease-oriented" campaigns.

***Objectives:*** To explore examples of disease awareness campaigns by pharmaceutical companies in the Netherlands, by assessing their compliance with the World Health Organization (WHO) Ethical Criteria for medicinal drug promotion and the Dutch guidelines for provision of information by pharmaceutical companies.

***Methods:*** Materials referring to health/disease and treatments published in the most widely circulated newspapers and magazines were collected from March to May 2012. An evaluation tool was developed based on relevant underlying principles from the WHO ethical criteria and Dutch self-regulation guidelines. Collected disease awareness advertisements were used to pilot the evaluation tool and to explore the consistency of information provided with the WHO and Dutch criteria.

***Findings:*** Eighty materials met our inclusion criteria; 71 were published in newspapers and 9 in magazines. The large majority were news items but 21 were disease awareness advertisements, of which 5 were duplicates. Fifteen out of the 16 disease awareness campaigns were non-compliant with current guidelines mainly due to lack of balance (n = 12), absence of listed author and/or sponsor (n = 8), use of misleading or incomplete information (n = 5) and use of promotional information (n = 5). None mentioned a pharmaceutical product directly.

***Conclusion:*** Disease Awareness Campaigns are present in Dutch printed media. Although no brand names were mentioned, the lack of compliance of disease awareness campaigns with the current regulations is alarming. There were information deficiencies and evidence of information bias. A key concern is that the context in which the information is provided, mostly through indirect referral, is likely to support treatment with the sponsor's product.

**Editor:** Elisabeth Hildt, University of Mainz, Germany

**Funding:** The authors have no support or funding to report.

**Competing Interests:** The authors have declared that no competing interests exist.

* Email: A.K.Mantel@uu.nl

## Introduction

In 1988, the World Health Organization established the Ethical Criteria for Medicinal Drug Promotion, defining promotion as "all informational and persuasive activities of manufacturers and distributors that affect the prescription, supply, purchase and/or use of medicinal drugs" [1]. While not legally binding, these criteria include a set of guiding principles that can be adapted to national circumstances.

Advertising of prescription drugs to the public – also known as direct-to-consumer advertising (DTCA) – is controversial and only allowed in the United States and New Zealand. European legislation prohibits advertising of products that have prescription-only status, aiming to protect public health. Despite this prohibition, however, manufacturers are using an increasing array of techniques to advertise these medicines to the public both directly and indirectly [2].

Media and communication channels are key influencers of consumer decisions, helping to shape consumers' information and options, also on health and treatment [3]. Media can also exert a powerful influence over human behaviours and public policy [4]. Health topics are often covered in printed media and they can include factual information on diseases and conditions but also treatment information of promotional nature [5,6].

In Europe, pharmaceutical companies are explicitly allowed to provide general information to the public on human health and diseases, as long as there is no reference, even indirectly, to a specific medicinal product [7]. This provision enables companies to run unbranded 'disease-awareness' or 'help-seeking' advertisements [8]. These materials draw viewers' attention to certain health conditions by focusing on symptoms and suggesting the public to 'ask their doctors' for newly available treatment information [9]. Such campaigns are not subject to any specific regulations governing pharmaceutical promotion, nor pre-clearance. They represent a grey area in regulation since regulators are reluctant to consider them to be product-specific promotion unless they include explicit links to branded information [10].

Disease awareness campaigns (DACs) can educate the public about disease, make consumers aware of untreated health problems and lead them to seek effective care at earlier stage, thus leading to better health [11]. Advocates consider disease awareness campaigns to be particularly important for under-diagnosed diseases [12]. However, concerns have been raised about the quality and nature of the information being provided to the public in disease awareness campaigns [13]. Proponents of direct to consumer advertising claim that it empowers consumers by stimulating discussions with physicians, enabling patients to obtain needed treatment at an earlier stage and improving adherence. Evidence shows, nevertheless, that exposure to advertisements increases prescribing volume and patient demand and that it shifts prescribing into less cost-effective choices. In addition, there is no evidence of improved adherence, nor treatment quality or early provision of needed care [14]. In a similar trend, albeit scarce, there is evidence that disease awareness campaigns can lead to increases in consultation rates and prescriptions for the advertisers' product [15]. If campaigns support use of newer, more expensive products with least well understood benefit-harm profiles, over cheaper, well-known, older medicines, they can lead to increases in consultations, inappropriate prescribing and more adverse drug reactions and drug-induced harm, as well as increases in hospitalisations, thus affecting both quality and costs of care [9]. While much research has been done in other areas of traditional drug promotion, far less is known about how these campaigns influence both physicians and the public, or on their compliance with the current regulatory framework [16].

In the Netherlands, a self-regulatory approach is used to oversee medicines' advertising [17]. In April 2011, the Foundation for the Medicinal Products' Advertising Code (CGR) published a set of guidelines on the provision of disease and treatment information about prescription-only medicines by pharmaceutical companies to the public, thus aiming to define the boundary between information and advertising [18].

Nevertheless, there is no instrument available to assess the compliance of disease awareness campaigns with the provisions included in the WHO Ethical Criteria for Medicinal Drug Promotion or in the Dutch self-regulation guidelines.

Evaluating the quality and nature of the information provided in disease awareness campaigns is very relevant to policy discussions at European level. The proposal for a European directive on information to the general public on medicinal products subject to medical prescription, presented by the European Commission in December 2008, foresaw changes to the regulations on advertising. It contemplated an expanded role for the pharmaceutical industry in the provision of information on prescription medicines directly to the public [19]. This study aims to inform future European policies regulating the dissemination of disease and treatment information to the public by the pharmaceutical industry. This article assesses the frequency of occurrence of disease awareness campaigns in printed media in the Netherlands and measures their compliance with current guidelines.

## Objectives

The aim of our research was threefold:

1. To assess the frequency of occurrence of medicines' promotion and disease awareness campaigns in printed media in the Netherlands.
2. To develop a user-friendly instrument to assess the compliance of disease information campaigns.
3. To use this instrument to measure compliance of disease information campaigns, including those disseminated by pharmaceutical companies, in Dutch printed media.

## Methods

### 1. Assessing disease-awareness campaign frequency in major print media

We examined high-circulation print media, which included three paid daily newspapers, three free daily newspapers and eight paid monthly magazines [20]. Data collection took place over three months (March to May 2012 inclusive). The three free newspapers were collected at train stations whereas the 14 paid publications were accessed in public libraries. Two authors (AMF and TLA) independently selected materials based on the inclusion criteria outlined below. If there were disagreements, these were to be resolved by consensus. Consensus was reached in all cases.

Our **inclusion criteria** were based on an interpretation of legal provisions, which prohibit direct and/or indirect reference to a pharmaceutical product. Firstly, we included all materials which addressed health and treatment issues. Materials on nutraceuticals, homeopathic products, over-the-counter medicines and vaccines were excluded, as they are governed by different legislation. Secondly, we selected all materials which covered one or more of the following four sets of linked information: (1) symptoms/health issues (for prevention purposes)/diseases/conditions AND a specific prescription-only medicine or a therapeutic drug class; (2) symptoms/health issues (for prevention purposes)/diseases/conditions AND a doctor or website referral/a description of a drug's mechanism of action or a suggestion to seek further treatment; (3) name or the logo of a pharmaceutical company AND mention of a symptom/problem/condition or referred to a website; and (4) reference to disease management programmes and discussion of adding another medical product to the ongoing treatment regimen. Finally, materials were then separated into two groups: disease awareness campaigns (Group I) – which included no author and were to be assessed using the instrument – and news items (Group II) – editorial content which included an author or was attributable to the news desk.

Additional descriptive data which were also recorded included: type of publication where materials were found (Paid or Free); printed media frequency; topic; reference to non-pharmaceutical interventions; reference to changes in the quality of life (either positive or negative); referral to visit a physician; reference to a clinical expert; referral to a website; reference to a patient organization or support group; reference to a brand-name, use of company's name or logo, and reference to the availability of a new medicine or treatment option.

### 2. Instrument development

The instrument (originally developed in Dutch and then translated into English) is based on seven relevant criteria from

**Table 1.** Overlap between relevant provisions within the WHO Ethical Criteria for Medicinal Drug Promotion and the CGR Guidelines for provision of information on prescription medicines.

| WHO Ethical Criteria | CGR Guidelines | Relevant criteria identified |
|---|---|---|
| Article 6. Definition of promotion: "all informational and persuasive activities by manufacturers and distributors, the effect of which is to induce the prescription, supply, purchase and/or use of medicinal drugs." | Introduction. Definition of promotion: "all informational and persuasive activities by manufacturers and distributors, the effect of which is to induce the prescription, supply, purchase and/or use of medicinal drugs." | Promotional information |
| Article 7. "Promotional material should not be designed so as to disguise its real nature." | Introduction. "Instances whereby prescription medication or pills are being mentioned without indicating the drug's brand name or company name" are considered indirect reference, for example when naming the active ingredients or the drug's mechanism of action. | |
| Article 9. "Scientific and educational activities should not be deliberately used for promotional purposes." | Article 5. "Information may not encourage irrational use of prescription medicines nor the search for unnecessary treatment." | |
| Article 14b. "Advertisements to the public should not generally be permitted for prescription drugs or to promote drugs for certain serious conditions that can be treated only by qualified health practitioners." | Article 6. "Information may not directly or indirectly lead to the choice of a particular medicine from different available treatments." | |
| Article 7. "Advertisements may claim that a drug can cure, prevent, or relieve an ailment only if this can be substantiated. ... All promotion-making claims concerning medicinal drugs should be reliable, accurate, truthful, informative, balanced, up-to-date, capable of substantiation and in good taste. They should not contain misleading or unverifiable statements or omissions likely to induce medically unjustifiable drug use or to give rise to undue risks." | Article 3. "Information may not be misleading. The information provided must comply with the most recent evidence and practice standards. The information must be factually correct and may not contain any misleading elements." | Misleading or incomplete information |
| | Article 17. "No comparison is allowed between relevant treatments and medicines that suggests that the effects of a treatment with a prescription drug are better or equal than those of another relevant treatment or drug." | |
| | 21.2 b) "No single option for treatment is to be highlighted, for instance by using words, colours or images, different font types, markings or any other elements. " | |
| | Article 21.2 d) "Treatments should be cathegorised based on acceptable formats. For instance using therapeutic classes or categories, or through therapeutic guidelines. Using expressions such as "most recent, or new is better, most commonly used, is not allowed." | |
| | Article 23. "Information should be displayed objectively and neutrally and must not contain information which relates directly to a specific treatment. When reference is made to specific treatment guidelines, the source must be listed... References to scientific literature should also be published..." | |
| Article 14: "While they [advertisements] should take account of people's legitimate desire for information regarding their health, they should not take undue advantage of people's concern for their health." | Article 9."Information should not aim nor encourage the public to seek unnecessary treatment, advice or further examination; nor on the other hand refrain the public from seeking treatment, advice or further examination." | Use of Fear |
| | Article 5. "Information may not encourage irrational use of prescription medicines nor the search for unnecessary treatment." | |
| Article 15. "Language which brings about fear or distress should not be used." | Article 4. "Information should not boost or amplify feelings of fear and superstition and should be displayed realistically." | |
| | Article 20. "The information may not be unjustified, unnecessarily alarming or misleading images of changes to the human body resulting from illness or disease." | |
| Article 29. "The wording ...if prepared specifically for patients, should be in lay language on condition that the medical and scientific content is properly reflected." | Article 7. "Information should be tailored to the average consumer and have understandable language. Medical and scientific terms should be avoided as much as possible, to avoid confusion." | Inadequate Language |
| Article 7. "All promotion-making claims concerning medicinal drugs should be reliable, accurate, truthful, informative, balanced, up-to-date, capable of substantiation and in good taste. They should not contain misleading or unverifiable statements or omissions likely to induce medically unjustifiable drug use or to give rise to undue risks... Comparison of products should be factual, fair and capable of substantiation". | Article 9."Information should not aim nor encourage the public to seek unnecessary treatment, advice or further examination; nor on the other hand refrain the public from seeking treatment, advice or further examination." | Lack of Balance |

**Table 1.** Cont.

| WHO Ethical Criteria | CGR Guidelines | Relevant criteria identified |
|---|---|---|
| | Article 17. "No comparison is allowed between relevant treatments and medicines that suggests that the effects of a treatment with a prescription drug are better or equal than those of another relevant treatment or drug." | |
| | Article 21. "Information should be as balanced and complete as possible. It should reflect the state-of-the-art. When providing information, all relevant factors should be taken into account. All information should be equally displayed both in content and layout, with the same amount of detail." | |
| | Article 21.2 c) "The positive and negative effects of a treatment are not to be emphasized in such a way that the pros or the cons of a given treatment are highlighted". | |
| | Article 21.2 d) Information about different therapeutic interventions can be provided. In that case, all relevant treatments should be named, including pharmacotherapy and other interventions, such as adjustments to lifestyle, nutrition and habits. Relevant treatments are the standard of care provided, as per treatment guidelines. Completeness ensures that no information is deliberately omitted. When enumerating all the pharmacotherapeutic options for treatment, all the relevant prescription drugs for the specific treatment are to be mentioned." | |
| Article 7. "Promotional material should not be designed so as to disguise its real nature." | Article 18. "Testimonials should portray the opinion or experience of the user truthfully (not that of a professional or any other public figure). They should not include any comparison of the user's situation before and after drug treatment...Before/after testimonials are not allowed because they can lead the public into false expectations regarding the speed of the treatment's effects". | Testimonials |
| Article 9. "Scientific and educational activities should not be deliberately used for promotional purposes." | | |
| Article 7. "Advertisements may claim that a drug can cure, prevent, or relieve an ailment only if this can be substantiated. ... All promotion-making claims con cerning medicinal drugs should be reliable, accurate, truthful, informative, balanced, up-to-date, capable of substantiation and in good taste. They should not contain misleading or unverifiable statements or omissions likely to induce medically unjustifiable drug use or to give rise to undue risks." | Article 22. "Each message is to contain the name of the person responsible for the information". | Absence of Source/Author |
| | Article 23. "Information may refer to scientific studies and results...The source must always be included. The studies and the results that are mentioned must always come from other sources than the medicine's producer and should be verifiable..." "Information should be displayed objectively and neutrally and must not contain information which relates directly to a specific treatment. When reference is made to specific treatment guidelines, the source must be listed... References to scientific literature should also be published..." | |

the WHO Ethical Criteria for Medicinal Drug promotion [1] and the KOAG/CGR guidelines [17]. These were identified by overlapping the relevant provisions within the two sets of regulatory guidelines that can be used to judge the content and quality of disease-oriented information (Table 1). These are promotional information, misleading or incomplete information, use of fear, inadequate language, lack of balance, use of testimonials and absence of listed author and/or sponsor. These criteria were translated into evaluation statements to judge whether or not a principle is being adequately applied (compliant, non-compliant and not applicable). An option to insert additional comments was also included. A reference to a company's name or logo in a disease awareness campaign was not considered sufficient for a material to be deemed non-compliant.

Three external reviewers (pharmaceutical policy researchers) tested the instrument using three examples of disease awareness campaigns by the pharmaceutical industry, previously published in European printed media. As a result, five statements were altered. Changes included merging, division or rewording of statements. The final instrument is included as Table S1.

## 3. Assessing compliance of disease awareness campaigns with guidelines

As the instrument is based on legal guidelines, the existence of a single non-compliant statement is sufficient to consider the material to be non-compliant. Two authors (TLA and AMF) independently assessed each of the seven criteria for all disease awareness campaigns and differences in scoring were discussed

**Table 2.** Material Characteristics.

| Type of publication | Group 1 Disease awareness campaigns (n = 21) (% within group) | Group 2 News items (n = 59) (% within group) | Risk Ratio (95% CI) |
|---|---|---|---|
| *All publications* | | | |
| Paid | 5 (24%) | 43 (73%) | |
| Free | 16 (76%) | 16 (27%) | **2.8 (1.7; 4.5)** |
| *Publication frequency* | | | |
| Daily | 5 (24%) | 38 (64%) | |
| Weekly | 2 (9%) | 3 (5%) | |
| Monthly | 0 (0%) | 4 (7%) | |
| Occasionally | 14 (67%) | 14 (24%) | |
| *Health Supplements* | 15 (71%) | 13 (22%) | **3.4 (1.9; 5.6)** |
| *Information included* | **Group 1 Disease awareness campaigns (n = 21) (% within group)** | **Group 2 News items (n = 59) (% within group)** | **Risk Ratio (95% CI)** |
| Non-pharmaceutical interventions in addition to therapy | 5 (31%) | 19 (32.2%) | 0.9 (0.4; 2.2) |
| Suggestion to visit the general practitioner | 6 (37%) | 10 (17%) | 2.21 (0.9; 5.1) |
| Reference to a Clinical expert | 3 (19%) | 14 (24%) | 0.8 (0,3; 2.4) |
| Website | 13 (81%) | 9 (15%) | **5.3 (2.8; 10.1)** |
| Patient or support group | 6 (37%) | 9 (15%) | 2.45 (1.0; 5.9) |
| Pharmaceutical company | 6 (37%) | 8 (8%) | **2.8 (1.1; 6.8)** |
| Brand name | 0 (0%) | 10 (17%) | **0.3* (0.0; 2.2)** |
| New medicine or treatment option | 2 (12%) | 15 (25%) | 0.5 (0.1; 1.9) |

* RR calculated by adding 0.5 to all cells.

and resolved by consensus. Any remaining disagreements were then adjudicated to a third author (AMT). The frequencies of the information provided in both groups were measured using the risk ratio (RR). When information was absent, a cell in Table 2 obtained a zero and no RR could be calculated. This was dealt by adding 0.5 to every cell in Table 2 to be able to calculate an estimate of the RR [21]. Whenever possible, data analysis was conducted using SPSS version 20.0 (SPSS Inc. Chicago, Illinois, USA).

## Results

### 1. Assessing disease-awareness campaign frequency

On average six materials covering disease and treatment information were published per week. A total of 80 materials were collected, 59 of which were news items (73,8%), whereas 21 were disease awareness campaigns (26.3%) (Table 2). Five of these disease awareness campaigns were duplicates - published in different printed media - leaving 75 materials for further description and 16 materials for the compliance analysis.

Overall (n = 80) the seven most commonly mentioned conditions were: allergies and respiratory diseases (n = 22; 28%), diabetes (n = 7; 9%), cardiovascular diseases (n = 5; 6%), cancer (n = 5; 6%), contraception (n = 4; 5%), Attention Deficit Hyperactivity Disorder (ADHD) (n = 4; 5%) and pain (n = 4; 5%). Within disease awareness campaigns, allergies and respiratory diseases, and contraception were common topics. Most notably, all the disease awareness duplicates regarded allergies and respiratory diseases. One disease awareness campaign was sponsored by a patient organisation.

Disease awareness campaigns were significantly more frequent in free publications (RR = 2.8, 95% CI 1.7; 4.5) and in health-related supplements (RR = 3.4, 95% CI 1.9; 5.6). When comparing news to disease awareness campaigns as to the information provided, the latter were more likely to mention a pharmaceutical company (RR = 2.8, 95% CI 1.1; 6.8), a website (RR = 5.3, 95% CI 2.8; 10.1) or a visit to the general practitioner (RR = 2.2, 95% CI 0.9; 5.16) but less likely to include a brand-name (RR = 0.3, 95% CI 0.04; 2.2) (Table 2).

### 2. Assessing compliance of DACs with guidelines

The initial inter-rater agreement in the assessment of overall compliance was of 88%; disparities between assessors were arbitrated by the fourth author. Fifteen out of the sixteen materials assessed were non-compliant with the guidelines. Non-compliance was more frequent due to lack of balance, absence of listed author and/or sponsor, use of promotional information or use of misleading or incomplete information (Table 3, Figure 1). Interestingly, most instances of non-compliance with the misleading or incomplete information criterion involved a lack of references.

Most notably, five out of the sixteen materials included the logo or name of a pharmaceutical company, referred to a particular condition and mentioned a treatment indirectly. Other four materials discussed a condition and indirectly a treatment, while including a referral to a website sponsored by a pharmaceutical company. Table 3 provides examples of non-compliance aggregated per key criteria and disease awareness campaign topic.

## Discussion

In this study we have shown that there is a focus on disease and treatment information in printed media in the Netherlands, both through news items and disease awareness campaigns. The majority of disease awareness campaigns identified during our

**Table 3.** Examples of non-compliance per key criteria from the disease awareness campaigns.

| KEY criteria | Problem identified | Example *(CONDITION)* |
|---|---|---|
| **Promotional information** | Reference to pharmaceutical products to treat a condition or disease in combination with: the name, logo and website of a pharmaceutical company; or a website for a disease awareness campaign; or quick response codes to dedicated websites. | "We are an international company with expertise in lung diseases…we develop innovative pharmaceutical solutions…" *(Respiratory diseases)* |
| | | A dedicated website is mentioned in big and bold typeface, as well as the name, logo and website of a pharmaceutical company. *(Contraception)* |
| | | "X strives respond to challenging medical conditions through innovative approaches. Pain treatment is one of our priorities… physical and emotional challenges borne by pain patients are key. Our R&D programme seeks alternative solutions to fight pain." *(Pain)* |
| | | "Our website helps you to choose the best treatment for your lifestyle. You will be able to find information about all therapies…and also do a test to help you select a suitable treatment." *(Kidney Failure)* |
| | | "Do you have, or someone close to you has, urinary incontinence? Have a look at our different links: (company) website; your digital logbook for your mobile phone; your online digital logbook to share with your doctor." *(Urinary incontinence)* |
| **Misleading or incomplete information** | No reference is provided on the sources of information provided about prevalence of disease. | "One out of every 8 adults in the Netherlands has high cholesterol". *(Cardiovascular diseases)* |
| | | "One out of each 10 Dutch has asthma …"one out of every 5 Dutch has hay fever". *(Allergies)* |
| | | "More than 5000 people get post-traumatic dystrophy every year." *(Post-traumatic dystrophy)* |
| | | "Approximately 40.000 Dutch suffer from renal disease. There are several treatments available for this debilitating disease." *(Kidney Failure)* |
| | | "One third of those who suffer from migraine in the Netherlands do not get the appropriate treatment…2.5 million Dutch suffer from migraine." *(Migraine)* |
| **Use of fear** | Reference to disability caused by the disease, either through text or picture. | An image of a disabled hand is used. *(Post-traumatic dystrophy)* |
| | | "Besides the pain…migraine also has implications for society…it costs the Netherlands 1.7 billion per year… I have seen people who cannot fulfil their dreams…. That is terrible… *(Migraine)* |
| **Inadequate language** | Uses medical terminology | "Perinasal inflammation…abscesses…metabolic diseases…" *(Alarm signals)* |
| **Lack of balance** | More emphasis on the benefits of pharmaceutical treatment than risks. Symptoms are accentuated by layout and/or enumeration. Risk factors are portrayed as diseases. Treatment is accentuated. | "This disease can have a great impact on the individual and its environment. It disturbs your daily life. It is important to diagnose it at an earlier stage, so that treatment can begin quickly. Therapy includes anti-inflammatory drugs and painkillers." *(Post-traumatic dystrophy)* |
| | | "These symptoms can seem mild, but they can have a great impact on your daily life, at school or at work, and even disturb your sleep patterns". |
| | | "Symptoms such as shortness of breath, cough and wheeziness result in an asthma attack…Red and itchy eyes, running nose, stuffy nose, sneezes and tiredness can have serious implications." *Allergies)* |
| | | Symptoms are referred to in headings in big and bold typeface. *(Allergies) (Alarm signals) (Urinary incontinence)* |
| | | "…when you have high cholesterol, you have a higher risk of developing cardiovascular diseases… you can reduce that risk by…treating your high cholesterol levels. Have a look at our new website about healthy living with lower cholesterol". *(Cardiovascular diseases)* |
| | | "Now women are able to choose a pill that contains a natural hormone and a progestogen. This natural hormone is easily absorbed by the body…this pill has a neutral effect on acne, weight-gain and blood pressure…your periods will be shorter and lighter…" *(Contraception)* |
| | | Contraception is mentioned on six occasions in big and bold typeface. *(Contraception)* |
| | | The sentence: "I (do not) want a pill" and the address of a dedicated website are included in big and bold typefaces. *(Contraception)* |
| | | "…suffering from migraine, days in a row, a pain impossible to bear…with nausea, and sensitivity to light and noises…seek a good treatment…Medicines play an important role…we advise patients to try two different triptans…" *(Migraine)* |
| **Use of testimonials** | Specialist mentions treatment and specific drug classes | "The doctor can prescribe anti-histamines…or corticosteroids… immunotherapy can be considered an option". *(Allergies)* |

**Table 3.** Cont.

| KEY criteria | Problem identified | Example *(CONDITION)* |
|---|---|---|
| | A comparison is made of the patient's experience before and after treatment with a specific drug. | "I had tummy and back aches with another pill. I visited my doctor and together we have chosen a new pill with a different ingredient. That has helped". " The first pill I took caused weight-gain and emotional changes. My GP then prescribed a lighter pill and I am feeling fine". *(Contraception)* |
| **Absence of author and/or sponsor** | No author and/or sponsor identified. | *(Allergies), (Alarm signals), (Cardiovascular diseases), (Contraception), (Migraine)* |

study period did not comply with the WHO ethical criteria nor with the current Dutch self-regulation guidelines.

Most collected materials on health and treatment were news items (74%). On average there were at least five news items published every week and seven disease-awareness campaigns published every four weeks. Our results seem to indicate that pharmaceutical companies often opt to reach a wider audience by publishing their unbranded product advertisements in free media outlets, most notably in dedicated health-supplements. The frequency of occurrence of disease awareness campaigns observed in our study is consistent with the results of an Australian study, where a total of sixty campaigns were identified in popular women's magazines over eleven months [22]. From these, fifteen contained a corporate brand or logo – a result also similar to ours.

The findings on low compliance are worrying, since serious information deficiencies in disease awareness campaigns result in information bias. A key concern is that the context in which the information is provided will be biased towards supporting treatment with the sponsor's product. One third of the disease awareness campaigns in our study referred readers to their physicians. Disease awareness campaigns can stimulate patients' intentions to make requests to doctors for prescription medicines products, increase consultation rates as well as prescriptions for the advertiser's product [15,23]. A survey in Australia has shown that 26,9% of the 800 patients enquired had approached their GP to discuss a treatment they had heard about in the media. Half of the patients reported that their inquiry had resulted in a treatment; more than forty-eight percent of those receiving treatment, reported being prescribed a medicine [5]. This has serious implications for general practitioners and regulators.

There is evidence that self-regulation of drug promotion is ineffective. A recent Swedish study demonstrated an overall system failure compounded by lax oversight, regulation lags, and low fines for violations [24]. The authors concluded that the current regulatory regimes have failed to deter industry from providing unreliable information. Researchers have raised concerns in the United States about the effects of indirect medical advertising, claiming that medical decisions based on such influences, as manipulated by advertisers, are likely to result in worse outcomes for patients, and have called for indirect advertising to be curtailed [25].

In contrast, researchers in Australia have concluded that the value of disease awareness campaigns could be improved if regulations and guidelines stipulated disease information requirements [23]. Our research suggests that in the Netherlands – where such guidelines do exist – pharmaceutical companies are aware of

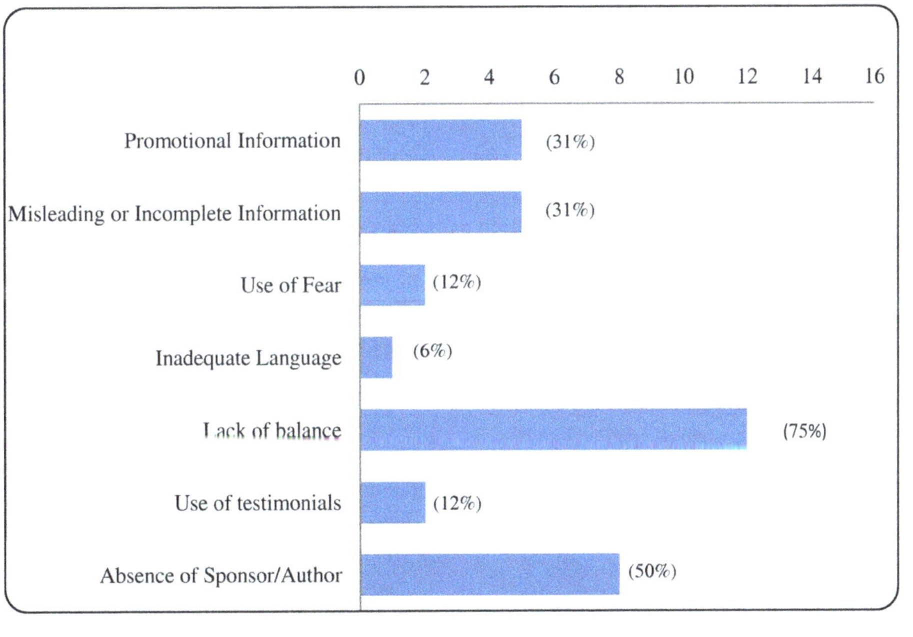


**Figure 1. Non-compliance of disease awareness campaigns (n = 16) per key criteria.** Fifteen out of the sixteen materials assessed were non-compliant with the guidelines. Non-compliance was more frequent due to lack of balance, absence of listed author and/or sponsor, use of promotional information and use of misleading or incomplete information.

the regulatory grey area that disease awareness campaigns represent – and of their subsequent limited regulatory response – thus circumventing the law and exploring new avenues in unbranded product advertising.

The indirect reference to a treatment in association with the name or the logo of a pharmaceutical company – observed in five disease awareness campaigns – constitutes unbranded product advertisement and seems to be in contravention of European law [7,17]. Our results are consistent with those of a 2009 study in the Netherlands which analysed 41 websites offering health information in the Dutch language: 32 were either hosted or sponsored by a pharmaceutical company, and 23 (72%) contravened national regulations by referring directly or indirectly to a specific prescription medicine [26].

The absence of an identifiable advertiser or sponsor was one of the main factors of non-compliance in our sample. This might be deliberate, as pharmaceutical companies face a real threat of litigation from unsubstantiated marketing claims. Their goal is to raise awareness about a condition and the availability of a treatment, but to leave the responsibility for a decision to the patient, who should "talk to the doctor the advantages and disadvantages of this new therapy" [27]. There is evidence that the rate of diagnoses of specific conditions increases during associated advertising campaigns [14]. A randomized controlled trial using standardized patients found that if patients requested an advertised brand, they were as likely to receive a prescription whether they had the condition that the product treated, depression, or milder life problems not requiring a medicine ('adjustment disorder') [28].

More than half of the disease awareness campaigns in our study (62%) referred to websites, some of which seemed independent at first glance, but were sponsored and/or maintained by one or more pharmaceutical companies. Bearing in mind the growing interest in online health information and that consumers are more likely to seek out more prescription drug information after exposure to advertising, as well as to engage in more communication with doctors about prescription drugs, the evaluation of the content and quality of disease awareness websites should also be envisaged [29].

Disease awareness campaigns have been identified as a form of disease mongering or "widening the boundaries of treatable illness in order to expand markets for those who sell and deliver treatments." [30,31] A recent commentary by Schwartz and Woloshin provides a template for how disease awareness campaigns work, using three basic strategies: lowering the bar for diagnosis (turning ordinary life experiences into conditions that require medical diagnoses), raising the stakes so that people want to get tested, and spinning the evidence about drug benefits and harms [16].

While seasonality might have influenced the conditions being mentioned in the materials – namely allergies and respiratory diseases - it is unlikely that it would have affected their quality. Contraception was one of the key topics covered in disease awareness campaigns. A new contraceptive pill was launched into the EU market in May 2012 [32]. This might indicate a potential marketing strategy of the marketing authorisation holder to draw attention to their new product. Newspaper readers were also amply exposed to information on diabetes. This might have been related with the inclusion of linagliptine into the Dutch reimbursement list [33].

One of the main limitations of our study has been the small sample of unique advertisements, due to the monitoring and inclusion process. A longer data collection window of a full calendar year would have allowed better sampling and extended statistical analysis.

The dynamics of disease awareness campaigns are intricate and deserve closer scrutiny by physicians, consumers and regulators [27,34]. While our proposed instrument has not been systematically evaluated, it represents an attempt to translate the relevant provisions included in the WHO Ethical Criteria for Medicinal Drug Promotion and the Dutch self-regulation guidelines into measurable operational components [1,17,18]. Further validation and testing are needed, to verify our tool's consistency and reliability.

## Conclusions

We have demonstrated that disease awareness campaigns are present in Dutch printed media. Their compliance with current self-regulation guidelines is low, which warrants the need for further research into the effects of these campaigns. The use of our instrument could help identify disease awareness campaigns of promotional nature and further encourage effective monitoring and implementation of the regulation by competent authorities.

## Acknowledgments

Barbara Mintzes for providing valuable guidance on the design and methods of this study and for reviewing this article.

## Author Contributions

Conceived and designed the experiments: TLA AMF MVE. Performed the experiments: AMF TLA. Analyzed the data: TLA AMF AMT MVE. Contributed reagents/materials/analysis tools: AMT. Wrote the paper: AMT MVE AMF TLA.

## References

1. World Health Organization (1988) Ethical Criteria for Medicinal Drug Promotion. Geneva: World Health Organization.
2. Mintzes B (1998) Blurring the Boundaries: New trends in drug promotion (HAI-Europe): Amsterdam: Health Action International.
3. Haimowitz IJ (2011) Healthcare relationship marketing: strategy, design and measurement. Great Britain: Gower Publishing Limited.
4. Harrabin R, Coote A, Allen J (2003) Health in the news: risk, reporting and media influence. Discussion Paper. United Kingdom: King's Fund Publications.
5. Hogue M-CB, Doran E, Henry DA (2012) A Prompt to the Web: The Media and Health Information Seeking Behaviour. PLOS ONE 7(4): e34314.
6. Cassels A, Hughes MA, Cole C, Mintzes B, Lexchin J, et al. (2003) Drugs in the news: an analysis of Canadian newspaper coverage of new prescription drugs. CMAJ 168 (9).
7. European Parliament and Council (2004) Directive 2004/27/EC of the European Parliament and the Council of 31 March 2004 amending Directive 2001/83/EC on the Community code relating to medicinal products for human use. Article 86 (2). European Parliament and Council (31 March).
8. Leonardo Alves T, Mintzes B (2007) A regulatory no man's land: Unbranded advertising of prescription drugs to the public in Europe. Poster presented at the Geneva Health Forum. Geneva: Geneva Health Forum.
9. Castleberry SB, Bayuk K, O'Brien AM (2008) We've got a cure for you! Disease Awareness Campaigns. Journal of Business Case Studies Feb 4; 2.

10. Vitry A, Mintzes B (2012) Disease Mongering and low testosterone in men: the tale of two regulatory failures. Med J Aust 196 (10): 619–621.
11. Tiner R (2002) The industry works to develop drugs, not diseases [letter].BMJ Jul 27;325(7357):216.
12. Wielondek M (2005) Can direct-to-consumer advertising help in reinventing the image of the pharmaceutical industry instead of eroding its credibility? J Med Mark 5:264–273.
13. Nuland S, van Eijk M, van Brakel RC (2009) Public information as a Marketing Tool, promotion of diseases and medicines. Netherlands: Gezonde scepsis.
14. Mintzes B (2012) Advertising of Prescription-Only Medicines to the Public: Does Evidence of Benefit Counterbalance Harm? Ann Rev Public Health 33: 259–77.
15. 't Jong GW, Stricker B, Sturkenboom M (2004) Marketing in the lay media and prescriptions of terbinafine in primary care: Dutch cohort study. BMJ. April 17; 328(7445): 931.
16. Schwartz LM, Woloshin S (2013) Low "T" as in "Template": How to Sell Disease: Comment on "Promoting 'Low T'". JAMA Intern Med:1–3.
17. Keuringsraad Openlijke Aanprijzing Geneesmiddelen (2013) Code voor de Publieksreclame voor Geneesmiddelen. Available: http://keuringsraad.brabers.nl/Keuringsraad/media/KoagKag/Downloads/Code-voor-de-Publieksreclame-voor-Geneesmiddelen-%28CPG%29.pdf. Accessed on 28 January 2014.
18. Stichting CGR (2011) Leidraad Informatie UR geneesmiddelen. Available: http://www.cgr.nl/Gedragscode-Geneesmiddelenreclame/Leidraad-Informatie-UR-geneesmiddelen. Accessed on 28 January 2014.
19. European Commission (2008) Proposal for a Directive of the European Parliament and of the Council amending, as regards information to the general public on medicinal products subject to medical prescription, Directive 2001/83/EC on the Community code relating to medicinal products for human use. Brussels: European Commission.
20. Instituut voor Media Auditing (2011) Harde Cijfers Jaar 2011. Netherlands. Available: http://www.hoi-online.nl/322346/HOI-HARDE-CIJFERS-JAAR-2011.pdf. Accessed on 22 February 2012.
21. Agresti A (2007) An introduction to categorical data analysis. 2 ed. Hoboken, New Jersey: John Wiley & Sons Inc.
22. Hall DK, Jones CJ, Iverson DC (2009) Content analysis of disease awareness advertisements in popular Australian women's magazines. Med J Aust 191(11–12):625–9.
23. Hall DK, Jones CJ, Iverson DC (2011) Disease Awareness advertising: women's intentions following exposure. Australian Family Physician 40: 143–147.
24. Zetterqvist AV, Mulinari S (2013) Misleading Advertising for Antidepressants in Sweden: A Failure of Pharmaceutical Industry Self-Regulation. PLoS ONE 8(5): e62609. doi:10.1371/journal.pone.0062609
25. Trafimow D (2013) Augmenting the Argument Against Indirect Medical Advertising. American Journal of Bioethics, 13(5), 21–23. doi: 10.1080/15265161.2013.776131
26. Nuland S, van Brakel RC (2009) Informatieaanbod op internet. Utrecht: Gezonde scepsis. 96 p. Dutch.
27. Braun S (2013) Promoting "Low T, a medical writer's perspective. JAMA Intern Med 12;173(15):1458-60. doi: 10.1001/jamainternmed.2013.6892
28. Kravitz RL, Epstein RM, Feldman MD, Franz CE, Azari R, et al. (2005) Influence of patients' requests for direct-to-consumer advertised antidepressants: a randomized controlled trial. JAMA 293(16):1995–2002.
29. Huh J, DeLorme D, Reid L (2005) Factors Affecting Trust in online prescription drug information and impact of trust on behavior following exposure to DTC advertising. Journal of Health Communication 10(8):711–31.
30. Moynihan R, Health I, Henry D (2002) Selling sickness: the pharmaceutical industry and disease mongering. BMJ 324: 886–891.
31. Woloshin S, Schwartz LM (2006) Giving Legs to Restless Legs: A Case Study of How the Media Helps Make People Sick. PLoS Med 3(4): e170. doi:10.1371/journal.pmed.0030170
32. European Medicines Agency Committee for medicinal products for human use (2011) Zoely, nomegestrol acetate/estradiol. Summary of opinion (initial authorisation. Available: http://www.ema.europa.eu/docs/en_GB/document_library/Summary_of_opinion_-_Initial_authorisation/human/001213/WC500103879.pdf. Accessed on 30 June 2012.
33. Koninklijke Nederlandse Maatschappij ter bevordering der Pharmacie (2012) Vergoeding voor linagliptine. Pharmaceutisch weekblad. Netherlands. Available: http://www.pw.nl/nieuws/nieuwsberichten/2012/vergoeding-voor-linagliptine. Accessed on 28 January 2014.
34. Quick J, Hogerzeil HV, Rágo L, Reffi V, Joncheere K (2003) Ensuring ethical drug promotion—whose responsibility? The Lancet, Volume 362, Issue 9385, Page 747, 30 August.

# 3

# Multidimensional Poverty in Rural Mozambique: A New Metric for Evaluating Public Health Interventions

**Bart Victor[1,2], Meridith Blevins[2,3], Ann F. Green[2], Elisée Ndatimana[6], Lázaro González-Calvo[6], Edward F. Fischer[7], Alfredo E. Vergara[2,4¤], Sten H. Vermund[2,5,6], Omo Olupona[8], Troy D. Moon[2,5,6]***

**1** Owen Graduate School of Management, Vanderbilt University, Nashville, Tennessee, United States of America, **2** Vanderbilt Institute for Global Health, Vanderbilt University, Nashville, Tennessee, United States of America, **3** Department of Biostatistics, Vanderbilt University School of Medicine, Nashville, Tennessee, United States of America, **4** Department of Preventive Medicine, Vanderbilt University School of Medicine, Nashville, Tennessee, United States of America, **5** Department of Pediatrics, Vanderbilt University School of Medicine, Nashville, Tennessee, United States of America, **6** Friends in Global Health, Maputo, Mozambique, **7** Vanderbilt Center for Latin American Studies and Department of Anthropology, Vanderbilt University, Nashville, Tennessee, United States of America, **8** World Vision International, Maputo, Mozambique

## Abstract

***Background:*** Poverty is a multidimensional phenomenon and unidimensional measurements have proven inadequate to the challenge of assessing its dynamics. Dynamics between poverty and public health intervention is among the most difficult yet important problems faced in development. We sought to demonstrate how multidimensional poverty measures can be utilized in the evaluation of public health interventions; and to create geospatial maps of poverty deprivation to aid implementers in prioritizing program planning.

***Methods:*** Survey teams interviewed a representative sample of 3,749 female heads of household in 259 enumeration areas across Zambézia in August-September 2010. We estimated a multidimensional poverty index, which can be disaggregated into context-specific indicators. We produced an MPI comprised of 3 dimensions and 11 weighted indicators selected from the survey. Households were identified as "poor" if were deprived in >33% of indicators. Our MPI is an adjusted headcount, calculated by multiplying the proportion identified as poor (headcount) and the poverty gap (average deprivation). Geospatial visualizations of poverty deprivation were created as a contextual baseline for future evaluation.

***Results:*** In our rural (96%) and urban (4%) interviewees, the 33% deprivation cut-off suggested 58.2% of households were poor (29.3% of urban vs. 59.5% of rural). Among the poor, households experienced an average deprivation of 46%; thus the MPI/adjusted headcount is 0.27 ( $= 0.58 \times 0.46$). Of households where a local language was the primary language, 58.6% were considered poor versus Portuguese-speaking households where 73.5% were considered non-poor. Living standard is the dominant deprivation, followed by health, and then education.

***Conclusions:*** Multidimensional poverty measurement can be integrated into program design for public health interventions, and geospatial visualization helps examine the impact of intervention deployment within the context of distinct poverty conditions. Both permit program implementers to focus resources and critically explore linkages between poverty and its social determinants, thus deriving useful findings for evidence-based planning.

**Editor:** Spencer Moore, University of South Carolina, United States of America

**Funding:** The Ogumaniha-SCIP baseline survey was supported by the United States Agency for International Development (USAID)–Mozambique (Award No. 656-A-00-09-00141-00) through a sub-grant from World Vision, Inc. Funding support for the secondary data analysis is from Vanderbilt University through the endowment of the Amos Christie Chair in Global Health. The funders had no role in study design, data collection and analysis, decision to publish, or preparation of the manuscript.

* Email: troy.moon@vanderbilt.edu

¤ Current address: US Centers for Disease Control and Prevention, Maputo, Mozambique

## Background

In the last two decades, the world's governments have generated unprecedented support for a comprehensive list of global development aims, of which the Millennium Development Goals (MDGs) are an integral part. [1–4] One of the most significant outcomes of these joint efforts has been the prioritization of poverty reduction at the center of national and international policy agendas. In fact, the first goal of the MDGs is to reduce by half the global proportion of people living in extreme poverty by 2015. Three additional MDGs target public health interventions that reduce child mortality, improve maternal health, and combat HIV/AIDS, malaria and other disease [1–4]. Understanding the link between poverty and the public health interventions employed in the developing world is among the most difficult yet important problems faced today [5,6].

Increasingly the effectiveness of public health interventions is recognized as being closely tied to the impact of other efforts such as economic development, education, agriculture programs and improvements in infrastructure (including water and sanitation), shelter and security. While each intervention area brings an emphasis and focus on distinct needs, there are significant interactions and co-dependencies between areas. For example, it is generally accepted that poverty is closely associated with the availability and quality of health service, but this relationship is far from simple. There is a complex mutual causation: poor health services contribute to poverty, which in turn negatively influences the ability to access and utilize health services. To determine the impact of public health interventions on poverty reduction, it is necessary to define an appropriate framework for poverty measurement. By creating an evaluation paradigm that establishes an index of "poverty" as the primary outcome measure, yet which can be further disaggregated based on the contributions of its defined dimensions such as health, education, and living standard; we get the added value of being able to evaluate each dimension independently while simultaneously learning from the interactions and co-dependencies between areas that subsequently impact the effectiveness of the interventions employed to address them.

Traditional standards for measuring poverty are ever more criticized for their potential to both "mis-measure" and more importantly, misunderstand the true drivers of poverty. [7] Per capita income is a unidimensional measure that categorizes a person as poor if their income falls below a particular "poverty line", now frequently defined as less than $1.25 a day. [8–10] Unidimensional measures have been extensively critiqued in terms of their validity and precision and have proven inadequate to the challenge of assessing the extent and dynamics of poverty in the world. [7] Critique has been mostly directed toward use of unidimensional measurements for national policy and global comparison purposes. However, this argument is perhaps even more compelling when directed at interventions or public health programming aimed to improve well-being. An alternative approach derived from the work of Amartya Sen, introduces the idea that there are multiple dimensions of poverty [9–12].

The International Fund for Agriculture Development (IFAD) and the Sustainable Coffee Partnership, for example, have each developed sophisticated multi-criteria models that take into account many dimensions when measuring their intervention's success or not. [13] This approach for measuring many dimensions is not the same as measuring multidimensionality. In practice, extant models measure many dimensions, but most do not produce an integrated multidimensional model. One notable exception has been the work of the Oxford Poverty and Human Development Initiative (OPHI). [14] Working within the OPHI framework, Alkire and Foster have developed a method for calculating dimensional weights and cut-offs that integrate a number of dimensions into a combined metric [15].

International development organizations, researchers, and an increasing number of national governments are beginning to adopt multidimensional measures of national poverty. [14,16] The United Nations Development Program's (UNDP) Human Development Index (HDI) includes not only measures of Gross National Product (GNP) per head, but also incorporates indicators related to education and health in order to produce a composite index. Some program monitoring and evaluation efforts have also begun to incorporate multiple measures.

The three main objectives of this paper are 1) to demonstrate how multidimensional measures of poverty can be utilized in the planning and evaluation of large scale public health and development interventions; 2) to utilize the Alkire and Foster method for multidimensional poverty measurement in Zambézia Province, an extremely rural, infrastructure-depleted region of north-central Mozambique, to establish a baseline poverty index from which future comparisons will be conducted in order to measure the impact of interventions in the province; and 3) to create geospatial maps of poverty deprivation at baseline, providing program implementers a visual needs assessment that characterizes the geographic differences of each target district and aids in prioritizing program planning.

## Methods

### Study Context

In 2009, World Vision International was awarded a United States Agency for International Development (USAID) grant called Strengthening Communities through Integrated Programming (SCIP) for a 5-year multi-sector program aimed at improving the health and livelihoods of children, women, and families in Zambézia Province, Mozambique. Known locally as the *Ogumaniha* project, which means "united for a common purpose" in the local language of Echuabo, SCIP is based on a consortium of five international non-governmental organizations led by World Vision. The broad goals of the 5-year project are to: 1) reduce poverty in Zambézia Province by pursuing the consolidation of an integrated, innovative, and sustainable community-based program in the province; and 2) integrate current and future United States Government (USG) investments in Zambézia Province in the areas of health, HIV/AIDS, water and sanitation, income generation, and institutional capacity building.

In 2012, Mozambique ranked 185 of 187 nations on the UNDP's HDI, and the gross national income was estimated at US $906 per capita [8], with male and female life expectancies of 47 and 51 years, respectively, in 2009 [17]. Although Mozambique's health expenditure has risen substantially over the past 10 years, as a proportion of total GDP it was only 6.6% in 2011 (66 USD per capita). [18] Mozambique is one of the sub-Saharan African countries most affected by the HIV/AIDS epidemic, with a national adult HIV prevalence of 11.5% in 2009. [19] Nationally, 12% of children were considered orphans or vulnerable children, and only 43% of households had access to clean drinking water in 2009 [20].

The magnitude of poverty is especially evident in Zambézia Province, Mozambique's second largest province and home to about 4 million persons (Figure 1). [21,22] While Mozambique ranks among the poorest of the poor nations, Zambézia consistently ranks among Mozambique's lowest performing provinces with low literacy rates, poor maternal and child health (MCH) indices, high rates of tuberculosis and malaria infections, and high levels of malnutrition. [20,23,24] Zambézia Province is overwhelmingly rural and depends almost entirely on subsistence farming and fishing. The province has the highest estimated number of persons living with HIV in the country (~275,000 or nearly 20% of Mozambique's HIV-infected population) as of 2009 [19,25] and yet only 31 of Zambézia's 214 health facilities provided antiretroviral therapy (ART) as of December 2012. This is partially because Zambézia Province housed much of the armed conflict in Mozambique's 16-year civil war (1976–1992) and suffered disproportionately in destruction of its healthcare infrastructure [21,22].

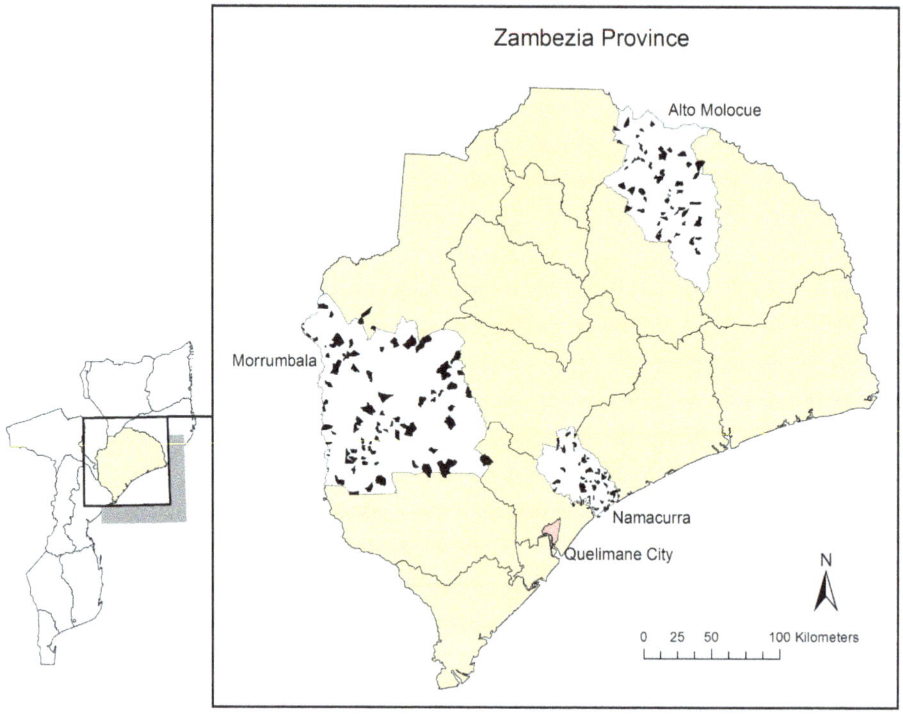


**Figure 1. Map of Mozambique, Zambézia Province, with Enumeration Areas Highlighted in Three Focus Districts, Namacurra, Morrumbala, and Alto Molócuè.**

## Study Design

Integral to *Ogumaniha's* design is a strong monitoring system and project evaluation based on performance indicators agreed upon with USAID and the provincial government. Because the project involves multi-sectoral interventions and an interdisciplinary approach to implementation, the consortium opted for a multidisciplinary evaluation design. A survey instrument used at *Ogumaniha's* initiation (baseline survey in 2010) and at the project's end (final survey implemented June 2014) was designed based on the human development theory originated by Sen (1999) and further developed by researchers from OPHI. This instrument uses multiple dimensions to measure poverty including health, education, and income; access to goods and services; and self-empowerment. The vision of this pre-post project evaluation is that the information collected can provide a more thorough and holistic measure of the impact of this large-scale, multi-sector intervention on the overall health and well-being of the households in Zambézia Province, more so than analysis of the individual sector specific measures when viewed in isolation.

The *Ogumaniha* survey tool collects information on over 500 variables in 8 dimensions and was developed by a multi-disciplinary team of researchers including staff, faculty, and graduate students from Vanderbilt University and the Universidade Eduardo Mondlane. To design the survey, we used many questions and validated scales from previous national surveys in Mozambique, including various National Institute for Statistics (*Instituto Nacional de Estatísticas* [INE]) surveys focusing on poverty and economic status; and other international surveys such as the Demographic Health Survey (DHS) and the Multiple Indicator Cluster Survey (MICS). The survey was designed to collect household information from the female head of household, defined as the principal wife of the nuclear family (polygamy is common practice), because she is thought to be most familiar with the majority of topics of interest. Survey questions covered household demographics; economic status; health knowledge, attitudes and practices; access to health and HIV-related services and products; access to improved water and sanitation; nutritional intake; and others.

The poverty index used to identify households or areas of poverty in the province following baseline survey data collection, was modeled after the Multidimensional Poverty Index (MPI) founded on the OPHI methodology which calculates the quantity of defined "poor" (the headcount), multiplied by their average amount of deprivation, called the Adjusted Headcount Ratio [15].

## Data Collection

Mobile survey teams conducted interviews with 3,916 (98%) of 3,960 planned female heads of households in 259 Enumeration Areas (EAs) across 14 of Zambézia's 17 districts. Complete data for analysis was available from 3,749 (96%) of the interviews conducted. EA selection was not stratified by district, thus 3 districts were randomly excluded from the province-wide sample. Interviews were conducted either in Portuguese or in one of the five predominant tribal languages of the province (Cisena, Elomwe, Echuabo, Cinyanja, and Emakhuwa), and data were collected using mobile cell phones. Interviewers received intensive training on the use of mobile phones for data collection prior to implementation. Satellite and census maps were used to locate the EAs. Initial plans for household selection included administering questionnaires at 15 household structures identified through a color threshold algorithm and randomly selected on the satellite map; however, the actual implementation resulted in division of the EA into four quadrants and collecting 3–4 interviews starting at the household nearest the center of each quadrant (household selection paper in preparation). In a subset of 95 randomly selected EAs, anthropometric measures of a random selection of children

**Table 1.** Ogumaniha Multidimensional Poverty Index (MPI) adapted from the Oxford Poverty and Human Development Initiative (OPHI).

| **OPHI Model** | | *Ogumaniha* **MPI** | | | **Districts of Alto Molócuè, Morrumbala and Namacurra** |
|---|---|---|---|---|---|
| **Dimension** | **Indicator** | **Deprivation cut-off (poverty line)** | **Weight** | **Deprivation** | **Percent of households deprived per indicator (95% CI)[1]** |
| Education | | | | | |
| | Years of Schooling | Literacy score<16 and numeracy score<5 | 1/6 | Low literacy | 14.7% (11.9, 17.5) |
| | Child Enrollment | Child in household = "Yes"+age ">6" or age "<15"+attending school = "No" | 1/6 | School-aged child is not attending school | 17.6% (15.5, 19.7) |
| Health | | | | | |
| | Child Mortality | Fever last 30 d = "Yes", Diarrhea last 30 d = "Yes" or Difficulty breathing last 30 d = "Yes" | 1/6 | Child with acute illness | 21.5% (18.5, 24.6) |
| | Nutrition | Household dietary diversity score<4 | 1/12 | Low dietary diversity | 15.4% (13.1, 17.6) |
| | | Lack of food episode during last month = "Yes" | 1/12 | Lack of food episode during last month | 30.4% (27.7, 33.1) |
| Standard of living | | | | | |
| | Electricity | Electricity = "No" | 1/18 | No electricity | 95.1% (93.7, 96.5) |
| | Water | Water source is river = "True", OR time to water = ">30 min", AND mode of transport to water = "On foot" | 1/18 | Water source is river or more than 30 minutes away on foot | 29.7% (25.6, 33.8) |
| | Sanitation | Household uses latrine = "No" | 1/18 | No use of latrine | 75.6% (72.4, 78.8) |
| | Flooring | Roof type = "grass/cane/leaves/straw" | 1/18 | Poor housing material (grass roof) | 92.5% (90.9, 94.0) |
| | Cooking Fuel | Type of fuel household uses = "Wood" | 1/18 | Poor cooking fuel (wood) | 95.9% (94.5, 97.2) |
| | Assets | Sum of radio = "Yes"+television = "Yes"+bicycle = "Yes" = <1 | 1/18 | Low assets (no radio, television, bike) | 43.2% (40.7, 45.8) |

[1]Weighted percentages include 95% confidence intervals that incorporate the effects of stratification and clustering due to the sample design.

under 5-years residing in participating households were also included. In these EA's, households with one or more children aged 0–12 months, one child was randomly selected for weight and height measurements. Similarly, for households with one or

**Table 2.** Use of the Oxford Poverty and Human Development Initiative (OPHI) Method for Monitoring and Evaluation.

| **Advantages of the OPHI Method for Monitoring and Evaluation** |
|---|
| -Expands dimension measures in critical areas including health |
| -Incorporates program specific detail in comparative evaluation |
| -Uses national comparisons for benchmarking and scale, and efficiency |
| -Isolates where the greatest impact is (and potentially unintended) |
| -Detects indirect benefits in poverty reduction from specific interventions |
| -Facilitates the collaboration between development policy makers who are increasingly measuring multidimensional poverty and development practitioners on the ground |
| -Allows for temporal and geographic comparisons |

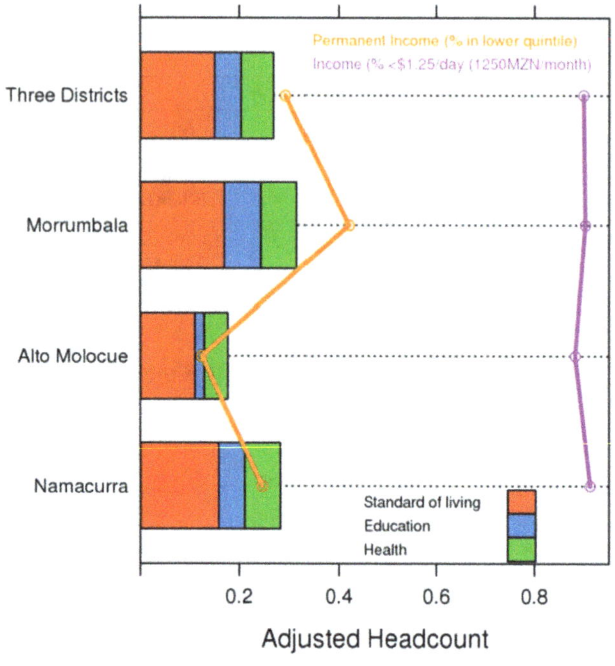


**Figure 2. Decomposition by District and Broken Down by Dimension in the Three Focal Districts, *Ogumaniha* 2010. Legend:** The adjusted headcount is decomposed by dimension for Morrumbala, Alto Molócuè, Namacurra and all three districts combined. Data that are overlaid include percent of households in the lowest quintile for permanent income wealth and % of households making less than USD$1.25/day. MZN = Metical.

more children aged 13–59 months, one child was randomly selected for height and weight measurements.

Baseline survey data were collected between August and September, 2010. Fourteen teams of five female surveyors were recruited, each with prior experience in survey work. The teams were assigned by language proficiency to a specific region, working under the supervision of a regional supervisor, and were trained on general aspects of survey conduct.

Mozambique's 2007 census served as the sampling frame. To appropriately capture *Ogumaniha's* public health and development interventions without increasing the sample size and survey costs, data were collected in two phases; a concentrated sample of 2,878 households in 193 EAs in three selected focal districts (Namacurra, Alto Molócuè, and Morrumbala) (Figure 1) and a smaller sample of 871 households in 66 EA from the remaining districts. These three districts were selected because they represent 3 distinct geographical regions, and *Ogumaniha* interventions were anticipated in each, allowing future analysis of intervention impact on poverty. We provide the sample size justification online: http://globalhealth.vanderbilt.edu/manage/wpcontent/uploads/Ogumaniha_SampleSize_20100613.pdf.

## Alkire and Foster Method

Methods to identify and aggregate the poor using multiple dimensions have mathematical properties that allow for decomposition of poverty indices by subgroups or by indicators. [15] The Alkire and Foster method was used to construct three key poverty indices: headcount, average poverty gap, and adjusted headcount (called the *Ogumaniha* MPI). Application of this method is detailed elsewhere (see http://www.ophi.org.uk/research/multidimensional-poverty/how-to-apply-alkire-foster/); briefly, the steps for identification and aggregation of households include:

**Table 3.** Poverty Distribution of Zambézia Province, Districts of Morrumbala, Namacurra, and Alto Molócuè.

| Poverty cut-off (Minimum deprivation) | Headcount (95% CI) (n = 2,878) |
|---|---|
| 11.1% | 99.2% (98.5, 99.8) |
| 16.7% | 97.7% (96.6, 98.8) |
| 22.2% | 91.4% (89.8, 93.0) |
| 25% | 77.4% (75.0, 79.8) |
| 27.8% | 75.6% (73.1, 78.2) |
| 30.6% | 64.2% (61.3, 67.1) |
| 33.0% | 58.2% (55.0, 61.4) |
| 36.1% | 52.2% (48.9, 55.5) |
| 38.9% | 44.9% (41.6, 48.3) |
| 41.7% | 35.9% (33.0, 38.8) |
| 44.4% | 33.5% (30.5, 36.4) |
| 47.2% | 25.1% (22.6, 27.7) |
| 50% | 21.0% (18.5, 23.5) |
| 52.8% | 17.0% (14.6, 19.5) |
| 55.5% | 11.5% (9.2, 13.7) |
| 58.3% | 8.9% (7.3, 10.4) |
| 61.1% | 6.9% (5.4, 8.3) |
| 63.9% | 4.7% (3.5, 5.9) |
| 66.7% | 3.6% (2.7, 4.5) |

**Table 4.** Respondent and Household Characteristics by Multidimensional Poverty Status, *Ogumaniha* 2010.

| Variables[a] | Non-poor | Poor | Total[d] | P-value[c] |
|---|---|---|---|---|
| | (n = 1196) | (n = 1682) | (n = 2878) | |
| Household size (n = 2878) | 4 (3–6) | 5 (3–6) | 4 (3–6) | <0.001 |
| Children under 5 (n = 2878) | 1 (0–1) | 1 (0–2) | 1 (0–2) | <0.001 |
| Age of respondent (n = 2425) | 30 (23–40) | 32 (25–41) | 32 (24–41) | <0.001 |
| Education (n = 2878) | 2 (0–4) | 0 (0–2) | 0 (0–3) | <0.001 |
| *Distance of EA from health facility (km) (n = 2878) | 6.8 (3.8–10.8) | 7.8 (4.5–12.2) | 7.5 (4–11.7) | <0.001 |
| Urban/rural (n = 2878) | | | | <0.001 |
| Rural | 40.5% | 59.5% | 95.7% | |
| Urban | 70.7% | 29.3% | 4.3% | |
| Length of residency (years) (n = 2785) | 6 (3–18) | 6 (3–15) | 6 (3–17) | 0.997 |
| Primary language of household (n = 2873) | | | | <0.001 |
| Cinyanja | 23.2% | 76.8% | 0.8% | |
| Cisena | 33.7% | 66.3% | 44.3% | |
| Echuabo | 39.8% | 60.2% | 25.6% | |
| Elomwe | 55.7% | 44.3% | 27.6% | |
| Emakhuwa | 45.4% | 54.6% | 0.3% | |
| Portuguese | 73.5% | 26.5% | 1.3% | |
| Respondent understands Portuguese (n = 2876) | 54.7% | 45.3% | 27.5% | <0.001 |
| Marital status (n = 2878) | | | | 0.035 |
| Married/Common Law | 42.8% | 57.2% | 72.9% | |
| Divorced/Separated | 29.5% | 70.5% | 3.4% | |
| Single | 43.0% | 57.0% | 17.5% | |
| Widowed | 34.0% | 66.0% | 6.2% | |
| Religion (n = 2598) | | | | <0.001 |
| Catholic | 48.0% | 52.0% | 45.7% | |
| Protestant | 41.2% | 58.8% | 10.7% | |
| Evangelical and Pentecostal | 39.6% | 60.4% | 14.3% | |
| Other Christian[b] | 37.1% | 62.9% | 4.5% | |
| Muslim | 41.1% | 58.9% | 8.5% | |
| Non-Christian Eastern | 37.8% | 62.2% | 4.3% | |
| Other[b] | 34.2% | 65.8% | 11.9% | |
| **Monthly household income, Meticais (n = 2691) | 150 (0–500) | 0 (0–300) | 150 (0–500) | <0.001 |
| No household income (n = 2691) | 33.4% | 66.6% | 48.8% | <0.001 |
| Household member has a farm (n = 2856) | 41.6% | 58.4% | 90.7% | 0.408 |
| Permanent income (n = 2878) | 0.6 (0.3–0.8) | 0.3 (0–0.5) | 0.4 (0.1–0.7) | <0.001 |
| Ever accessed health facility (n = 2878) | 45.4% | 54.6% | 57.4% | <0.001 |
| Ever accessed pharmacy (n = 2878) | 46.5% | 53.5% | 18.1% | 0.004 |
| Ever accessed traditional healer (n = 2878) | 43.8% | 56.2% | 39.7% | 0.579 |
| ***Ever accessed VCT (n = 2878) | 55.1% | 44.9% | 10.7% | <0.001 |
| ****Accessed ANC last pregnancy (n = 2457) | 44.7% | 55.3% | 41.8% | 0.001 |

[a]Continuous variables are reported as weighted estimates of median (interquartile range] and categorical variables are reported as weighted percentages, with each observation being weighted by the inverse of the household sampling probability.

[b]'Other Christian' includes LDS Mormon and Jehovah's Witness. 'Other' includes Spiritual, Traditional Religions, and Agnostic or Atheist.

[c]Tests of associations (continuous) include Wilcoxon rank sum (continuous) and chi-squared test (categorical).

[d]All percentages in the cross tabulations are row percentages. The final column presents column (overall) percentages.

*EA = enumeration area.

**Approximate exchange rate as of October 2013: $1 USD = 30 Meticais.

***VCT = voluntary counseling and testing (for HIV).

****ANC = antenatal clinic.

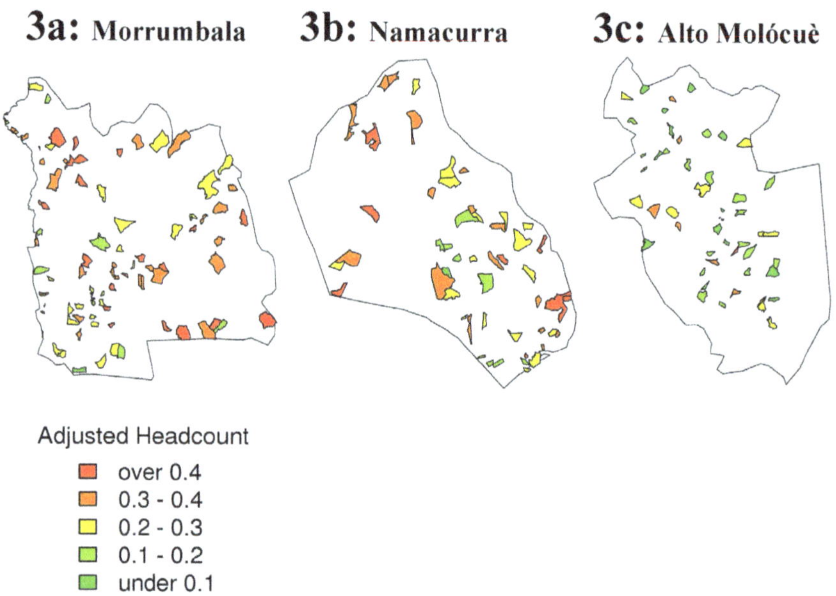


**Figure 3. Enumeration Area Distribution in Three Focus District by Adjusted Headcount: Morrumbala, Namacurra and Alto Molócuè.** *Enumeration area representations of poverty by adjusted headcount with green being less deprived and red.

1. Creation of a listing of **dimensions** and corresponding **indicators** collected from the household survey. (Table 1, columns 1–2)
2. Setting **poverty lines** at values where a person is identified as deprived or non-deprived for each indicator. (Table 1, column 3)
3. Setting **weights** for contribution of each indicator to the overall metric. (Table 1, column 4)
4. Determining the poverty cut-off for **identification**. (Table 2, row 7)
5. Performing **robustness** checks of the cut-off. (Table 2)
6. Estimating across group or dimension using **aggregation**:

a. Headcount (H): proportion of households that are identified as poor.
b. Average Poverty Gap (A): weighted average deprivation experienced by poor.
c. Adjusted Headcount (called the *Ogumaniha* MPI): multiply headcount by average poverty gap to reflect the breadth of deprivations. Thus, MPI = HxA.

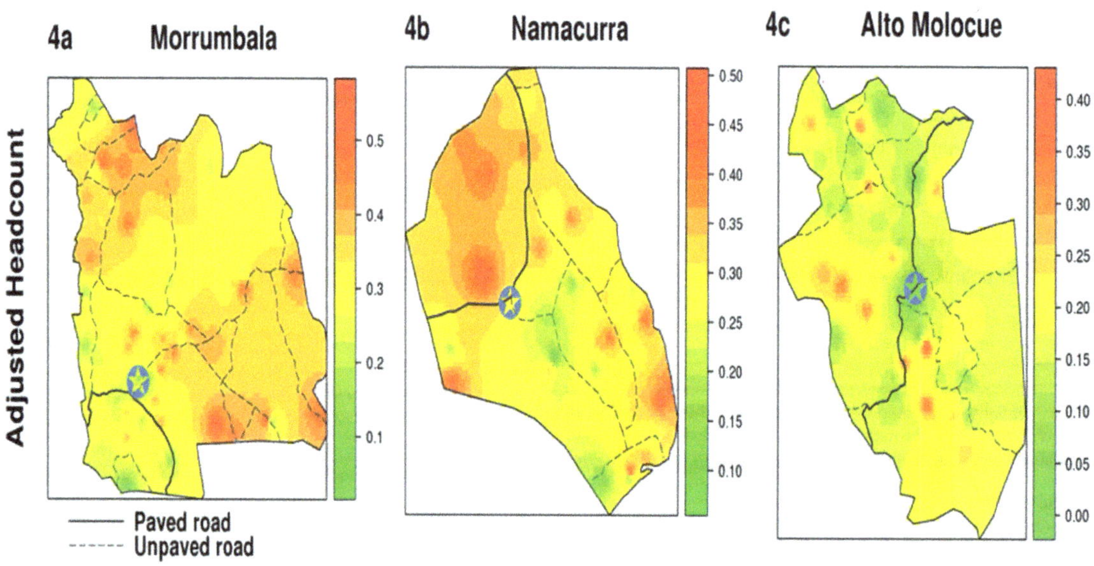


**Figure 4. Smoothed Heat Map of Three Focus Districts: Morrumbala, Namacurra, and Alto Molócuè.** *Figures 4a, 4b, and 4c show heat map geographical representations of poverty by adjusted headcount with green being less deprived and red most deprived. (Circled Star represents location of district capital).

Proportions include 95% confidence intervals that incorporate the effects of stratification and clustering due to the sample design. [26] Descriptive analysis of continuous variables includes weighted estimates of median, 25th and 75th quantiles (interquartile range). Categorical variables are reported as weighted percentages, with each observation being weighted by the inverse of the household sampling probability. Tests of association by poverty ignore effects of clustering, and they include Wilcoxon rank sum (continuous) and chi-square (categorical) tests.

### Map generation

Using Esri shape files provided by INE to identify EA boundaries, a basic heat-map of poverty metrics was generated for the three focus districts. To enhance readability of the maps, ordinary kriging was used to predict poverty metrics for unsampled areas, assuming only spatial correlation. The 'krige' function is in the gstat package of R, which uses generalized least squares prediction with spatial covariances to produce smoothed geospatial representations of poverty. [27] R-software 2.15.1 (www.r-project.org) was employed for all data analyses; analysis scripts are available online at (http://biostat.mc.vanderbilt.edu/ArchivedAnalyses).

### Description of permanent income

The measurement of household income is particularly problematic in high poverty areas. [28] In the current sample, 49% report no monetary income whatsoever. Increasingly in economics and development, monetary income is no longer the preferred measure. Instead, a "permanent income", [29] or wealth measure based upon ownership of selected assets is employed. Poverty stemming from lack of resources is associated with low income, but it is perhaps more closely related to low wealth. Low wealth individuals always have low income, but not all low income individuals have low wealth. In that sense, wealth and poverty are more closely related than income and poverty. We applied a measure of permanent income developed by the World Bank. [28] Briefly, a series of 37 asset and other indicator variables were used in a dichotomous hierarchical ordered probit model to derive a latent variable which denotes the permanent income of household to be incorporated into the *Ogumaniha* MPI (Figure 2, orange line) [12].

### Ethical Considerations

Participation in the household survey was completely voluntary, no incentive was provided for participation. At enrollment written informed consent was obtained. The protocol for data collection and consent forms were approved by the Mozambican National Bioethics Committee for Health (*Comité Nacional de Bioética em Saúde* [CNBS]) and the Institutional Review Board of Vanderbilt University.

## Results and Discussion

Results are presented in two sections. Section 1 describes the methodology we employed to define our metric, the *Ogumaniha* MPI, and demonstrates its usefulness to planning and evaluation of large scale public health and development interventions. Section 2 applies the *Ogumaniha* MPI to households and EAs in the three focus districts by utilizing data collected in the *Ogumaniha* baseline survey, in order to establish baseline multidimensional poverty estimates in Mozambique's Zambézia Province.

### Section 1 - Defining the Ogumaniha Multidimensional Poverty Index (MPI)

We employ a method of monitoring and evaluation that looks at the analysis of development interventions in holistic terms, producing an aggregate metric that can be disaggregated by dimension (education, health, and living standard) and further disaggregated by subgroups (e.g., urban/rural, Portuguese proficiency). In the OPHI model, the 3 dimensions were further disaggregated into 10 indicators, weighted evenly within dimension such that each dimension had equal weight, and then a person was defined as poor if they were "deprived" in more than 33% of the indicators (Table 1). We used dimensional weighting similar to the OPHI model that would produce a comparable aggregate metric that could be used to compare across projects while incorporating national norms. Our method allows the isolation of the relative impact of specific inputs on overall well-being, and thus target areas for effective interventions.

This method goes beyond multiple measures and generates a true MPI. Specifically, it 1) uses intentionally selected dimensions of poverty to capture relevant functioning and capability deficits; 2) calculates deficit cut points based on comparative conditions; 3) applies differential weighting of deficits that contribute to poverty level; and 4) combines calculated poverty measures to produce a single metric for comparative purposes (Table 2).

An advantage of the *Ogumaniha* MPI includes its basis on survey data, which takes into account community level impact, perceptions, and buy-in. Additionally, survey data were collected utilizing a low-cost cell phone technology that reduced data entry costs and errors. The *Ogumaniha* MPI may be used for planning purposes to identify areas with high frequency of poor, intense poverty, or both. In being able to isolate not only the direct impact of a particular intervention but also the effect of inputs on other dimensions and overall well-being, this model can also serve as a useful tool in assessing return on investment and cost-benefit analyses.

### Section 2 - Identifying Poverty by Household and Enumeration Area

Building upon the OPHI MPI, we maintained the same 3 dimensions (education, health, and living standard), but defined 11 indicators rather than the 10 utilized in the OPHI model. When possible, the same OPHI indicators were used; however, some were adapted for best fit based on the questions asked in the baseline survey. Table 1 shows the OPHI Model in comparison to our adapted *Ogumaniha* MPI with the "weight" column representing the contribution of each indicator to multidimensional poverty. The rightmost column (Table 1) reports the proportion of households that are deprived in each indicator.

Of 2,878 female heads of household interviewed in the three focal districts, the median age was 32 years. The median household size was four persons and the median number of children <5 years old in the home was one. Choosing to maintain the same OPHI poverty definition cut-off, in which the "poor" must be deprived in at least 33% of the indicators, a headcount of 58.2% of our provincially representative sample met that definition and were identified as poor. The highest cut-off would identify 3.6% of households as poor whereas the lowest cut-off would identify 99.2% of households as poor. If the poor were deprived in 50% or more deprivations, then the headcount is 20% (Table 3). Approximately 96% of households lived in an EA designated as rural by INE, of which 59.5% met the criteria for being defined poor, compared to 29.3% of urban households. Looking at the relationship of poverty to the primary language spoken in the household, 26.5% of Portuguese speaking households and 58.6% of households speaking one of the other five local languages were considered poor (Table 4).

Once identified as poor, if the intensity of deprivation increases for a household (say from 33% to 60% of weighted indicators), the headcount remains unchanged. As such, robust models must be able to adjust for changes in both headcount and the average deprivation; this MPI is called adjusted headcount. Using the 33% deprivation cut-off from the OPHI method, we estimated a headcount of 58.2% of the three focal districts sample to be poor; among these, households experienced an average deprivation of 46%; thus the adjusted headcount (= 0.58×0.46) is 0.27 (95% CI: 0.25–0.29). The headcounts for the three focal districts (Morrumbala, Namacurra, Alto Molócuè) plus all three combined are 0.67, 0.60, 0.42, and 0.58, respectively. The average deprivation for the three focal districts, plus all three combined, are 0.48, 0.47, 0.42, and 0.46. Analyzed separately, Morrumbala has the greatest breadth of poverty with an index of 0.32 (0.29–0.34), followed by Namacurra at 0.28 (0.26–0.31), and the least deprived being Alto Molócuè with an index of 0.18 (0.15–0.21). Additionally, the *Ogumaniha* MPI can be further broken down revealing the weight of each dimension's contribution to that index. In all three districts, living standard was the most dominant dimension deprived, followed by health, and then education (Figure 2).

Following calculation of the *Ogumaniha* MPI for each of the 193 EAs in three focal districts, geospatial maps were created that allow for visualization of the dispersion of EAs throughout the three districts (Figure 3) and provide smoothed estimates of poverty at baseline (Figure 4). The mapping of poverty deprivation at baseline provides program implementers a visual needs assessment that characterizes the geographic differences of each target district and aids in prioritizing program planning. Additionally, going forward we can overlay maps depicting the location and intensity of the various *Ogumaniha* sector interventions in the target districts (which were not uniformly implemented) and evaluate the impact of those interventions, or the combination of interventions. This is possible for measured outcomes in the specific individual-level locations in which interventions were implemented and also for a broader area-level evaluation or "neighborhood effect" that interventions may or may not have on nearby locales and/or the district as a whole.

In Morrumbala (Figure 4a), there are two geographic areas of high poverty deprivation, one in the extreme northwest of the district and the other in the southeastern region. Areas of least poverty deprivation, tend to focus around the main transportation corridor in the south, around the district capital and extends to the northeast through the center of the district. The area of high poverty deprivation in the northeast is fairly isolated, and difficult to reach (can take up to 5 hours to reach by car from the district capital). Morrumbala suffers from flooding of the Zambezi and Chire rivers each year. Flood zones are located in the southwest region and extending north along the western border of the district.

In Namacurra (Figure 4b), the largest geographic area of high poverty deprivation is in the northwest side of the district with pockets of high poverty deprivation distributed throughout the southeast. The southern parts of Namacurra can be difficult to reach with roads that flood, cutting them off from the rest of the district during the rainy season. However this area has some of the more fertile farm-land. Furthermore, the southernmost tip of Namacurra is coastal (one of only a handful of natural deep water ports on the eastern African coastline). This port is slated for large investments in infrastructure over the next 5–10 years, and may become an economic hub for the north-central provinces of Mozambique.

Alto Molócuè (Figures 4c) is one of the more economically developed districts with several commercial factories. The national highway cuts across the district and connects Alto Molócuè with commercial centers in the south and Nampula Province to the north. Pockets of high deprivation tend to be located in areas farthest away from transportation corridors.

## Conclusions

We seek innovative approaches to conducting evaluation research in public health. [30] Baseline assessments of poverty that are more valid can improve our program planning as well as evaluation of interventions. Advancement in evaluation is increasingly critical due to the pressures created by the burdens of disease in the developing world, and even more so by the increasing complexity of interventions. In developing the measurement and evaluation tools reported here we employ the most current understanding of the crucial interdependency between conditions of poverty and both the need for and effectiveness of public health interventions. However, significant obstacles still limit the potential utility of this new approach to public health program evaluation. While measures taking multidimensionality into account have already been adopted by the Mozambican government, its meaning and use remains relatively unfamiliar. In our sample, relatively few households sampled came from urban areas as the make-up of Zambézia Province is predominantly rural. In our context we feel the MPI measure accurately captures a relevant view of the condition of poverty across the province. However, a limitation to this approach is that if applied to a predominantly urban area, the indicators used to assess poverty may overestimate households as non-deprived based on a lack of dirt floor for example, despite the fact that they may live in a poorly quality structures with crowded conditions and limited space. As a result, analysis must take into account context for what is considered deprived or not. Additionally, the logistics, manpower, and costs of implementing such a large population-based survey at program's beginning and end may limit the accessibility of this approach to only governments, donor agencies, and/or larger multi-sector public health development projects whose outcomes of interest are not isolated to the individual sector specific program indicators.

In this paper, we have reported the estimated baseline MPI for Zambézia Province at initiation of a large scale USAID funded, 5-year multi-sector grant. We believe that our estimates of poverty are a conservative minimum, as our results show that greater than half of our representative sample is poor (based on the 33% deprivation standard), and one-fifth or more are deprived in 50% of indicators. We found that living standard was the dominant dimension of poverty, followed by health and then education. By avoiding a unidimensional income measure, which in the Zambézia context classifies >90% of households as poor based on the generic < $1.25/day standard (Figure 2), the *Ogumaniha* MPI reveals a more nuanced and differentiated view of the conditions of poverty in an area that frequently employs non-monetary economic structures and is reliant on subsistence farming and fishing. This will assist in setting priorities for development in an area of near-universal poverty, as the neediest persons and regions can be differentiated from the less needy.

The implications of this work apply to both program planning and research. The integration of multidimensional poverty measures into planning and implementation design and the use of geospatial visualization of the relationships between interventions and distinct conditions of poverty at baseline have great utility and added value to the field of public health. Geospatial mapping, for instance, can dramatize variations of poverty in microenvironments, helping set program intervention priorities. Key to meeting the twin demands of greater impact and greater efficiency for public health interventions is recognizing and responding to the challenges created by the interdependencies between public health and other dimensions of poverty. Such interdependencies are rarely incorporated into program evaluation, thus leaving public health implementers and researchers struggling to understand both the positive and negative outcomes of interventions.

The MPI technique allows public health professionals and agencies to better target their resources by accounting for variation. With respect to research, we demonstrate how a robust multidimensional measurement can explore the linkages between poverty and health differentials in a population and derive useful inferences for further evidence-based planning. When repeated in Zambézia at the end of the 5-year program, evaluators will be permitted to not only observe the relative impact of *Ogumaniha's* intervention intensity, duration, and composition, but also analyze factors that drive or inhibit direct effectiveness and interaction effects, at both the micro/household level as well as a more macro/provincial level. This work demonstrates the distinctive and highly valuable insights that are created by applying a multidimensional measure of poverty to the evaluation of a complex, large scale public health intervention such as the *Ogumaniha*-SCIP project.

## Acknowledgments

We acknowledge the members of the Ogumaniha monitoring and evaluation team including: Jeff Weiser, Lara Vaz, Iranett Manteiga, Ofelia Santiago, Faride Mussagy, Aurélio André Andate, Luciano Bene and Reginaldo Muluco. We give special thanks to the whole OPHI organization for providing excellent instruction to an investigator (MB) at the 2011 OPHI-HDCA Summer School in Delft, Netherlands at Delft University of Technology (course content available online at http://www.ophi.org.uk/resources/online-training-portal). We also thank Spencer James, Post-Bachelor Fellow of University of Washington for sharing his analysis code to estimate permanent income.

## Author Contributions

Conceived and designed the experiments: BV MB AG SV AV EF OO TM. Performed the experiments: EN LG AV. Analyzed the data: BV AG MB TM EF OO. Contributed to the writing of the manuscript: BV MB AG SV TM.

## References

1. The United Nations Development Agenda: Development for all. Available: http://www.un.org/esa///devagenda/UNDA_BW5_Final.pdf. Accessed 2014 Sep 5.
2. Fanzo JC, Pronyk PM (2011) A review of global progress toward the Millennium Development Goal 1 Hunger Target. Food Nutr Bull, 32: 144–158.
3. Dodd R, Cassels A (2006) Health, development and the Millennium Development Goals. Ann Trop Med Parasitol, 100: 379–387.
4. Gaffikin L, Ashley J, Blumenthal PD (2007) Poverty reduction and Millennium Development Goals: recognizing population, health, and environment linkages in rural Madagascar. Medscape Gen Med, 9: 17.
5. Anand S, Sen A Concepts of human development and poverty: A multidimensional perspective. Available: http://clasarchive.berkeley.edu/Academics/courses/center/fall2007/sehnbruch/UNDP%20Anand%20and%20Sen%20Concepts%20of%20HD%201997.pdf. Accessed 2014 Sep 5.
6. Saith A (2011) Inequality, imbalance, instability: reflections on a structural crisis. Dev Change, 42: 70–86.
7. Sen A (2000) A decade of human development. J Hum Dev, 1: 17–23.
8. International Human Development Indicators - UNDP: Mozambique. Available: http://hdr.undp.org/en/countries/profiles/MOZ. Accessed 2014 Sep 5.
9. Bourguignon F, Chakravarty SR (2003) The measurement of multidimensional poverty. Journal of Economic Inequality, 1: 25–49.
10. Guedes GR, Brondizio ES, Barbieri AF, Anne R, Penna-Firme R, et al (2012) Poverty and inequality in the rural Brazilian Amazon: A multidimensional approach. Hum Ecol, 40: 41–57.
11. Deutsch J, Silber J (2005) Measuring multidimensional poverty: An empirical comparison of various approaches. Rev Income Wealth, 51: 145–174.
12. Victor B, Fischer EF, Cooil B, Vergara A, Mukolo A, et al (2013) Frustrated freedom: The effects of agency and wealth on wellbeing in rural Mozambique. World Dev, 47: 30–41.
13. The multidimensional poverty assessment tool (MPAT): A new approach for measuring rural poverty. Available: http://www.ifad.org/mpat/. Accessed 2014 Sep 5.
14. Alkire S, Santos ME (2011) Acute multidimensional poverty. A new index for developing countries (2011). In Proceedings of the German Development Economics Conference, Berlin, No. 3.
15. Alkire S, Foster J (2011) Counting and multidimensional poverty measurement. J Public Econ, 95: 476–487.
16. Sagar AD, Najam A (1998) The human development index: a critical review. Ecol Econ, 25: 249–264.
17. Country Health Profile of Mozambique - WHO Regional Office for Africa. Available: http://www.afro.who.int/en/mozambique/country-health-profile.html. Accessed 2014 Sep 5.
18. WHO World Health Statistics 2011. Available: http://www.who.int/whosis/whostat/2011/en/index.html. Accessed 2014 Sep 5.
19. INSIDA 2009, Inquérito Nacional de Prevalência, Riscos Comportamentais e Informação sobre o HIV e SIDA em Moçambique. Available: http://www.measuredhs.com/pubs/pdf/AIS8/AIS8.pdf. Accessed 2014 Sep 5.
20. Multiple Indicator Cluster Survey (2008). Available: http://www.unicef.org/mozambique/MICS_Summary_English_201009.pdf. Accessed 2014 Sep 5.
21. Moon TD, Burlison JR, Sidat M, Pires P, Silva W, et al (2010) Lessons learned while implementing an HIV/AIDS care and treatment program in rural Mozambique. Retrovirology: Research and Treatment, 3: 1–14.
22. Moon TD, Burlison JR, Blevins M, Shepherd BE, Baptista A, et al (2011) Enrolment and programmatic trends and predictors of antiretroviral therapy initiation from president's emergency plan for AIDS Relief (PEPFAR)-supported public HIV care and treatment sites in rural Mozambique. Int J STD AIDS, 22: 621–627.
23. Cook RE, Ciampa PJ, Sidat M, Blevins M, Burlison J, et al (2011) Predictors of successful early infant diagnosis of HIV in a rural district hospital in Zambézia, Mozambique. J Acquir Immune Defic Syndr, 56: e104–109.
24. Ciampa PJ, Vaz LME, Blevins M, Sidat M, Rothman RL, et al (2012) The association among literacy, numeracy, HIV knowledge and health-seeking behavior: a population-based survey of women in rural Mozambique. PloS One, 7: e39391.
25. Ministério da Saúde-Moçambique: HIV/SIDA. Available: http://www.misau.gov.mz/index.php/hiv-sida. Accessed 2014 Sep 5.
26. Lumley T (2004) Analysis of complex survey samples. Journal of Statistical Software, 9(1): 1–19.
27. Pebesma EJ (2004) Multivariable geostatistics in S: the gstat package. Comput Geosci, 30: 683–691.
28. Ferguson J (1999) *Expectations of modernity: Myths and meanings of urban life on the Zambian copperbelt*. Berkeley: University of California Press.
29. Friedman M (1957) *A Theory of the Consumption Function*, Princeton: Princeton University Press.
30. Editorial (2010) Evaluation: the top priority for global health. The Lancet, 375: 526.

4

# Mobile Phones: The Next Step towards Healthcare Delivery in Rural India?

**Sherwin I. DeSouza**[1]*, **M. R. Rashmi**[1,2], **Agalya P. Vasanthi**[1], **Suchitha Maria Joseph**[1], **Rashmi Rodrigues**[1]

**1** St. John's National Academy of Health Sciences, Bangalore, India, **2** Department of Community Medicine, Saveetha Medical College, Thandalam, Chennai, Tamil Nadu, India

## Abstract

***Background:*** Given the ubiquity of mobile phones, their use to support healthcare in the Indian context is inevitable. It is however necessary to assess end-user perceptions regarding mobile health interventions especially in the rural Indian context prior to its use in healthcare. This would contextualize the use of mobile phone communication for health to 70% of the country's population that resides in rural India.

***Objectives:*** To explore the acceptability of delivering healthcare interventions through mobile phones among users in a village in rural Bangalore.

***Methods:*** This was an exploratory study of 488 mobile phone users, residing in a village, near Bangalore city, Karnataka, South India. A pretested, translated, interviewer-administered questionnaire was used to obtain data on mobile phone usage patterns and acceptability of the mobile phone, as a tool for health-related communication. The data is described using basic statistical measures.

***Results:*** The primary use of mobile phones was to make or receive phone calls (100%). Text messaging (SMS) was used by only 70 (14%) of the respondents. Most of the respondents, 484 (99%), were willing to receive health-related information on their mobile phones and did not consider receiving such information, an intrusion into their personal life. While receiving reminders for drug adherence was acceptable to most 479 (98%) of our respondents, 424 (89%) preferred voice calls alone to other forms of communication. Nearly all were willing to use their mobile phones to communicate with health personnel in emergencies and 367 (75%) were willing to consult a doctor via the phone in an acute illness. Factors such as sex, English literacy, employment status, and presence of chronic disease affected preferences regarding mode and content of communication.

***Conclusion:*** The mobile phone, as a tool for receiving health information and supporting healthcare through mHealth interventions was acceptable in the rural Indian context.

**Editor:** Christian Lovis, University Hospitals of Geneva, Switzerland

**Funding:** The authors have no support or funding to report.

**Competing Interests:** The authors have declared that no competing interests exist.

* Email: desouza.sherwin@gmail.com

## Introduction

Wireless technologies now cover 96% of the global population and penetrate all walks of life. With 6.8 billion mobile-cellular subscriptions worldwide [1], the technology has successfully bridged gaps in communication and ignited economic growth and development globally [2]. It has also found a strong foothold within the healthcare sector in the emerging field of 'mHealth'. 'mHealth' or 'Mobile Health' is healthcare supported by mobile technology, such as mobile phones, personal digital assistants and other wireless devices [3]. The emerging use of this technology in healthcare for treatment compliance, emergency management, mobile telemedicine, health promotion and community mobilization, are currently being researched or implemented globally [3].

### India and mobile communication technology

With 877 million wireless subscribers, India has the second largest wireless communication subscriber base in the world [4]. Wireless subscribers comprise 96% of telecom subscribers in India and contribute to an urban wireless tele-density fourfold that of rural India [4].

One of the reasons for the popularity of mobile phones in India is the low call tariff. At 1.6 USD/month, India has one of the lowest mobile call tariffs globally [5]. This makes mobile phone communication economical in the Indian context. Further, the average expenditure on mobile phones in rural households is an estimated five INR/month, while the same is 37 INR/month in urban poor households. More recent studies indicate that majority of the urban poor households in India spend approximately 3% of their monthly income on mobile communication [5]. Given the overwhelming popularity of mobile phone communication, at low cost, mHealth in the Indian context holds promise.

Research studies have explored the acceptability of mHealth interventions for supporting adherence to antiretroviral therapy in South India and for healthcare consultation in rural North India [6,7]. The potential of mHealth is being harnessed by the Indian government in the 'Mother and Child Tracking System' (MCTS) within the 'National Rural Health Mission' (NRHM) [8,9]. The MCTS gathers health information from antenatal and postnatal women in an attempt to ensure healthcare delivery to these women and to under-five children. Text messaging or Short Message Service (SMS) technology is also used to communicate with 3.2 million Indian central government employees under the Central Government Health Scheme (CGHS). Plans for its use in adolescent health, reproductive health and family planning, substance abuse and non-communicable disease prevention and treatment, are underway [10]. Given that the use of mobile phones, as a mode of communication in healthcare is inevitable, it is necessary to assess rural end-user perceptions and experiences with the technology. This would help contextualize healthcare delivery via mobile phones to 70% of the country's population residing in rural India.

We undertook this study to explore the acceptability of delivering healthcare interventions via mobile phones in a village in South India. Information obtained with this study could aid the development of appropriate user-friendly applications contextualized to the health needs of the population they target.

## Methods

This is an exploratory study done at a village, 52 kilometres from Bangalore, Karnataka State, South India between March 2009 and 2010. Karnataka state has a total population of 61 million. With 29,098 villages, the state has a rural population of 37,469,335 (61%). The Government provides primary healthcare to the rural population at no cost through a network of sub-centres, primary healthcare centres and community health centres. Additionally, healthcare can be availed at any of the several private facilities that may cater to the rural population for a fee. Healthcare at the village where the study was conducted, is available through a public primary healthcare facility and a private non-profit, faith-based secondary healthcare facility. This private healthcare facility supports research and medical internship training for medical interns from St. John's Medical College, Bangalore, South India, the academic institution that the researchers are affiliated with. The hospital also provides a base for some of the research work undertaken by the institution.

The village has an agrarian economy and is easily accessible by road via the national highway. It has a total population of 3,180 persons belonging to 608 households. Our survey covered all households in the village. Data was collected by door-to-door visits by trained members of the research team. A consenting participant above the age of 15 years, who owned a mobile phone, was enrolled in the study from each household visited. Those households found locked when visited, were excluded from the study.

An interviewer-administered questionnaire was developed. Some questions were adapted from the HIVIND study questionnaire that explored mobile phone usage in people living with HIV/AIDS at an infectious disease clinic in Bangalore, India [7]. The questionnaire was pretested in the local language i.e. Kannada and suitably modified based on feedback from the respondents to improve comprehension. The questionnaire assessed the respondent's demographic profile, mobile phone usage patterns and the acceptability of healthcare interventions delivered via mobile phones. The questionnaire included five domains (i) basic functionality of the mobile phone (ii) delivery and acceptability of health information via mobile phones (iii) use of mobile phones in the management of chronic illnesses (iv) use of mobile phones in the management of acute illnesses and (v) acceptability of usage of cell phones for health promotion.

### Data Analysis

Data was analysed using IBM-SPSS version 20. Frequencies, means, and standard deviation were used to describe the variables. Chi-square, Kruksal Wallis test and bivariate logistic regression models (standard LR) were used to study associations between demography and outcome variables, i.e. (i) preference for voice call to SMS reminders, (ii) more frequent versus less frequent medication reminders in chronic illnesses and (iii) preference for calling a doctor over the mobile phone in times of acute illnesses.

### Ethics statement

Ethical clearance for the study and its informed consent procedures was obtained from the Institutional Ethics Committee, St. John's Medical College, Bangalore, India, a private, non-profit, tertiary level, teaching, healthcare institution, to which the researchers were affiliated. Verbal consent was obtained from all potential participants or their guardians (for those <18 years of age) in the presence of a witness who endorsed the process. In addition, assent to participate in the study was obtained from participants below 18 years of age. Verbal consent was uniformly administered to all potential participants, some of who were illiterate, to ensure participation from those hesitant to sign the consent form but willing to participate in the study. This enabled representation of all demographic subgroups in the study.

## Results

Of the 608 households, 558 were available and willing to participate in the study, of these only 488 owned a mobile phone and were enrolled. The demographic details of the participants who owned a mobile phone are described in table 1. Those who owned a mobile phone had a larger median family than those who did not (Median family size 5; IQR 2 versus 4; IQR 2, p-value Kruksal Wallis test <0.004).

### Basic functionality of mobile phones

All the 488 respondents routinely used their phones for making and receiving calls. On average, the respondents received four calls, while six outgoing calls were made in a day. Additionally, 70 (14%) used their mobile phones for text messaging, 56 (11%) for setting alarms, 337 (69%) for listening to music, 72 (15%) for playing games, 22 (4.5%) for photography and five (1%) for accessing the Internet. Those who were literate in English and 40 years of age or less were more likely to use the text messaging function than those who were not (unadjusted OR = 7.5, CI = 3.69, 15.14).

Of the 488 respondents who owned mobile phones, 484 (99%) were willing to make an appointment at the doctor's clinic via the mobile phone and 467 (96%) were willing to share their mobile number with their doctor. The 21 (4%) respondents who declined to share their phone number did so for fear of misuse of contact details or apprehension with regard to speaking with their doctor over the phone. Others preferred to meet the doctor in person.

### Mobile phones in health promotion

Of 488 respondents, 484 (99%) were open to receiving health information on mobile phones. Topics that participants preferred information on included healthy living, nutrition, maternal and

**Table 1.** Demographic characteristics of the study population **(n = 488)**.

| | **Total (%) (n = 488)** | **Female (%) (n = 360)** | **Male (%) (n = 128)** |
|---|---|---|---|
| **Age** | | | |
| Median (Inter Quartile Range) | 30 (25–40) | 30 (25–37) | 33 (25–45) |
| <20 yrs | 30 (61) | 28 (7) | 2 (2) |
| 20–40 yrs | 328 (67) | 254 (70) | 74 (57) |
| >40 yrs | 130 (27) | 78 (22) | 52 (4) |
| **Formally education**# | | | |
| No | 29 (6) | 21 (6) | 8 (6) |
| Yes | 360 (74) | 339 (94) | 120 (9) |
| **Literate in English** | 46 (9) | 26 (7) | 20 (16) |
| **Currently employed** | | | |
| No | 299 (61) | 297 (83) | 2 (2) |
| Yes | 189 (39) | 63 (17) | 126 (98) |
| **Landline** | 40 (8) | 27 (7) | 13 (10) |
| **Expenditure on mobiles** Median (IQR) | 100 (IQR: 50–200) | 100 (50–200) | 100 (52–200) |
| **Socio economic status (n = 192)**$ | | | |
| High | 12 (6) | 9 (7) | 3 (4) |
| Middle | 93 (48) | 62 (50) | 31 (46) |
| Low | 87 (45) | 53 (43) | 34 (50) |
| **Family's with children** | 84 (44) | 50 (59) | 34 (40) |
| **Chronic illness reported** | | | |
| No | 448 (92) | 336 (93) | 112 (88) |
| Yes | 40 (8) | 24 (7) | 16 (13) |

#Formal education i.e. school and college education.
$Socio economic status as defined by Parasuraman et al (1999).

child health, vaccination, self-care in chronic illnesses and information on infectious disease epidemics, (Figure 1).

Of the 484 respondents willing to receive health information via mobile phones, 218 (45%) preferred to receive the information daily, 223 (46%) weekly, and 42 (9%) monthly. A majority 371 (76%) preferred to receive vaccination reminders a day earlier to the date of vaccination, 73 (15%) on the vaccination day itself and 42 (9%) from a week to a month prior to the date of vaccination.

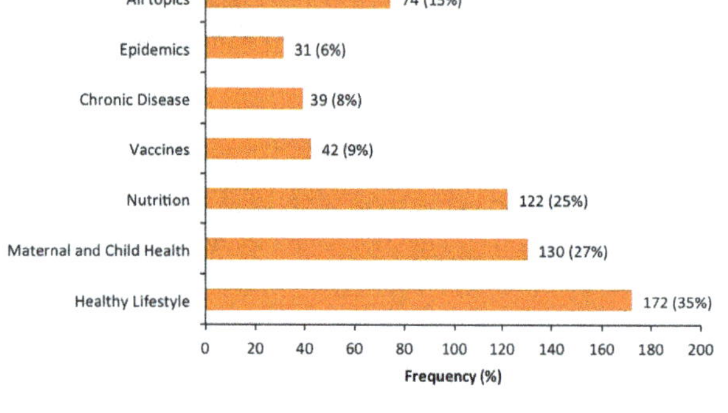


**Figure 1. Type of health information requested over mobile phone (n = 488).** (Uploaded as Figure 1 in TIFF format).

## Mobile phones in the management of chronic illnesses (table 2 and 3)

For the management of chronic illness, 479 (98%) respondents preferred to receive medication adherence reminders via mobile phones. Those who refused reported that they remembered to take their medication without reminders. From among those who preferred reminders, 424 (89%) preferred only voice calls, 45 (9%) preferred text messages and 11 (2%) had no specific preference. Most respondents preferred voice calls (419; 86%) and SMSs (319; 65%) in the local language i.e. Kannada. With every year increase in age, the preference for SMSs was less likely in comparison to voice calls (adjusted OR = 0.951, CI = 0.917, 0.987). Those who were literate in English (adjusted OR = 4.579, CI = 2.111, 9.933) and those currently employed (OR = 2.628, CI = 1.209, 5.714) were more likely to prefer SMSs alone or SMS and voice calls in comparison to those who were not literate in English and those unemployed.

Medication reminders were preferred as often as the medication was to be taken by 163 (34%), daily by 129 (27%), biweekly by 22 (5%) and weekly by 165 (34%). Respondents who were literate in English were twice more likely to prefer more frequent reminders (adjusted OR = 2.264, CI = 1.050, 4.886), while those who suffered from chronic illnesses were less likely to prefer more frequent reminders (adjusted OR = 0.459, CI = 0.227, 0.930). We also found that men were almost twice more likely to prefer more frequent medication reminders in comparison to women (unadjusted OR = 1.868, CI = 1.203, 2.902), as were respondents who

**Table 2.** Preference for daily or less frequent medication reminders compared to demographic characteristics **(n = 479)**.

| | Prefer less frequent reminders (%) (n = 187) | Prefer more frequent reminders (%)(n = 292) | Unadjusted OR | Adjusted OR |
|---|---|---|---|---|
| **Age** | 31.5±9.91 | 33.13±11.09 | 1.014 (0.997, 1.032) | 1.014(0.995, 1.033) |
| **Sex** | | | | |
| Female | 151 (43) | 202 (57) | | |
| Male | 36 (29) | 90 (71) | 1.868 (1.203, 2.902) | 1.502 (0.780, 2.892) |
| **Formally educated#** | | | | |
| No | 8 (28) | 21 (72) | | |
| Yes | 179 (40) | 271 (60) | 0.578 (0.250, 1.330) | 0.589 (0.250, 1.391) |
| **Literate in English** | | | | |
| No | 176 (40) | 259 (60) | | |
| Yes | 11 (25) | 33 (75) | 2.038 (1.003, 4.141) | 2.264 (1.050, 4.886) |
| **Currently Employed** | | | | |
| No | 129 (44) | 165 (56) | | |
| Yes | 58 (31) | 127 (69) | 1.712 (1.163, 2.250) | 1.198 (0.670, 2.143) |
| **Chronic disease** | | | | |
| No | 168 (38) | 274 (62) | | |
| Yes | 19 (51) | 18 (49) | 0.581 (0.296, 1.138) | 0.459 (0.227, 0.930) |

Logistic Regression Model p-value <0.001.
#Formal education indicates education that includes school.

**Table 3.** Preference for voice calls only and SMS with or without voice call reminders compared to demographic characteristics **(n = 480)**.

| | Prefer voice calls only (%) (n = 424) | Prefer SMS or SMS + voice calls* (%) (n = 56) | Unadjusted OR | Adjusted OR |
|---|---|---|---|---|
| **Age** | 33.19±10.85 | 27.48±7.64 | 0.937 (0.905, 0.970) | 0.951 (0.917, 0.987) |
| **Sex** | | | | |
| Female | 314 (88) | 40 (12) | | |
| Male | 110 (87) | 16 (13) | 1.142 (0.615, 2.120) | 0.534 (0.230, 1.243) |
| **Formally educated#** | | | | |
| No | 26 (90) | 3 (10) | | |
| Yes | 398 (88) | 53 (12) | 1.154 (0.337, 3.944) | 0.575 (0.158, 2.091) |
| **Literate in English** | | | | |
| No | 395 (91) | 37 (9) | | |
| Yes | 29 (60) | 19 (40) | 8.196 (4.131, 16.25) | 4.579 (2.111, 9.933) |
| **Currently Employed** | | | | |
| No | 271 (92) | 24 (8) | | |
| Yes | 153 (83) | 32 (17) | 2.361 (1.342, 4.156) | 2.628 (1.209, 5.714) |
| **Presence of chronic disease** | | | | |
| No | 396 (89) | 48 (11) | | |
| Yes | 28 (78) | 8 (22) | 2.270 (0.981, 5.248) | 1.661 (0.642, 4.296) |

Logistic Regression Model p-value <0.001.
#Formal education indicates education that includes school.
*This category includes those who preferred the SMS alone or both SMS and voice calls.
AIC: 312.7853, BIC: 342.002.

were currently employed (unadjusted OR = 1.712, CI = 1.163, 2.250).

### Mobile phones in the management of acute illness

Of the 488 respondents, 367 (75%) were willing to call their doctor using their mobile phones for the management of an acute illness and 487 (99.7%) would call their doctor with their mobile phones in a medical emergency. Respondents with a formal education were 6 times more likely to call their doctor over the mobile phone in an acute illness (adjusted OR = 6.866, CI = 3.080, 15.30) as opposed to those literate in English who did not prefer calling the doctor (adjusted OR = 0.114, CI = 0.055, 0.236), (table 4). Further, men were less likely to prefer calling their doctor in the management of an acute illness in comparison to women (unadjusted OR = 0.606, CI = 0.388, 0.948).

Respondents who did not prefer using their mobile phones in an emergency, did not do so, either due to the proximity of the hospital or because they preferred to consult a doctor in person.

### Challenges to the use of mobile phones in healthcare

From among 488 respondents, 475 (97%) felt that receiving health information via mobile phones was not an intrusion into their lives. On the contrary, 345 (70%) felt that calling their doctor over the phone would disturb the doctor at work.

Prejudice that the mobile phone was a bad influence on the youth and concerns about the health hazards of mobile phone usage, expressed by 2 of the respondents, were potential barriers to their use in healthcare.

## Discussion

Rapid advances in mHealth call for the development of end-user friendly mobile phone applications that may be used for healthcare delivery. These applications should be simple, minimally intrusive and ensure confidentiality of personal information. It is equally important to contextualize every planned intervention to the population for which it is intended. With the Indian government's new impetus to use mobile phone technology in healthcare, mHealth services are expected to have a vast rural outreach. Given the immense potential for mHealth in India, we chose to explore experiences and perceptions of rural Indian mobile phone users towards using mobile phone technology in healthcare.

### Mobile phone-based reminders

A majority of respondents expressed interest in receiving medication adherence reminders for chronic illnesses. Forgetfulness, a barrier to medication adherence [11], can be minimised with the use of reminders. Medication reminders can be sent via mobile phones. Such reminders have been found effective in improving medication adherence, in chronic non-communicable disease and communicable diseases like tuberculosis and HIV infection [12–18].

Further, our respondents also expressed an interest in receiving appointment reminders and vaccination reminders. Reviews indicate appointment reminders via SMS improve attendance in primary care clinics, chronic disease follow up, family planning clinics and ophthalmology clinics [19,20]. A study from rural Haryana, reported using mobile phones to obtain appointments for outpatient visits [21]. The probable reduction in clinic waiting time is assumed to have made the concept more appealing to our respondents.

### Preferred type of communication: *SMS versus Voice calls*

The second global survey on eHealth reported that SMS reminders were preferred to voice calls, globally [3]. However, most of our respondents preferred voice calls to text messages. Employed or English-literate respondents were more likely to

**Table 4.** Preference for calling the doctor over the mobile phone for acute illnesses compared to demographic characteristics (n = 488).

| | Did not prefer calling the doctor (%) (n = 121) | Preferred calling the doctor (%) (n = 367) | Unadjusted OR | Adjusted OR |
|---|---|---|---|---|
| **Age** | 31.89±10.68 | 32.72±10.64 | 1.007 (0.988, 1.027) | 1.00 (0.979, 1.025) |
| **Sex** | | | | |
| Female | 80 (22) | 280 (78) | | |
| Male | 41 (32) | 87 (68) | 0.606 (0.388, 0.948) | 1.073 (0.527, 2.183) |
| **Literate in English** | | | | |
| No | 89 (20) | 353 (80) | | |
| Yes | 32 (70) | 14 (30) | 0.110 (0.056, 0.218) | 0.114 (0.055, 0.236) |
| **Formally educated#** | | | | |
| No | 17 (59) | 12 (41) | | |
| Yes | 104 (23) | 355 (77) | 4.835 (2.238, 10.450) | 6.866 (3.080, 15.30) |
| **Currently Employed** | | | | |
| No | 57 (19) | 242 (81) | | |
| Yes | 64 (34) | 125 (66) | 0.460 (0.303, 0.698) | 0.593 (0.307, 1.143) |
| **Chronic disease** | | | | |
| No | 108 (24) | 342 (76) | | |
| Yes | 13 (34) | 25 (66) | 0.607 (0.300, 1.228) | 0.822 (0.366, 1.844) |

Logistic Regression Model p-value <0.001.
#Formal education indicates education that includes school.

prefer SMS communication. The employed respondents, probably due to lesser personal time and privacy at work, preferred reading an SMS at their own convenience as opposed to answering a phone call.

A study from Mumbai, India reported that only a few women at an urban antenatal clinic reported using the SMS facility. Their reasons included low literacy levels and even among the literates, difficulty in articulating text messages [22]. Similarly, technical difficulties in responding to both IVR calls and SMS reminders have been reported from South Africa [23]. Voice calls may be more useful in a population with minimal expertise in mobile phone operation or for health conditions that require more direct interaction e.g. suicide hotlines, HIV helplines, contraceptive hotlines [24–26]. The preference for voice calls among older respondents indicates a probable discomfort in operating mobile phones to access an SMS or a difficulty with reading SMSs. It is likely that some of our respondents also found SMS technology cumbersome to use. While SMS technology may have greater appeal among the English literate, maintaining communication in the local language could make them more accessible to those literate only in the local language. It is also worth noting that though the language maybe different, the script of communication is frequently English. This may continue to be a barrier to the use of SMS technology. Studies on HIV-infected populations in our setting (South India) have reported similar preferences for voice calls and an association with English language literacy and the preference for voice calls [7,18,27].

Despite SMS not being preferred in our setting, it has been found acceptable and effective elsewhere. Hospital attendance rates of patients receiving SMS reminders were comparable with those receiving voice call reminders, with lower cost per attendance [28]. Vaccination reminders (text messages) were found more acceptable than phone calls and letters among Latino mothers in New York City [29] and improved influenza vaccination rates in children and adolescents in low-income urban populations in USA [30]. In populations with low literacy, the possibility of using pictorial SMS reminders that use standard symbols e.g. ASCII art, could be explored [31]. It is therefore our recommendation that in the Indian context, voice calls would be the best form of communication. Failing this option, pictorial text messages using universally understood symbols maybe used in an effort to abstain from using the English script.

## Frequency of reminders

While language and format are obvious issues, increased frequency of reminders is a significant cause of intervention-fatigue and therefore needs attention [32,33]. Respondents literate in English were twice more likely to prefer more frequent reminders. This may be explained by the fact that they were also more likely to be employed ($p<0.001$) or involved in completing their education and therefore likely to forget their medication and would benefit from frequent reminding. By similar reasoning, men and those employed were also more likely to prefer more frequent reminding in comparison to women and those unemployed. Respondents with chronic disease may have already become accustomed to maintaining a medication schedule without any assistance, therefore requiring less frequent reminders.

## Use of mobile phones in behaviour change communication

Mobile phones have been used in creating health awareness and bringing about behavioural change [12,34]. SMS has been successfully used to improve physical activity and reduce the number of servings of red meat in middle-aged men in Australia [35] and receiving information on lifestyle modification lowered the incidence of diabetes in men (30–35 years of age) with impaired glucose tolerance in India [36]. A majority of our respondents also consider the mobile phones an acceptable tool for health education. Mobile phone based communication therefore provides an opportunity to promote a healthy lifestyle while satiating the desire for health information in our study population [37].

Our respondents also expressed interest in information on maternal health and child. Studies exploring an SMS intervention to promote healthy behaviour during pregnancy showed improved birth-preparedness and healthy attitudes to alcohol consumption in a pilot study in Virginia, USA [38]. SMSs were also considered acceptable for sexual health promotion in different settings [39,40]. Similar communication to educate women about antenatal care, maternal nutrition, necessity of iron and folic acid (IFA) tablet consumption and newborn care could be explored in the rural Indian context. The possibility of improving adherence of IFA tablets and maintaining obstetric appointments through reminders should also be considered.

Health information could be made available passively through text and automated voice calls or a system where people call a phone number, select the type of information they want by keying in codes for a particular topic and listen to pre-recorded information regarding the same. Such automated systems may however be difficult to operate [23]. Live helplines could provide real-time assistance in addition to a personal touch. Reports of switching from automated HIV helplines to those manned by personnel are available from Bangalore, India [41]. However, establishing and maintaining them is resource-intensive, in comparison to automated communication systems [25].

## Use of mobile phones in acute care and epidemics

A study from Washington, D.C. reported participants' willingness to send photographs of their wounds to physicians for diagnosis and recommendations [42]. Majority of our respondents were willing to communicate with healthcare providers via mobile phones in an emergency. However, their limited use of phone camera (4.5%) and phone-based Internet (1%) minimises the possibility of using photographs, Internet and MMS. A study from Nakuru, Kenya demonstrated that mobile phones were useful in facilitating communication and decision-making in reproductive health [40]. This may be due to quicker communication and easier access to information in an emergency. Such use of mobile phones could especially benefit rural India, where frequently, patients must travel long distances to meet a doctor, not only for their most basic health requirements but also in emergencies. The possibility of using emergency helplines that either provide verbal basic or professional assistance could also be explored in this setting. However for the population in our study, accessing healthcare in an emergency may not pose a significant issue given the presence of a primary and a secondary level healthcare facility in the village.

In our study, those with formal education were more likely to contact their doctor via mobile phone, for acute and emergency care. It is possible that this group had better health literacy [43] than the others because of their education. They were likely to understand the importance of health personnel and urgent intervention in the management of emergencies. However, those literate in English were less likely to contact their doctor in an emergency. The reasons for this association need to be determined.

A study in China used mobile phone technology in a disaster management setting for detecting and controlling disease outbreaks [44]. Data gathering via mobile phones, was done effectively in malaria epidemics in Sub-Saharan Africa [45]. A study from Ivory Coast, Africa reported the use of mobile phone-based one-to-one communication to create awareness and control epidemics [46]. Our respondents were also open to such usage of mobile phones in the setting of infectious epidemics. However, care must be taken to ensure communication is informative while not creating panic regarding the epidemic.

### Privacy and related concerns

While most participants were open to using mobile phones for health-related issues, those who were not, generally preferred face-to-face interactions with their healthcare provider. A substantial proportion felt they would be invading their doctors' privacy by calling him or her on the mobile phone. Some of our respondents expressed concern with sharing their phone number with the doctors' clinic. However, we did not assess specific privacy and confidentiality concerns. Studies report minimal privacy concerns for communicating laboratory results to HIV patients and wound images for acute healthcare [42]. Universally acceptable guidelines addressing confidentiality, privacy and ethical concerns applicable to mHealth and adaptable to local contexts need to be developed.

### Women, health and mobile phones

A large proportion of the respondents in our study were women with access to mobile phones. In the Indian context, women are often responsible for the health and hygiene in their family. They are primarily involved in cooking, cleaning and caring for children and elderly in their households [47]. It is therefore not surprising that nutrition and maternal and child health were popular among information requested. The existing experience with caregiving within families may have resulted in women preferring less frequent adherence reminders in our study. Women were also less likely to be employed making their schedules more flexible and conducive to ensuring better medication adherence in comparison to men [32]. Our finding that women were more likely to communicate directly with their doctor in the management of an acute illness may indicate that they had lesser knowledge about health issues and needed assistance. It is also noteworthy that they were able to take cognizance of a situation where they were out of their depth, and were willing to assume responsibility in procuring the necessary expertise required.

Thus, while reduced autonomy among majority of Indian women is likely to adversely affect health-seeking behaviour; our findings indicate that mobile phones may serve to enable women to actively participate not only in their own healthcare and but also that of their families [47]. Our study was able to capture the opinions of women, a group largely underrepresented in research, since the interviews were conducted primarily during working hours. Given that the women in our study have access to mobile phones, both the women and the healthcare system have an opportunity to communicate with each other, which can be exploited to improve the population's health.

### Methodological issues

Our study assessed the usage and acceptability of mobile phones in healthcare in a rural setting approximately 52 kilometres from Bangalore city. It is possible that participant responses may not be entirely representative of other rural settings in India, given the proximity of our study setting to Bangalore city.

Healthcare personnel, who routinely administer services to the concerned community, were responsible for data collection. Therefore the possibility of social desirability bias or acquiescence must be considered. Further, as most of the interviews were conducted during the day, the opinions of those who are regularly away during these hours may not be adequately reflected. This also explains the large proportion of women in our study. Keeping in mind that we tried to evaluate the acceptability of a new form of communication; we must consider, having included the opinions of more forthcoming respondents, as a possible bias. No specific data on the type of mobile phones or privacy concerns with mobile healthcare communication was obtained in our study. Though the acceptability of reminders for supporting medication adherence was assessed, we did not assess their acceptability for supporting adherence to prescribed diet and exercise. Further, as missing data on socio-economic status reduced the size of the dataset this variable was excluded from the analysis.

## Conclusion

Our study sought an answer to the question of whether mobile phones would be an acceptable next step towards improving healthcare delivery in India. Our findings have generally corroborated the acceptability of mHealth interventions and may even direct future endeavours in this area.

mHealth interventions such as reminders and information disseminating applications via mobile phone were acceptable in our study. The voice call was the preferred mode of communication in our setting, and needs to be considered in light of the popularity of SMSs globally. Attention to factors such as English literacy, education, employment status, and sex of the end user would only serve to improve the efficacy of mhealth. Healthcare communication directed at women via mobile phones, could empower them with the necessary knowledge to promote not only their own health but also the health of their families. While these findings are encouraging to further the development and deployment of mHealth interventions in rural India, the interventions designed should be acceptable to the targeted population and minimally intrusive while ensuring the privacy of the end user.

## Supporting Information

**Annexure S1 Questionnaire - Mobile phones in health care in rural India.** This is the questionnaire that was developed for the purpose of the study.

## Acknowledgments

The authors would like to thank Dr. Sr. Cristeena J, Dr. Sr. Anngrace, Dr. Sr. Roselet and the staff at Snehalaya Hospital, Solur for supporting the research team during the study.

## Author Contributions

Conceived and designed the experiments: APV SMJ RR. Performed the experiments: APV SMJ. Analyzed the data: SID MRR APV SMJ RR. Wrote the paper: SID RR.

## References

1. Union IT (2013) The world in 2013: ICT facts and figures. Place des Nations, 1211 Geneva 20 - Switzerland: International Telecommunication Union. Available: http://www.itu.int/en/ITU-D/Statistics/Documents/facts/ICTFactsFigures2013-e.pdf. Accessed 2013 Dec 29.
2. Aker JC, Mbiti IM (2010) Mobile phones and economic development in Africa. Journal of Economic Perspectives 24: 207–232. Available: http://sites.tufts.edu/jennyaker/files/2010/09/aker_mobileafrica.pdf. Accessed 2013 Dec 29.

3. World Health Organisation (2011) mHealth: new horizons for health through mobile technologies: second global survey on eHealth 20 Avenue Appia, 1211 Geneva 27, Switzerland. Global Observatory for eHealth series. Available: http://www.who.int/goe/publications/goe_mhealth_web.pdf. Accessed 2014 Jul 25.
4. Telecom Regulatory Authority of India (2013) Highlights on Telecom Subscription Data as on 31st August, 2013. Government of India. Available: http://www.trai.gov.in/WriteReadData/WhatsNew/Documents/PR-TSD-Aug, 13.pdf. Accessed 2013 Nov 4.
5. Telecom Regulatory Authority of India (2013) Telecom sector in India: A decadal profile. New Delhi: Government of India. Available: http://www.trai.gov.in/WriteReadData/Publication/Document/201304121052403536675NCAER-Report08june12.pdf. Accessed 2013 Nov 1.
6. Bali S, Singh AJ (2007) Mobile phone consultation for community health care in rural north India. Journal of Telemedicine Telecare 13: 421–424. Available: http://jtt.sagepub.com/content/13/8/421. Accessed 2014 Jul 25
7. Shet A, Arumugam K, Rodrigues R, Rajagopalan N, Shubha K, et al. (2010) Designing a mobile phone-based intervention to promote adherence to antiretroviral therapy in South India. AIDS Behav 14: 716–720. Available: http://link.springer.com/article/10.1007%2Fs10461-009-9658-3. Accessed 2014 Jul 25.
8. Department of Health and Family Welfare, Government of India MCTS. Available: http://nrhm-mcts.nic.in/. Accessed 2013 Dec 30.
9. Chib A, Cheong YJ, Lee LCL, Ng CHC, Tan CK, et al. (2012) The hope of mobile phones in Indian rural healthcare. Journal of Health Informatics in Developing Countries 6: 406–421. Available: http://www.jhidc.org/index.php/jhidc/article/view/81. Accessed 2013 Dec 29.
10. Ministry of Health and Family Welfare, Government of India (2012) India is the second-kargest mobile phone user in world. Available: http://pib.nic.in/newsite/erelease.aspx?relid = 85669. Accessed 2013 Dec 29.
11. Vervloet M, Linn AJ, JC vW, de Bakker DH, Bouvy ML, et al. (2012) The effectiveness of interventions using electronic reminders to improve adherence to chronic medication: A systematic review of the literature. Am Med Inform Assoc 19: 696–704 Available: http://www.ncbi.nlm.nih.gov/pubmed/22534082.
12. Horvath T, Azman H, Kennedy GE, Rutherford GW (2012) Mobile phone text messaging for promoting adherence to antiretroviral therapy in patients with HIV infection. The Cochrane database of systematic reviews 3: CD009756. Available: http://onlinelibrary.wiley.com/store/10.1002/14651858.CD009756/asset/CD009756.pdf?v = 1&t = hs5pxxyu&s = ec18131db26079828068ddfacab31977b5821268. Accessed 2014 Jul 25.
13. Vervloet M, van Dijk L, Santen-Reestman J, van Vlijmen B, Bouvy ML, et al. (2011) Improving medication adherence in diabetes type 2 patients through Real Time Medication Monitoring: a randomised controlled trial to evaluate the effect of monitoring patients' medication use combined with short message service (SMS) reminders. BMC health services research 11: 5. Available: http://www.ncbi.nlm.nih.gov/pubmed/21219596.
14. Park LG, Howie-Esquivel J, Chung ML, Dracup K (2013) A text messaging intervention to promote medication adherence for patients with coronary heart disease: A randomized controlled trial. Patient education and counseling. Available: http://www.ncbi.nlm.nih.gov/pubmed/24321403.
15. Nglazi MD, Bekker LG, Wood R, Hussey GD, Wiysonge CS (2013) Mobile phone text messaging for promoting adherence to anti-tuberculosis treatment: a systematic review protocol. Syst Rev 2: 6. Available: http://www.ncbi.nlm.nih.gov/pmc/articles/PMC3564775/pdf/2046-4053-2-6.pdf.
16. Mbuagbaw L, Thabane L, Ongolo-Zogo P, Lester RT, Mills EJ, et al. (2012) The Cameroon Mobile Phone SMS (CAMPS) trial: a randomized trial of text messaging versus usual care for adherence to antiretroviral therapy. PLoS One 7: e46909. Available: http://www.ncbi.nlm.nih.gov/pmc/articles/PMC3516507/pdf/pone.0046909.pdf.
17. Lester RT, Ritvo P, Mills EJ, Kariri A, Karanja S, et al. (2010) Effects of a mobile phone short message service on antiretroviral treatment adherence in Kenya (WelTel Kenya1): a randomised trial. Lancet 376: 1838–1845. Available: http://www.ncbi.nlm.nih.gov/pubmed/21071074.
18. Rodrigues R, Shet A, Antony J, Sidney K, Arumugam K, et al. (2012) Supporting adherence to antiretroviral therapy with mobile phone reminders: results from a cohort in South India. PLoS One 7: e40723. Available: http://www.ncbi.nlm.nih.gov/pubmed/22952574.
19. Car J, Gurol-Urganci I, de Jongh T, Vodopivec-Jamsek V, Atun R (2012) Mobile phone messaging reminders for attendance at healthcare appointments. The Cochrane database of systematic reviews 7: CD007458. Available: http://onlinelibrary.wiley.com/store/10.1002/14651858.CD007458.pub2/asset/CD007458.pdf?v = 1&t = hs5pnigz&s = a203eabd12b628093edf9b5c33160c5fd7d7fa9d. Accessed 2014 Jul 25.
20. Klasnja P, Pratt W (2012) Healthcare in the pocket: mapping the space of mobile-phone health interventions. Journal of biomedical informatics 45: 184–198. Available: http://www.ncbi.nlm.nih.gov/pmc/articles/PMC3272165/pdf/nihms323686.pdf. Accessed 2014 Jul 25.
21. Bali S, Singh AJ (2007) Mobile phone consultation for community health care in rural north India. Journal of Telemedicine and Telecare 13: 421–424. Available: http://jtt.sagepub.com/content/13/8/421. Accessed 2014 Jul 25.
22. Niranjan P, Pradnya S, Shailesh K, Nandanwar YS, Hegde A, et al. (2013) Using Automated Voice Calls to Improve Adherence to Iron Supplements During Pregnancy: A Pilot Study. ICTD 2013. Cape Town, South Afrca. Available: http://dx.doi.org/10.1145/2516604.2516608. Accessed 2014 Jul 25.
23. Haberer JE, Kiwanuka J, Nansera D, Wilson IB, Bangsberg DR (2010) Challenges in using mobile phones for collection of antiretroviral therapy adherence data in a resource-limited setting. AIDS and behavior 14: 1294–1301. Available: http://www.ncbi.nlm.nih.gov/pubmed/20532605.
24. Alexander G, Kanth C, Thomas R (2011) A Descriptive Study on the Users and Utility of HIV/AIDS Helpline in Karnataka, India. IJCM 36: 17–20. Available: http://www.ncbi.nlm.nih.gov/pubmed/21687375. Accessed 2014 Jul 25.
25. Urban Health Initiative (2010) Expanding Contraceptive Use in Urban Uttar Pradesh: Telephone Helplines. Available: http://www.uhi-india.org/index.php?option = com_docman&task = doc_download&gid = 362&Itemid = .
26. Knox KL, Kemp J, McKeon R, Katz IR (2012) Implementation and early utilization of a Suicide Hotline for veterans. Am J Public Health 102 Suppl 1: S29–32. Available: http://www.ncbi.nlm.nih.gov/pubmed/22390596. Accessed 2014 Jul 25.
27. Sidney K, Antony J, Rodrigues R, Arumugam K, Krishnamurthy S, et al. (2012) Supporting patient adherence to antiretrovirals using mobile phone reminders: patient responses from South India. AIDS Care 24: 612–617. Available: http://www.ncbi.nlm.nih.gov/pubmed/22150088. Accessed 2014 Jul 25.
28. Perron NJ, Dao MD, Righini NC, Humair J-P, Broers B, et al. (2013) Text-messaging versus telephone reminders to reduce missed appointments in an academic primary care clinic: a randomized controlled trial. BMC Health Services Research 13: 125. Available: http://www.biomedcentral.com/1472-6963/13/125. Accessed 2013 Dec 29.
29. Hofstetter AM, Vargas CY, Kennedy A, Kitayama K, Stockwell MS (2013) Parental and provider preferences and concerns regarding text message reminder/recall for early childhood vaccinations. Preventive medicine 57: 75–80. Available: http://www.sciencedirect.com/science/article/pii/S0091743513001163. Accessed 2014 Jul 25.
30. Stockwell MS, Kharbanda EO, Martinez RA, Vargas CY, Vawdrey DK, et al. (2012) Effect of a text messaging intervention on influenza vaccination in an urban, low-income pediatric and adolescent population: a randomized controlled trial. JAMA: the journal of the American Medical Association 307: 1702–1708. Available: http://www.ncbi.nlm.nih.gov/pubmed/22535855.
31. Rodrigues R, Shet A, Antony J, Sidney K, Arumugam K, et al. (2011) Supporting Adherence to Antiretroviral Therapy with Mobile Phone Reminders: Results from a Cohort in South India. PLoS one. Available: http://www.plosone.org/article/info:doi/10.1371/journal.pone.0040723. Accessed 2014 Jul 25.
32. Huang HL, Li YC, Chou YC, Hsieh YW, Kuo F, et al. (2013) Effects of and satisfaction with short message service reminders for patient medication adherence: a randomized controlled study. BMC medical informatics and decision making 13: 127. Available: http://www.ncbi.nlm.nih.gov/pubmed/24238397. Accessed 2014 Jul 25.
33. Pop-Eleches C, Thirumurthy H, Habyarimana JP, Zivin JG, Goldstein MP, et al. (2011) Mobile phone technologies improve adherence to antiretroviral treatment in a resource-limited setting: a randomized controlled trial of text message reminders. Aids 25: 825–834. Available: http://www.ncbi.nlm.nih.gov/pubmed/21252632. Accessed 2014 Jul 25.
34. Free C, Phillips G, Galli L, Watson L, Felix L, et al. (2013) The effectiveness of mobile-health technology-based health behaviour change or disease management interventions for health care consumers: a systematic review. PLoS medicine 10: e1001362. Available: http://www.ncbi.nlm.nih.gov/pmc/articles/PMC3548655/pdf/pmed.1001362.pdf. Accessed 2014 Jul 25.
35. Duncan MJ, Vandelanotte C, Rosenkranz RR, Caperchione CM, Ding H, et al. (2012) Effectiveness of a website and mobile phone based physical activity and nutrition intervention for middle-aged males: trial protocol and baseline findings of the ManUp Study. BMC public health 12: 656. Available: http://www.ncbi.nlm.nih.gov/pmc/articles/PMC3507858/pdf/1471-2458-12-656.pdf. Accessed 2014 Jul 25.
36. Ramachandran A, Snehalatha C, Ram J, Selvam S, Simon M, et al. (2013) Effectiveness of mobile phone messaging in prevention of type 2 diabetes by lifestyle modification in men in India: a prospective, parallel-group, randomised controlled trial. The Lancet 1: 191–198.
37. Yoo HJ, Park MS, Kim TN, Yang SJ, Cho GJ, et al. (2009) A Ubiquitous Chronic Disease Care system using cellular phones and the internet. Diabetic medicine: a journal of the British Diabetic Association 26: 628–635. Available: http://www.ncbi.nlm.nih.gov/pubmed/19538239. Accessed 2014 Jul 25.
38. Evans WD, Wallace JL, Snider J (2012) Pilot evaluation of the text4baby mobile health program. BMC public health 12: 1031. Available: http://www.ncbi.nlm.nih.gov/pmc/articles/PMC3570294/pdf/1471-2458-12-1031.pdf. Accessed 2014 Jul 25.
39. Gold J, Lim MS, Hellard ME, Hocking JS, Keogh L (2010) What's in a message? Delivering sexual health promotion to young people in Australia via text messaging. BMC public health 10: 792. Available: http://www.ncbi.nlm.nih.gov/pmc/articles/PMC3022861/pdf/1471-2458-10-792.pdf. Accessed 2014 Jul 25.
40. Ibembe JDB, Lagsten J (2011) Mobile phone use and Reproductive health care in Nakuru provincial hospital,Kenya. Department of informatics. Kenya: Örebro university. Available: https://spidercenter.org/sites/default/files/master_theses_sponsored/JohnDanielIbembe.pdf. Accessed 2014 Jul 25.
41. Alexander G, Kanth C, Thomas R (2011) A Descriptive Study on the Users and Utility of HIV/AIDS Helpline in Karnataka, India. Indian journal of community medicine: official publication of Indian Association of Preventive

& Social Medicine 36: 17–20. Available: http://www.ncbi.nlm.nih.gov/pubmed/21687375.

42. Sikka N, Carlin KN, Pines J, Pirri M, Strauss R, et al. (2012) The use of mobile phones for acute wound care: attitudes and opinions of emergency department patients. Journal of health communication 17 Suppl 1: 37–42; quiz 42–33. Available: http://www.ncbi.nlm.nih.gov/pubmed/22548597. Accessed 2014 Jul 25.

43. (2004) Health Literacy: A Prescription to End Confusion. The National Academies Press. Available: http://www.nap.edu/openbook.php?record_id = 10883. Accessed 2014 Jul 25.

44. Yang C, Yang J, Luo X, Gong P (2009) Use of mobile phones in an emergency reporting system for infectious disease surveillance after the Sichuan earthquake in China. Bull World Health Organ 87: 619–623. Available: http://www.ncbi.nlm.nih.gov/pubmed/19705013. Accessed 2014 Jul 25.

45. Mueller DH, Abeku TA, Okia M, Rapuoda B, Cox J (2009) Costs of early detection systems for epidemic malaria in highland areas of Kenya and Uganda. Malaria journal 8: 17. Available: http://www.ncbi.nlm.nih.gov/pmc/articles/PMC2636824/pdf/1475-2875-8-17.pdf. Accessed 2014 Jul 25.

46. Lima A, De Domenico M, Pejovic V, Musolesi M Exploiting Cellular Data for Disease Containment and Information Campaigns Strategies in Country-Wide Epidemics. School of Computer Science. United Kingdom: University of Birmingham. Available: http://www.cs.bham.ac.uk/~musolesm/papers/d4d.pdf.

47. Kishor S, Gupta K (2009) Gender Equality and Women's Empowerment in India. National Family Health Survey (NFHS-3), India, 2005–06. Mumbai: International Institute for Population Sciences; Calverton, Maryland, USA: ICF Macro.

# 5

# Caregivers' Health Literacy and Gaps in Children's Medicaid Enrollment: Findings from the Carolina Oral Health Literacy Study

**Jessica Y. Lee[1,2]*, Kimon Divaris[1,3], Darren A. DeWalt[4], A. Diane Baker[1], Ziya Gizlice[5], R. Gary Rozier[2], William F. Vann, Jr.[1]**

**1** Department of Pediatric Dentistry, School of Dentistry, University of North Carolina at Chapel Hill, Chapel Hill, NC, United States of America, **2** Department of Health Policy and Management, UNC Gillings School of Global Public Health, University of North Carolina at Chapel Hill, Chapel Hill, NC, United States of America, **3** Department of Epidemiology, UNC Gillings School of Global Public Health, University of North Carolina at Chapel Hill, Chapel Hill, NC, United States of America, **4** School of Medicine and Cecil G. Sheps Center for Health Services Research, University of North Carolina at Chapel Hill, Chapel Hill, NC, United States of America, **5** Center for Health Promotion and Disease Prevention, University of North Carolina at Chapel Hill, Chapel Hill, NC, United States of America

## Abstract

***Background and Objectives:*** Recent evidence supports a link between caregivers' health literacy and their children's health and use of health services. Disruptions in children's health insurance coverage have been linked to poor health care and outcomes. We examined young children's Medicaid enrollment patterns in a well-characterized cohort of child/caregivers dyads and investigated the association of caregivers' low health literacy with the incidence of enrollment gaps.

***Methods:*** We relied upon Medicaid enrollment data for 1208 children (mean age = 19 months) enrolled in the Carolina Oral Health Literacy project during 2008–09. The median follow-up was 25 months. Health literacy was measured using the Newest Vital Sign (NVS). Analyses relied on descriptive, bivariate, and multivariate methods based on Poisson modeling.

***Findings:*** One-third of children experienced one or more enrollment gaps; most were short in duration (median = 5 months). The risk of gaps was inversely associated with caregivers' age, with a 2% relative risk decrease for each added year. Low health literacy was associated with a modestly elevated risk increase [Incidence Rate Ratio (IRR) = 1.17 (95% confidence interval (CI) 0.88–1.57)] for enrollment disruptions; however, this estimate was substantially elevated among caregivers with less than a high school education [IRR = 1.52 (95% CI 0.99–2.35); homogeneity $p<0.2$].

***Conclusions:*** Our findings provide initial support for a possible role of caregivers' health literacy as a determinant of children's Medicaid enrollment gaps. Although the association between health literacy and enrollment gaps was not confirmed statistically, we found that it was markedly stronger among caregivers with low educational attainment. This population, as well as young caregivers, may be the most vulnerable to the negative effects of low health literacy.

**Editor:** Gozde Ozakinci, University of St Andrews, United Kingdom

**Funding:** The Carolina Oral Health Literacy Study is supported by a grant from the National Institute of Dental and Craniofacial Research of the National Institutes of Health (RO1DE018045). The funders had no role in study design, data collection and analysis, decision to publish, or preparation of the manuscript.

**Competing Interests:** The authors have declared that no competing interests exist.

* Email: Jessica_Lee@unc.edu

## Introduction

### Health Insurance Coverage Affects Appropriate Health Care during the First Years of Life

Children's health insurance coverage is a major determinant of preventive and continuous health care [1–3]. Low-income children enrolled in Medicaid are more likely to receive timely preventive care, including well-child visits, compared with their counterparts without insurance coverage [4–8]. Nationally representative US data confirm that being uninsured is associated with low levels of adherence to professional recommendations for well-child visits, with the lowest rates found among children eligible but not enrolled in public insurance [9]. This is an important observation because well-child visits and preventive care during the first years of life have demonstrable benefits [10–12]. Similarly, continuity of care has been linked to favorable health outcomes, including lower emergency department utilization [13]. These observations are aligned with the concept of a 'medical home' which, according to the American Academy of Pediatrics, encompasses the characteristics of pediatric care considered essential for all children" and is defined as a "model of primary care that is accessible, continuous, comprehensive, family-centered, coordinated, compassionate, and culturally effective" [14–15].

Current legislation supports the expansion in Medicaid coverage in 2014 [16] and has the potential to benefit a large and vulnerable component of the US population. Insurance coverage is an important enabling factor for health care use overall and its absence leads to under-utilization and unmet medical needs [8]; however, its availability is not sufficient for enrollment or the establishment of a medical home [10]. To affect health outcomes, the expansion of coverage must be met with adequate enrollment.

## To What Extent are Disruptions in Health Insurance Detrimental for Children?

Current evidence demonstrates that disruptions ("gaps") in coverage are likely to decrease both access to a medical home and the likelihood of seeking routine care for young children [17–19]. A 2006 report [20] found that between 18–36% of children in four states had insurance gaps over a period of up to 2 years. Other recent studies confirmed that insurance gaps may be frequent, with 25% of children experiencing a gap in Medicaid enrollment over a 12-month period in Oregon [17], and 14–61% of children in five other states experiencing similar gaps over a 4-year period [21]. Because of its frequency and negative effects, unstable health insurance coverage is a phenomenon that needs further investigation as a risk factor for children's health [2,22–23].

## What is known about the Correlates of Health Insurance Enrollment Gaps?

State Medicaid programs have a compelling interest in enrolling and maintaining coverage for eligible children but there is a paucity of evidence to inform policy makers on relevant strategies and best practices to accomplish these goals [24]. Although state programs strive to keep enrollment and renewal procedures simple, most reports on enrollment gaps implicate caregiver-related factors. For example, studies by DeVoe et al. [17] and Satchell and Pati [22] relied upon nationally representative data and found that poverty and maternal education were the strongest correlates of enrollment gaps. Gaps may be attributed to changes in family circumstances that render parents and children ineligible; nevertheless, caregivers' difficulty in navigating the complex administrative processes can also explain why those eligible for public or private insurance are challenged to enroll and maintain enrollment. The challenges of the required forms and paperwork are well-documented [20,25–26]. As one example, recent findings indicate that Medicaid enrollment forms may be excessively demanding to read and comprehend [27]; in fact, most states fail to meet their self-established readability criteria [28].

## The Role of Health Literacy

A recent report [29] identified low health literacy as a risk factor for lack of adult health insurance and outlined the direct implications for the anticipated Medicaid expansion and implementation under the Affordable Care Act (ACA). Several studies have documented an association between caregiver health literacy and child health and services' use [30–33]. Health literacy's relationship to Medicaid enrollment gaps may offer one potential explanation of the relationship between parental health literacy and child health outcomes. To the best of our knowledge, no data exist to date regarding the possible association between caregivers' health literacy and gaps in their children's public health insurance enrollment. Our aims were to 1) describe and characterize gaps in Medicaid enrollment of young, low-income children of English-speaking families in North Carolina, and 2) identify caregiver factors associated with this phenomenon, including health literacy.

# Methods

## Ethics statement

Written consent and HIPPA approval were obtained by all participants and the study was approved by the Biomedical Institutional Review Board at the University of North Carolina-Chapel Hill (approval #07-0837).

## Parent study sampling frame

This investigation utilizes data obtained in the context of the Carolina Oral Health Literacy (COHL) Study, which initially enrolled 1,405 clients of the Special Supplemental Nutrition Program for Women, Infants and Children (WIC) in seven counties in NC: Brunswick, Buncombe, Burke, New Hanover, Orange, Robeson, and Wake [34]. The study's aim was to investigate the impact of caregivers' health literacy on their children's oral health and use of services. The study population consisted of low-income predominantly female caregivers who were 18 years of age or older, English-speaking, and the primary caregiver of a Medicaid-eligible healthy child. Purposeful quota sampling [35] was used to ensure adequate representation of African American (AA; 40%) and American Indian (AI; 20%) participants. Detailed descriptions of the study procedures, interview instruments and baseline outcomes have been reported previously [36–38]. In brief, non-random WIC sites were selected based on geographic region, rural or urban makeup, population demographics, existence of very active WIC clinics, and established working relationship with the investigators [34]. Consecutive WIC-attending clients were approached by study personnel while in the waiting areas and asked if they would to 8 questions included in the study's eligibility screener. Caregivers who were determined to be eligible and agreed to participate were accompanied to a private area to complete the in-person study interview. Of note, to qualify for WIC, caregivers must have an income <185 percent of the federal poverty level.

## Data Sources

Data were collected in 30-minute in-person interviews with one of the two trained study interviewers between July 2008-July 2009 in the domains of socio-demography, caregivers' self-reported personal and children's general and dental health status, dental knowledge and behaviors, quality of life, dental neglect, general self-efficacy, and health literacy. Study personnel screened eligible participants to ensure that unique children were enrolled in the cohort. In June 2011, we obtained Medicaid enrollment and claims files for children from the NC Division of Medical Assistance, ranging from January 2004 to December 2010, a period that covered the lifetime Medicaid enrollment history for all children up to the end of CY-2010. We merged these files with interview data that were obtained at baseline using the children's unique Medicaid identification number that was provided by the caregivers at study enrollment. All COHL children were Medicaid-eligible or enrolled at baseline, as per our inclusion requirements. Of the 1405 caregivers recruited, 1242 had children with a Medicaid identification number at the baseline interview. Children's unique Medicaid identification number was used to link interview and Medicaid claims data. Subsequently, we excluded dyads wherein children had no Medicaid data (n = 31; 2% of total), caregivers under 18 years old (n = 2; 0.2%), and one caregiver (0.1%) who had missing information on health literacy. Thus, the final analytical sample included 1208 child/caregiver dyads.

## Outcome Definition and Covariates

The study's primary analytical endpoint was the incidence of Medicaid enrollment disruptions or "gaps". During the study period (2004–2010) Medicaid eligibility criteria in NC, as well as procedures of enrollment and re-enrollment varied for different categories of child/caregiver dyads; however, these criteria included, among others, income, resources, residence, and proof of citizenship. Re-enrollment processes included periodic verifications of eligibility criteria at intervals ranging between 3–12 months, unless changes were self-reported by the beneficiaries. The current list of eligibility criteria and required documentation can be found at: http://www.ncdhhs.gov/dma/forms/famchld.pdf. For the purposes of this study we defined gap as a period during which a child was Medicaid-eligible but not enrolled, which was preceded *and* followed by periods of enrollment, as described by Copper et al. [39]. This definition of enrollment disruption was conservative, in a manner that prevented children with a permanent change in Medicaid-eligibility from being classified as having a gap. In such instances, there would be no subsequent re-enrollment in the NC files and the child would be labeled "lost to follow-up" rather than having an enrollment gap.

Apart from caregivers' difficulty with necessary forms and processes and administrative reasons, there are several other reasons why enrollment interruptions occur for children covered by Medicaid. Among others, these include: a child/family moving out of state, a child's acquisition of comprehensive private health insurance, a caregiver's request for termination of coverage, and family income changes. Any of these result in permanent eligibility changes without subsequent re-enrollment. We cannot ascertain with certainty the reason for permanent eligibility changes and some may be due to difficulty in processes/procedures; however, our goal for using a conservative definition of gaps was to ensure we were capturing administrative-related lapses due to parental actions that resulted in an interruption in enrollment.

Enumeration of enrolled/non-enrolled months began at the month of the baseline COHL interview and ended in December 2010. For each child, we identified and counted enrolled/non-enrolled periods and calculated their duration in months. We calculated 'enrollment proportion' as the ratio of months enrolled divided by months eligible with a range of 0–100. History of Medicaid enrollment was available from January 2004-December 2010, a period that included all available Medicaid data up to 2010 for all children. To further characterize patterns of Medicaid enrollment, we calculated periods of non-enrollment, enrollment gaps, and percent time enrolled both during the study duration and the entire period available.

We measured health literacy using a comprehension and numeracy-based instrument, the Newest Vital Sign (NVS). The NVS is a nutritional label accompanied by six questions, requiring approximately three minutes for completion. The NVS is a validated test with good psychometric properties and it has been used extensively since its introduction [40–41]. According to Weiss et al. [40] who developed and tested the NVS, the instrument is reliable (Cronbach alpha >0.76 in English), correlates with the test of functional health literacy in adults (TOFHLA), requires 3 minutes for administration and, thus, is suitable for use as a quick screening test for limited health literacy. According to Osborn et al. [42], the NVS is able to reliably identify individuals with limited literacy skills, which was the group of interest in this study (vs. the upper end of the literacy spectrum). In the context of our study, the NVS's Cronbach's *alpha* was 0.75. The NVS score ranges from 0–6, wherein values of 0–1 are indicative of "low", 2–3 "moderate" and 4–6 "higher health literacy" [42]. We used this 3-level categorical classification as well as a dichotomous one where NVS score 0–1: "low health literacy" and 2–6: "higher health literacy". The examination of the latter dichotomy was driven by our working hypothesis which considered low caregiver health literacy as a predictor of children's Medicaid enrollment gap; in this scenario, a contrast between the lowest category of the NVS index (containing individuals most likely to face difficulties with forms and administrative processes) and higher ones was the most meaningful one.

Socio-demographic covariates included caregivers' race, sex, age, education, marital status, number of children, and child's age. Race was self-reported and categorized as white, African American (AA), and American Indian (AI). Caregivers' age was measured in years and classified as a tertile-categorical variable for descriptive purposes and a continuous variable for analytical purposes. Education was grouped in four categories: less than high school (HS) education, HS/General Education Diploma (GED), some technical or college training, and college or higher education. Marital status was classified as single, married, and divorced/separated/other. Children's age was measured in months and was categorized in five groups: 0–11, 12–23, 24–25, 36–47, and 48–59 months.

As a measure of caregivers' self-perceived health status, we used the National Health and Nutrition Examination Study (NHANES) self-reported item containing five possible answers: excellent, very good, good, fair, and poor. For analytical purposes, the responses were converted to a dichotomous variable, excellent/very good/good *versus* fair/poor.

## Data availability

We have created and made available a de-identified dataset to accompany this manuscript, as supplemental material available online. This tab-delimited dataset (Dataset S1) contains all original and derived variables described and used for this study's analyses, including a data dictionary as a separate spreadsheet.

## Statistical Analyses

We used descriptive statistics for our initial data presentation and $\chi^2$ tests to compare the distribution of low/adequate health literacy and Medicaid enrollment gaps across strata of covariates. Because the occurrence of enrollment gaps is a time-dependent event, ignoring the time at-risk could introduce bias of substantial magnitude and unknown direction. For this reason, we used multivariate Poisson regression models that accounted for time at risk using months enrolled as the exposure and a log-link function. Although our modeling approach did not consider the length of each gap, we support that it is superior to the enumeration of months not enrolled due to reasons outlined above. To identify a final model, we employed a backward hierarchical variable selection strategy [43], starting with a full model that included all covariates and a $p<0.2$ criterion. We included caregivers' race, age, and general health status *a priori* in all models and obtained exponentiated model coefficients corresponding to Incidence Rate Ratios (IRR) and 95% confidence intervals (CI). For the interpretation of results, we followed an effect-estimation (estimation of the magnitude and precision of the association) *versus* hypothesis-testing (determination of the presence of an association or not) approach [44].

For sensitivity analysis, we developed a second identical model considering all Medicaid enrollment history available, prior to and after enrollment in the COHL study. All Medicaid enrollment history covered the lifetime period for all enrolled children, up to December 2010. In addition, to explore for potential vulnerable sub-groups, we conducted a *post hoc* homogeneity analysis to determine whether educational attainment and race modified the association between caregivers' health literacy and insurance gaps. To do so, we compared education level and race-specific estimates against the main effect estimate using a homogeneity $\chi^2$ test. Because these *post hoc* stratified analyses are *de facto* underpowered, we used an a priori p value criterion of <0.2 for the detection of heterogeneity [45]. We used Stata version 12.1 (StataCorp LP, College Station, TX) and SAS version 9.3 (SAS Institute, Cary, NC) software for data analyses.

## Results

The primary caregivers' socio-demographic characteristics and responses to the self-reported health status items, both overall and stratified by health literacy group, are presented in Table 1. There was a 2:2:1 distribution of white, AA, and AI participants with the vast majority of all participants being female. Caregivers' and children's mean age at the baseline interview was 27 years and 17 months, respectively. A small proportion (11%) of caregivers reported their general health as fair or poor. Fifteen percent of participants were classified as low health literacy based on their NVS score. This proportion was higher among AA and AI participants and among those who were younger, had lower educational attainment, and worse self-reported health status.

The median follow-up time was 25 months (mean = 24; range = 18–29), with 11% of children experiencing an interruption of Medicaid enrollment with no subsequent re-enrollment. This latter phenomenon was almost twice as high among children of caregivers with some technical/college or higher education *versus* those with less than high school education (15% *versus* 8%). Thirty percent of children experienced at least one enrollment gap (Table 2). Relative to gaps, the majority of the children (90%) experienced only one, 9% had two, and 1% had three. Twenty percent of these interruptions had duration of one month, 50% four months or less, while 21% were 12 months or longer. As anticipated, children with no gaps were enrolled longer, on average for six more months compared to those with gaps. Relative to bivariate associations, continuous enrollment was more frequent among children of older caregivers, older children, and those with more siblings (Table 2). Continuous enrollment was more frequent among children whose caregivers reported having better health but the difference was small (3%).

We present the final Poisson regression model (A) for enrollment gap incidence in Table 3. After adjusting for race, education, gender, and all other covariates, inclusion in the low health literacy group was associated with a modestly elevated risk for an enrollment gap (adjusted IRR = 1.17; 95% CI 0.89–1.54). The risk of gaps was inversely associated with caregivers' age, with a 2% relative risk decrease for each added year. An association between female gender and decreased risk of enrollment gaps was also noted; however, this finding was based on an analysis including only 46 male caregivers and thus should be viewed with caution. Stratified analyses (Table 4) revealed that educational attainment significantly modified the association between literacy and gaps (homogeneity p<0.2), with the highest risk estimates found among caregivers with less than high school education (IRR = 1.52; 95% CI 0.99–2.35). Race-stratified estimates did not depart substantially from homogeneity. Inspection of the exploratory models (B) that considered all available Medicaid enrollment history did not reveal any important differences compared to our main analyses.

## Discussion

In this study of approximately 1200 young children of low-income predominantly female caregivers enrolled in WIC, 30% had a gap in Medicaid enrollment over 25 months. Most experienced only one gap of short duration. Our findings revealed a weak association between caregivers' health literacy and their children's Medicaid enrollment gaps; in the entire cohort, independent of race, education, and age, low health literacy was associated with a non-significant gap risk increase of about 20%. Nevertheless, this effect was substantially elevated among caregivers with less than high school education compared to those with high school or higher education; caregivers with low education may be the most vulnerable to the effects of low health literacy. Moreover, above and beyond other caregiver factors, caregivers' age was inversely associated with the risk of gaps.

The concept of Medicaid's serving as a revolving-door for some children has been recognized and more steps must be taken by state Medicaid programs to alleviate this problem. While we cannot confirm it using our data, this phenomenon may be more closely related to administrative issues (i.e. difficulty with the enrollment and maintenance process) rather than eligibility disruptions. States are required to record and report on children's coverage stability but this has generally not been undertaken [46]. It is not uncommon for children who are uninsured for less than a full year to be reported as insured and this cohort of children has received less attention in public health research and policy discussions [23]. Olson [2] found that children insured for part of the previous year had higher proportions of delayed care and unmet medical care *versus* those uninsured for the full year. A similar finding was reported by DeVoe and colleagues [17], who compared children with gaps longer than six months *versus* those never insured.

Children from poor and near-poor families have been reported to be 4–5 times more likely to have lapsed coverage than those from high-income families [22]. At the same time, decreased preventive care utilization among children who had Medicaid insurance gaps was irrespective of their insurance status after discontinued enrollment [47]. Taken together, these findings underscore the dramatic effects that interruptions may have for children, their families, and the health care system. The association between Medicaid interruptions and subsequent children's health outcomes and related costs is fertile ground for future research.

As more health literacy findings are reported, the multi-level effects of health literacy are becoming increasingly evident. Health literacy is recognized already as having a pivotal role in numerous health outcomes [48–49], insurance status [29], and health disparities [50–51], and recently was termed the "sixth vital sign" [52]. Strategies that attempt to circumvent or mitigate the effects of low health literacy, such as the Federal Plain Language Act and simplification of enrollment procedures are promising [53], but more steps towards implementation are necessary. Although it is impossible to quantify the precise contributors to the relationship between health literacy and Medicaid enrollment gaps from our data, it appears that the readability of Medicaid forms [27] and user-friendliness of the enrollment renewal process [26,54–55] are potential targets for addressing literacy-sensitive concerns. This notion was recently mirrored by findings reported by Pati et al. [56] who found that mothers with inadequate health literacy were less likely to receive child care subsidy than those with adequate health literacy, implicating the application processes as health literacy-sensitive step.

Our findings on the incidence of enrollment gaps are consistent with previous reports of Medicaid insurance gaps among young children. Previously published estimates [20,46,57] of any gap of enrollment were 25% over a 12-month period in Oregon, 26–35% over 18 months in Ohio, 18% over a 2-year period in Louisiana,

**Table 1.** Distribution of Health Literacy Estimates (NVS) across Levels of Caregivers' Characteristics, in the COHL Study Follow-up Cohort, North Carolina, 2008–2010.

| | No.[a] (%) or mean (median) | Health Literacy (NVS) NVS score (95% CI) | Low n (row %) | Moderate n (row %) | Higher n (row %) | $\chi^2$; p |
|---|---|---|---|---|---|---|
| All | 1208 | 3.1 (3.0, 3.2) | 199 (16) | 508 (42) | 501 (41) | |
| **Race** | | | | | | <0.001 |
| White | 484 (40) | 3.8 (3.6, 3.9) | 45 (9) | 162 (33) | 277 (57) | |
| African American | 478 (40) | 2.7 (2.6, 2.9) | 96 (20) | 239 (50) | 143 (30) | |
| American Indian | 236 (20) | 2.8 (2.6, 3.0) | 51 (22) | 106 (45) | 79 (33) | |
| **Caregiver's sex** | | | | | | 0.6 |
| Male | 46 (4) | 3.3 (2.7, 3.8) | 9 (20) | 16 (35) | 21 (46) | |
| Female | 1162 (96) | 3.1 (3.0, 3.2) | 190 (16) | 492 (42) | 480 (41) | |
| **Caregiver's age** (years, tertiles; range) | | | | | | <0.001 |
| *Q1* (18.0, 23.0) | 20.8 (20.9) | 2.8 (2.7, 3.0) | 71 (18) | 202 (50) | 130 (32) | |
| *Q2* (23.1, 28.4) | 25.5 (25.3) | 3.4 (3.3, 3.6) | 51 (13) | 155 (38) | 197 (49) | |
| *Q3* (28.5, 65.6) | 35.0 (33.2) | 3.2 (3.0, 3.4) | 77 (19) | 151 (38) | 174 (43) | |
| **Education** | | | | | | <0.001 |
| Did not finish high school | 288 (24) | 2.2 (2.1, 2.4) | 87 (30) | 143 (50) | 58 (20) | |
| High school diploma or GED | 467 (39) | 3.0 (2.8, 3.1) | 80 (17) | 212 (45) | 175 (37) | |
| Some technical/college or higher | 453 (37) | 3.9 (3.8, 4.1) | 32 (7) | 153 (34) | 268 (59) | |
| **Marital status** | | | | | | <0.001 |
| Single | 772 (64) | 2.9 (2.7, 3.0) | 149 (19) | 363 (47) | 260 (34) | |
| Married | 316 (26) | 3.7 (3.5, 3.9) | 33 (10) | 103 (33) | 180 (57) | |
| Divorced/separated/other | 120 (10) | 3.5 (3.2, 3.8) | 17 (14) | 42 (35) | 61 (51) | |
| **Number of children** | | | | | | 0.6 |
| 1 | 479 (40) | 3.2 (3.1, 3.4) | 73 (15) | 204 (43) | 202 (42) | |
| 2 | 395 (33) | 3.1 (3.0, 3.3) | 62 (16) | 173 (44) | 160 (41) | |
| 3 | 196 (16) | 3.2 (2.9, 3.4) | 34 (17) | 76 (39) | 86 (44) | |
| ≥4 | 136 (11) | 2.9 (2.6, 3.2) | 29 (21) | 55 (40) | 52 (38) | |
| **Caregiver general health** | | | | | | 0.4 |
| Excellent/Very good/Good | 1076 (89) | 3.2 (3.1, 3.3) | 173 (16) | 451 (42) | 452 (42) | |
| Fair/Poor | 132 (11) | 2.9 (2.6, 3.2) | 26 (20) | 57 (43) | 49 (37) | |

*Note.* NVS = Newest Vital Sign; COHL = Carolina Oral Health Literacy; CI = Confidence Interval; HS = High School; GED = General Educational Development. The sample size was n = 1208.
[a]Column figures may not add up to total because of missing values.

25% over 12 months in Rhode Island, and 33% over an 18-month period in in Virginia. State, community, and local population-specific parameters may account for these relatively small variations. Our finding of increased risk for children's enrollment gaps among younger caregivers is a likely reflection of additional stressors and strains experienced by young parents/caregivers compared to older ones that could include education, employment, transportation, or others.

The finding of a weak association between enrollment gaps and literacy in the full cohort analysis requires further investigation. First, it must be acknowledged that in absence of statistical confirmation, an association may in fact be non-existent. Further, it is possible that the negative effects of low health literacy are manifested only among vulnerable subsets of the population, including those with low educational attainment, a scenario supported by our data. It is also possible that truly a weak association exists; this result might be a reflection of the NC Medicaid Program's success in addressing issues with the enrollment and maintenance processes and caregiver community support (i.e. an effect of WIC and practice health coordinators). In fact, while NC had the highest readability level goal (6–8 grade) for enrollment forms among all states with such guidelines, it was 40$^{th}$ in terms of actual readability level [28]. This parallels our finding of a 52% risk increase for enrollment gaps among caregivers in the lowest educational attainment group. Nevertheless, other differences in caregivers' age, family conditions, or children's health care needs may influence the likelihood to enroll in Medicaid and remain continuously enrolled. As an example, Cooper et al. [39] found that among children with asthma, those without insurance gaps had more hospitalizations compared with those with insurance gaps. This finding was a possible consequence of health

**Table 2.** Medicaid Enrollment Estimates (Children with and without Gaps in Enrollment) by Caregiver Characteristics among the COHL Study Follow-up Cohort during the Follow-up Period (Median 25 Months), North Carolina, 2008–2010.

| | No enrollment gap[a] | | | | One or more enrollment gaps[a] | | | |
|---|---|---|---|---|---|---|---|---|
| | | Enrollment (months) | | | | Enrollment (months) | | |
| | No.[b] (row %) | Mean | Median (range) | $\chi^2$; p[c] | No.[b] (row %) | Mean | Median (range) | Enrollment Proportion[d] (95% CI) |
| Total | 846 (70) | 24 | 25 (8–30) | | 362 (30) | 18 | 19 (1–29) | 0.71 (0.68–0.74) |
| **Race** | | | | 0.2 | | | | |
| White | 329 (68) | 25 | 25 (8–30) | | 155 (32) | 18 | 19 (2–29) | 0.71 (0.66–0.75) |
| African American | 334 (70) | 25 | 27 (18–30) | | 144 (30) | 18 | 19 (1–29) | 0.71 (0.66–0.75) |
| American Indian | 177 (75) | 22 | 21 (11–29) | | 579 (25) | 17 | 18 (4–29) | 0.76 (0.70–0.81) |
| **Caregiver's sex** | | | | .02 | | | | |
| Male | 25 (54) | 26 | 27 (18–30) | | 21 (46) | 17 | 17 (3–29) | 0.64 (0.51–0.78) |
| Female | 821 (71) | 24 | 25 (8–30) | | 341 (29) | 18 | 19 (1–29) | 0.71 (0.69–0.74) |
| **Caregiver's age** (tertiles) | | | | 0.03 | | | | |
| *Q1* | 264 (66) | 24 | 24 (18–30) | | 139 (34) | 19 | 20 (3–29) | 0.76 (0.72–0.80) |
| *Q2* | 284 (70) | 24 | 25 (8–30) | | 119 (30) | 17 | 18 (3–29) | 0.70 (0.65–0.75) |
| *Q3* | 298 (74) | 25 | 25 (18–30) | | 104 (26) | 17 | 18 (1–29) | 0.66 (0.60–0.71) |
| **Child's age** (months; at baseline interview) | | | | 0.05 | | | | |
| 0–11 | 347 (66) | 25 | 25 (18–30) | | 182 (34) | 17 | 18 (2–28) | 0.69 (0.65–0.73) |
| 12–23 | 177 (72) | 25 | 25 (11–30) | | 70 (28) | 19 | 20 (1–29) | 0.75 (0.69–0.81) |
| 24–35 | 154 (74) | 24 | 23 (8–30) | | 55 (26) | 18 | 20 (3–29) | 0.74 (0.68–0.81) |
| 36–47 | 146 (75) | 24 | 25 (18–30) | | 48 (25) | 17 | 17 (3–28) | 0.69 (0.62–0.76) |
| 48–59 | 22 (76) | 21 | 19 (18–30) | | 7 (24) | 16 | 17 (7–25) | 0.73 (0.50–0.95) |
| **Education** | | | | 0.8 | | | | |
| <HS | 204 (71) | 24 | 25 (8–30) | | 84 (29) | 19 | 21 (3–29) | 0.79 (0.74–0.84) |
| HS/GED | 330 (71) | 24 | 25 (18–30) | | 137 (29) | 18 | 19 (3–29) | 0.72 (0.68–0.77) |
| Some college/technical or more | 312 (69) | 25 | 25 (18–30) | | 141 (31) | 16 | 18 (1–29) | 0.65 (0.61–0.70) |
| **Marital status** | | | | 0.5 | | | | |
| Single | 537 (70) | 24 | 25 (8–30) | | 235 (30) | 19 | 20 (2–29) | 0.75 (0.72–0.78) |
| Married | 221 (70) | 24 | 25 (18–30) | | 95 (30) | 16 | 16 (2–29) | 0.63 (0.57–0.68) |
| Divorced/separated/other | 88 (73) | 24 | 25 (18–30) | | 32 (27) | 16 | 17.5 (1–26) | 0.67 (0.56–0.78) |
| **Number of children** | | | | 0.03 | | | | |
| 1 | 313 (65) | 24 | 24 (18–30) | | 166 (35) | 18 | 19 (2–29) | 0.71 (0.67–0.75) |
| 2 | 294 (74) | 25 | 25 (18–30) | | 101 (26) | 18 | 18 (1–29) | 0.72 (0.67–0.77) |
| 3 | 139 (71) | 24 | 25 (11–30) | | 57 (29) | 17 | 19 (3–29) | 0.69 (0.62–0.76) |
| ≥4 | 98 (72) | 25 | 26 (8–30) | | 38 (28) | 19 | 19.5 (6–29) | 0.74 (0.65–0.82) |

**Table 2.** Cont.

| | No enrollment gap[a] | | | | One or more enrollment gaps[a] | | | |
|---|---|---|---|---|---|---|---|---|
| | | Enrollment (months) | | | | Enrollment (months) | | |
| | No.[b] (row %) | Mean | Median (range) | $\chi^2$; p[c] | No.[b] (row %) | Mean | Median (range) | Enrollment Proportion[d] (95% CI) |
| **Caregiver general health** | | | | 0.4 | | | | |
| Excellent/Very good/Good | 758 (70) | 24 | 25 (8–30) | | 318 (30) | 18 | 19 (1–29) | 0.71 (0.69–0.74) |
| Fair/Poor | 88 (67) | 25 | 25 (18–30) | | 44 (33) | 17 | 17.5 (2–29) | 0.69 (0.61–0.77) |
| **Health Literacy** (NVS) | | | | 0.8 | | | | |
| Low[e] | 137 (69) | 24 | 24 (8–30) | | 62 (31) | 19 | 19 (4–29) | 0.77 (0.72–0.83) |
| Moderate[f] | 360 (71) | 24 | 25 (18–30) | | 148 (29) | 18 | 19 (1–29) | 0.71 (0.67–0.75) |
| Higher[g] | 349 (70) | 25 | 25 (11–30) | | 152 (30) | 17 | 18 (2–29) | 0.69 (0.65–0.73) |

*Note.* COHL = Carolina Oral Health Literacy; CI = Confidence Interval; HS = High School; GED = General Educational Development; NVS = Newest Vital Sign. The sample size was n = 1208.
[a] Enrollment gap was defined as any disruption in Medicaid enrollment within a period of eligibility, preceded and superseded by periods of enrollment.
[b] Column figures may not add up to total because of missing values.
[c] Corresponds to $X^2$ tests of the equality of distribution of participants with and without enrollment gap across categories of caregiver characteristics.
[d] Enrollment proportion was calculated for children with enrollment gaps as the ratio of months enrolled over months eligible.
[e] Defined as NVS score: 0–1.
[f] Defined as NVS score: 2–3.
[g] Defined as NVS score: 4–6.

**Table 3.** Results of Multivariate Poisson Regression Modeling of Medicaid Enrollment Gap Incidence on Caregiver and Child Characteristics, among the COHL Study Follow-up Cohort in North Carolina, during the Study Period (A) and Using all Available Medicaid History (B) between January 2004 and December 2010.

| | Model A[a]: COHL study follow-up period | | | Model B[a]: All available Medicaid history | | |
|---|---|---|---|---|---|---|
| | IRR | 95% CI | p | IRR | 95% CI | p |
| **Health literacy** (NVS) | | | | | | |
| Low[b] | 1.17 | 0.89–1.54 | 0.3 | 1.10 | 0.87–1.38 | 0.4 |
| Moderate-Higher[c] | 1.00 | *referent* | | 1.00 | *referent* | |
| **Race** | | | | | | |
| White | 1.00 | *referent* | | 1.00 | *referent* | |
| African American | 0.91 | 0.73–1.13 | 0.4 | 0.93 | 0.77–1.12 | 0.4 |
| American Indian | 0.86 | 0.64–1.15 | 0.3 | 0.94 | 0.75–1.18 | 0.6 |
| **Education** (ordinal categorical) | 1.10 | 0.96–1.26 | 0.2 | 1.08 | 0.96–1.21 | 0.2 |
| **Caregiver's sex** | | | | | | |
| Male | 1.00 | *referent* | | 1.00 | *referent* | |
| Female | 0.53 | 0.35–0.80 | 0.003 | 0.62 | 0.43–0.90 | 0.01 |
| **Caregiver's age** (years; continuous) | 0.98 | 0.96–1.00 | 0.01 | 0.98 | 0.96–0.99 | $<0.001$ |
| **Child's age** (years; ordinal categorical) | 0.93 | 0.86–1.02 | 0.1 | 0.99 | 0.93–1.06 | 0.9 |
| **Caregiver general health** | | | | | | |
| Excellent/Very good/Good | 0.83 | 0.61–1.12 | 0.2 | 0.88 | 0.69–1.14 | 0.3 |
| Fair/Poor | 1.00 | *referent* | | 1.00 | *referent* | |

*Note.* NVS = Newest Vital Sign; COHL = Carolina Oral Health Literacy; IRR = Incidence Rate Ratio; CI = Confidence Interval. The sample size was n = 1208.
[a]Variable selection was based on a backward hierarchical procedure starting from a full model and a $P<.2$ criterion; caregivers' race, age and general health were included a priori in the models; time at risk for a gap was considered time (months) of Medicaid enrollment.
[b]Defined as NVS score: 0–1.
[c]Defined as NVS score: 2–6.

**Table 4.** Estimates of the Association between Caregivers' Low Health Literacy (Defined as NVS Score of less than 2) and the Incidence of Children's Medicaid Enrollment Gaps, Overall and Stratified by Educational Attainment, among the COHL Study Follow-up Cohort in North Carolina, during the Study Period (A) and Using all Available Medicaid History (B) between January 2004 and December 2010.

| | Model A[a]: COHL study follow-up period | | Model B[a]: All available Medicaid history | |
|---|---|---|---|---|
| | IRR | 95% CI | IRR | 95% CI |
| **All** | 1.17 | 0.89–1.54 | 1.10 | 0.86–1.40 |
| **Race** | | | | |
| Whites | 1.23 | 0.73–2.06 | 1.29 | 0.85–1.96 |
| African American | 1.14 | 0.76–1.69 | 1.05 | 0.75–1.48 |
| American Indian | 1.18 | 0.64–2.16 | 0.96 | 0.58–1.57 |
| Homogeneity ($\chi^2$)[b] *P* | 0.97 | | 0.63 | |
| **Education** | | | | |
| Did not finish high school | 1.52 | 0.99–2.35 | 1.36 | 0.97–1.92 |
| High school diploma or GED | 1.07 | 0.68–1.69 | 1.07 | 0.73–1.58 |
| Some technical/college training or higher | 0.67 | 0.31–1.45 | 0.65 | 0.34–1.24 |
| Homogeneity ($\chi^2$)[b] *P* | 0.17 | | 0.13 | |

*Note.* NVS = Newest Vital Sign; COHL = Carolina Oral Health Literacy; IRR = Incidence Rate Ratio; CI = Confidence Interval; GED = General Educational Development. The sample size was n = 1208.
[a]Variable selection was based on a backward hierarchical procedure starting from a full model and a $P<.2$ criterion; caregivers' race, age and general health were included a priori in the models; time at risk for a gap was considered time (months) of Medicaid enrollment.
[b]Wald $\chi^2$ test of a common IRR (across-strata homogeneity).

problem-initiated and enrollment pattern driven care-seeking behavior.

Evidence supporting an association between parental health literacy and child health insurance status has been reported by large, rigorous studies, including those by Pati et al. [56] and Yin et al. [58]. Although these studies did not investigate enrollment gaps, they add to the growing evidence base linking health literacy with children's insurance status. The findings of the DeVoe et al. [17] and Satchell and Pati [22] studies underscored the importance of socio-economic stressors, including poverty and maternal education as strong predictors of enrollment gaps. This effect was reflected in our study's stratified analyses, wherein the effect of low health literacy varied significantly according to education level, with the largest estimates found among the lowest-educated caregivers.

Our findings have limitations. This WIC study cohort was not a probability sample, an important factor because WIC enrollment alone has been shown to confer benefits for child health behaviors and outcomes [59–60]. The WIC program is the largest public health nutrition program in the US and, as such, serves a large percentage of low-income children and their mothers. To put this in perspective, in fiscal year 2013, more than 2 million women and infants nationwide participated in WIC, whereas there were 264,000 WIC participants in North Carolina. Our sample size was modestly sized, including approximately 1,200 dyads and 199 caregivers with low health literacy; however, it must be noted to the best of our knowledge no other cohorts to-date exist with person-level data on parents' health literacy and children's Medicaid enrollment information. For many practical reasons, our population was limited to English-speaking caregivers over the age of 18, limiting the generalizability of our findings beyond that demographic group. Although there is a Spanish version of the NVS tool, most of our survey instruments at the time of the study had not been developed for or validated in Spanish. Because Hispanic children are often the most likely to have insurance gaps [22], the absence of this demographic group is an obvious study limitation. Future studies among these high-risk, vulnerable groups are warranted. Another limitation that must be pointed out is that NVS is only one of many available instruments available to assess health literacy; as a comprehension and numeracy-based test, it is not a comprehensive health literacy assessment.

Understanding Medicaid enrollment gaps is a complex issue. State differences in the enrollment and re-enrollment processes warrant the investigation of the association between health literacy and enrollment gaps in diverse population-based samples in different states. It is possible that enrollment and re-enrollment in Medicaid require cognitive and/or executive functioning skills not well-captured by the instrument used in this study. Prolonged interruptions could be due to changes in eligibility, but gaps can be due to administrative issues on both the program and the client's sides. Our data included rich information from the perspective of the client, but lacked information from the perspective of the program.

## Summary and implications

Health insurance gaps have been linked to increased health disparities [61], leading to a poorer quality of health care [62]. Accordingly, correcting problems with children's health insurance enrollment and coverage should be a priority for stakeholders. We found that 30% of young children experienced one or more enrollment gaps over a 2-year period. Our data did not reveal any important association between caregivers' health literacy and the incidence of these gaps; however, they indicated that low health literacy may be a risk factor for enrollment gaps among the lowest-educated caregivers, who may be the most vulnerable to its detrimental effects. Moreover, caregivers' young age showed an association with increased risk for enrollment gaps. Considering the economy of scale of the anticipated health insurance coverage expansion in 2014, insurance coverage and continuity issues are certain to become ever more important challenges. Because health literacy issues are, unlike many other social determinants, amenable to interventions, it is critical that they are kept on the agendas of policy makers. Although age is a non-intervenable factor, it may be pertinent to consider caregivers' (young) age as a possible additional risk factor for their children's public insurance enrollment disruptions.

The Congressional Budget Office projects that the currently 34 million people that are covered by Medicaid will increase to 47 million in 2014 with the implementation of the ACA [63]. Considering this huge expansion, health insurance coverage should be examined from a social and behavioral perspective to inform and guide states' actions in the implementation of the Medicaid coverage expansion [16,64–66]. Gaps in insurance coverage should be considered with a rigor similar to non-enrollment. More research is needed to comprehensively characterize health system and individual-level risk factors for public health insurance gaps; however, it must be acknowledged that population-wide, policy solutions such as continuous eligibility and automatic re-enrollment in public insurance may be more effective approaches compared to "individual risk factor" strategies. Beyond the obvious utility of identifying susceptible groups or individuals (i.e., young caregivers of children), it is critical that planned interventions are evidence-based with attention to the critical issues of health literacy and cultural appropriateness.

## Supporting Information

**Dataset S1 Tab-delimited dataset containing all original and derived variables described and used for this study's analyses, including a data dictionary as a separate spreadsheet.**

## Author Contributions

Conceived and designed the experiments: JYL DAD RGR WFV. Performed the experiments: ADB. Analyzed the data: KD ZG. Contributed reagents/materials/analysis tools: JYL KD ZG. Wrote the paper: KD WFV. Conceived the study: JYL. Overviewed the data analysis: JYL. Contributed to the interpretation of results: JYL. Assisted in preparation of the first draft of the manuscript: JYL. Conducted the data analysis: KD. Prepared the first draft of the manuscript: KD. Participated in the study design: DAD RGR. Participated in results interpretation: DAD RGR ADB. Participated in data collection: ADB. Critically revised the manuscript: ADB ZG. Participated in the data management and data analysis: ZG. Contributed to the critical interpretation of results: JYL KD DAD ADB ZG RGR WFV. Substantially revised the initial manuscript draft for content and accuracy, confirm that they are responsible for the reported research, and meet all criteria for authorship: JYL KD DAD ADB ZG RGR WFV.

## References

1. Chung PJ, Lee TC, Morrison JL, Schuster MA (2006) Preventive care for children in the United States: quality and barriers. Annu Rev Public Health 27: 491–515.

2. Olson LM, Tang SF, Newacheck PW (2005) Children in the United States with discontinuous health insurance coverage. N Engl J Med 353: 382–291.

3. Newacheck PW, Stoddard JJ, Hughes DC, Pearl M (1998) Health insurance and access to primary care for children. N Engl J Med 338: 513–519.
4. Fisher MA, Mascarenhas AK (2009) A comparison of medical and dental outcomes for Medicaid-insured and uninsured Medicaid-eligible children: a U.S. population-based study. J Am Dent Assoc 140: 1403–1412.
5. Fisher MA, Mascarenhas AK (2007) Does Medicaid improve utilization of medical and dental services and health outcomes for Medicaid-eligible children in the United States? Community Dent Oral Epidemiol 35: 263–271.
6. Freed GL, Clark SJ, Pathman DE, Schectman R (1999) Influences on the receipt of well-child visits in the first two years of life. Pediatrics 103: 864–869.
7. St Peter RF, Newacheck PW, Halfon N (1992) Access to care for poor children. Separate and unequal? JAMA 267: 2760–2764.
8. Newacheck PW, Halfon N (1988) Preventive care use by school-aged children: differences by socioeconomic status. Pediatrics 82: 462–468.
9. Selden TM (2006) Compliance with well-child visit recommendations: evidence from the Medical Expenditure Panel Survey, 2000–2002. Pediatrics 118: e1766–1778.
10. Starfield B, Shi L (2004) The medical home, access to care, and insurance: a review of evidence. Pediatrics 113: 1493–1498.
11. Savage MF, Lee JY, Kotch JB, Vann WF Jr (2004) Early preventive dental visits: effects on subsequent utilization and costs. Pediatrics 114: e418–423.
12. Hakim RB, Bye BV (2001) Effectiveness of compliance with pediatric preventive care guidelines among Medicaid beneficiaries. Pediatrics 108: 90–97.
13. Christakis DA, Wright JA, Koepsell TD, Emerson S, Connell FA (1999) Is greater continuity of care associated with less emergency department utilization? Pediatrics 103: 738–742.
14. Strickland BB, Jones JR, Ghandour RM, Kogan MD, Newacheck PW (2011) The medical home: health care access and impact for children and youth in the United States. Pediatrics 127: 604–611.
15. National Association of Pediatric Nurse Practitioners (2003) NAPNAP position statement on credentialing and privileging for pediatric nurse practitioners. J Pediatr Health Care 17: A22–23.
16. Landers RM (2012) The Dénouement of the Supreme Court's ACA Drama. N Engl J Med 367: 198–199.
17. DeVoe JE, Graham A, Krois L, Smith J, Fairbrother GL (2008) "Mind the Gap" in children's health insurance coverage: does the length of a child's coverage gap matter? Ambul Pediatr 8: 129–134.
18. Federico SG, Steiner JF, Beaty B, Crane L, Kempe A (2007) Disruptions in insurance coverage: patterns and relationship to health care access, unmet need, and utilization before enrollment in the State Children's Health Insurance Program. Pediatrics 120: e1009–1016.
19. Wise PH, Wampler NS, Chavkin W, Romero D (2002) Chronic illness among poor children enrolled in the temporary assistance for needy families program. Am J Public Health 92: 1458–1461.
20. Summer L, Mann C (2006) Instability of public health insurance coverage for children and their families: causes, consequences, and remedies. New York: The common wealth fund. Available: http://www.commonwealthfund.org/~/media/Files/Publications/Fund%20Report/2006/Jun/Instability%20of%20Public%20Health%20Insurance%20Coverage%20for%20Children%20and%20Their%20Families%20%20Causes%20%20Consequence/Summer_instabilitypubhltinschildren_935%20pdf.pdf. Accessed 2014 Sept 19.
21. Fairbrother GL, Emerson HP, Partridge L (2007) How stable is medicaid coverage for children? Health Aff (Millwood) 26: 520–528.
22. Satchell M, Pati S (2005) Insurance gaps among vulnerable children in the United States, 1999–2001. Pediatrics 116: 1155–1161.
23. Tang SF, Olson LM, Yudkowsky BK (2003) Uninsured children: how we count matters. Pediatrics 112: e168–173.
24. Wachino V, Weiss A (2009) Maximizing kids' enrollment in Medicaid and SCHIP: What works in reaching, enrolling, and retaining eligible children. National Academy for State Health Policy, Washington, DC. Available: http://nashp.org/sites/default/files/Max_Enroll_Report_FINAL.pdf?q=files/Max_Enroll_Report_FINAL.pdf. Accessed 2014 Sept 19.
25. Price J, Boswell J, Lessard M, Wood K (2006) Why Parents Disenroll Children from Public Health Insurance: The Case of Southeastern North Carolina. Journal of Applied Social Science 21: 92–106.
26. DeVoe JE, Westfall N, Crocker S, Eigner D, Selph S, et al. (2012) Why do some eligible families forego public insurance for their children? A qualitative analysis. Fam Med 44: 39–46.
27. Wilson JM, Wallace LS, DeVoe JE (2009) Are state Medicaid application enrollment forms readable? J Health Care Poor Underserved 20: 423–431.
28. Pati S, Kavanagh JE, Bhatt SK, Wong AT, Noonan K, et al. (2012) Reading level of medicaid renewal applications. Acad Pediatr 12: 297–301.
29. Sentell T (2012) Implications for reform: survey of California adults suggests low health literacy predicts likelihood of being uninsured. Health Aff (Millwood) 31: 1039–1048.
30. DeWalt DA, Hink A (2009) Health literacy and child health outcomes: a systematic review of the literature. Pediatrics 124 Suppl 3: S265–274.
31. Sanders LM, Federico S, Klass P, Abrams MA, Dreyer B (2009) Literacy and child health: a systematic review. Arch Pediatr Adolesc Med 163: 131–140.
32. Ferguson B (2008) Health literacy and health disparities: the role they play in maternal and child health. Nurs Womens Health 12: 286–298.
33. Sanders LM, Thompson VT, Wilkinson JD (2007) Caregiver health literacy and the use of child health services. Pediatrics 119: e86–92.
34. Lee JY, Divaris K, Baker AD, Rozier RG, Lee SY, et al. (2011) Oral health literacy levels among a low income population. J Public Health Dent 71: 152–160.
35. Kalton G (1983) Models in the practice of survey sampling. International Statistical Review 51: 175–188.
36. Lee JY, Divaris K, Baker AD, Rozier RG, Vann WF Jr (2012) The relationship of oral health literacy and self-efficacy with oral health status and dental neglect. Am J Public Health 102: 923–929.
37. Divaris K, Lee JY, Baker AD, Vann WF Jr (2011) The relationship of oral health literacy with oral health-related quality of life in a multi-racial sample of low-income female caregivers. Health Qual Life Outcomes 9: 108.
38. Vann WF Jr, Lee JY, Baker D, Divaris K (2010) Oral health literacy among female caregivers: impact on oral health outcomes in early childhood. J Dent Res 89: 1395–400.
39. Cooper WO, Arbogast PG, Hickson GB, Daugherty JR, Ray WA (2005) Gaps in enrollment from a Medicaid managed care program: effects on emergency department visits and hospitalizations for children with asthma. Med Care 43: 718–725.
40. Weiss BD, Mays MZ, Martz W, Castro M, DeWalt DA, et al. (2005) Quick assessment of literacy in primary care: the newest vital sign. Ann Fam Med 3: 514–522.
41. Welch VL, VanGeest JB, Caskey R (2011) Time, costs, and clinical utilization of screening for health literacy: a case study using the Newest Vital Sign (NVS) instrument. J Am Board Fam Med 24: 281–289.
42. Osborn CY, Weiss BD, Davis TC, Skripkauskas S, Rodrigue C, et al. (2007) Measuring adult literacy in health care: performance of the newest vital sign. Am J Health Behav 31 Suppl 1: S36–46.
43. Peixoto JL (1987) Hierarchical variable selection in polynomial regression models. The American Statistician 41: 311–313.
44. Gardner MJ, Altman DG (1986) Confidence intervals rather than P values: estimation rather than hypothesis testing. Br Med J (Clin Res Ed) 292: 746–750.
45. Greenland S, Rothman KJ (2008) Introduction to stratified analysis. In: Rothman KJ, Greenland S, Lash TL. Modern epidemiology. New York: Lippincott, Williams and Wilkins. pp. 258–282.
46. Fairbrother G, Madhavan G, Goudie A, Watring J, Sebastian RA, et al. (2011) Reporting on continuity of coverage for children in Medicaid and CHIP: what states can learn from monitoring continuity and duration of coverage. Acad Pediatr 11: 318–325.
47. Yu J, Harman JS, Hall AG, Duncan RP (2011) Impact of Medicaid/SCHIP disenrollment on health care utilization and expenditures among children: a longitudinal analysis. Med Care Res Rev 68: 56–74.
48. Sørensen K, Van den Broucke S, Fullam J, Doyle G, Pelikan J, et al. (2012) Health literacy and public health: a systematic review and integration of definitions and models. BMC Public Health 12: 80.
49. Berkman ND, Sheridan SL, Donahue KE, Halpern DJ, Crotty K (2011) Low health literacy and health outcomes: an updated systematic review. Ann Intern Med 155: 97–107.
50. Sentell TL, Halpin HA (2006) Importance of adult literacy in understanding health disparities. J Gen Intern Med 21: 862–866.
51. Parker RM, Ratzan SC, Lurie N (2003) Health literacy: a policy challenge for advancing high-quality health care. Health Aff (Millwood) 22: 147–153.
52. Heinrich C (2012) Health literacy: the sixth vital sign. J Am Acad Nurse Pract 24: 218–223.
53. Sheridan SL, Halpern DJ, Viera AJ, Berkman ND, Donahue KE, et al. (2011) Interventions for individuals with low health literacy: a systematic review. J Health Commun 16 Suppl 3: 30–54.
54. Flores G, Abreu M, Brown V, Tomany-Korman SC (2005) How Medicaid and the State Children's Health Insurance Program can do a better job of insuring uninsured children: the perspectives of parents of uninsured Latino children. Ambul Pediatr 5: 332–340.
55. Ross DC, Hill IT (2003) Enrolling eligible children and keeping them enrolled. Future Child 13: 81–97.
56. Pati S, Siewert E, Wong AT, Bhatt SK, Calixte RE, et al. (2014) The Influence of Maternal Health Literacy and Child's Age on Participation in Social Welfare Programs. Matern Child Health J 18: 1176–1189.
57. DeVoe JE, Krois L, Edlund T, Smith J, Carlson NE (2008) Uninsurance among children whose parents are losing Medicaid coverage: Results from a statewide survey of Oregon families. Health Serv Res 43: 401–418.
58. Yin HS, Johnson M, Mendelsohn AL, Abrams MA, Sanders LM, et al. (2009) The health literacy of parents in the United States: a nationally representative study. Pediatrics 124: S289–298.
59. Chatterji P, Brooks-Gunn J (2004) WIC participation, breastfeeding practices, and well-child care among unmarried, low-income mothers. Am J Public Health 94: 1324–1327.
60. Lee JY, Rozier RG, Norton EC, Kotch JB, Vann WF Jr (2004) Effects of WIC participation on children's use of oral health services. Am J Public Health 94: 772–777.
61. Lillie-Blanton M, Hoffman C (2005) The role of health insurance coverage in reducing racial/ethnic disparities in health care. Health Aff (Millwood) 24: 398–408.
62. Chassin MR, Galvin RW (1998) The urgent need to improve health care quality. Institute of Medicine National Roundtable on Health Care Quality. JAMA 280: 1000–1005.

63. Congressional Budget Office Bulletin (2012) "Updated Estimates for the Insurance Coverage Provisions of the Affordable Care Act". Available: http://cbo.gov/sites/default/files/cbofiles/attachments/03-13-Coverage%20Estimates.pdf. Accessed 2014 Sept 19.
64. Baicker K, Congdon WJ, Mullainathan S (2012) Health insurance coverage and take-up: lessons from behavioral economics. Milbank Q 90: 107–134.
65. Sommers BD, Tomasi MR, Swartz K, Epstein AM (2012) Reasons for the wide variation in Medicaid participation rates among states hold lessons for coverage expansion in 2014. Health Aff (Millwood) 31: 909–919.
66. Kronebusch K, Elbel B (2004) Simplifying children's Medicaid and SCHIP. Health Aff (Millwood) 23: 233–246.

# 6

# Knowledge, Attitude, Practice, and Determinants Emergency Contraceptive Use among Women Seeking Abortion Services in Dire Dawa, Ethiopia

**Meskerem Abate[1], Nega Assefa[2*], Tadesse Alemayehu[2]**

**1** Sabian Health Centre, Dire Dawa Health Office, Dire Dawa, Ethiopia, **2** College of Health and Medical Sciences, Haramaya University, East Harerge, Ethiopia

## Abstract

***Background:*** Unplanned pregnancy from casual sex, unplanned sexual activity, and sexual violence are increasing. Emergency Contraceptives (EC) are used to prevent unplanned pregnancies thereby preventing the occurrence and consequences of unplanned pregnancy. Emergency contraception is widely available in Ethiopia particularly in major cities. Yet the use of EC is very low and abortion rate in cities is high compared to the national average.

***Objectives:*** To assess knowledge, attitude and practice and determinants on the use of emergency contraception among women obtaining abortion service at selected health institutions in Dire Dawa, Eastern Ethiopia.

***Methods:*** A facility based cross-sectional study was conducted on 390 women selected by multi-stage random sampling technique. The samples were generated from government and private for non profit health facilities. Participant's knowledge and attitude towards emergency contraception were measured using composite index based on 7 and 9 questions, respectively and analyzed using mean score to classify them as knowledgeable or not, and have positive attitude or not. Practice was assessed if the women reported ever use of emergency contraception. Determinants of use of emergency contraception were analyzed using logistic regression.

***Result:*** Out of 390 women interviewed, 162 women (41.5%) heard about EC, only 133 (34.1%) had good knowledge, and 200 (51.3%) of the respondents had positive attitudes towards to EC. Ever use of EC was reported by 38 (9.7%). Age, living arrangement, education, marital status, religion were found to be significantly associated with the use of emergency contraceptives. Women with poor knowledge were less likely to use EC compared to the knowledgeable ones [AOR = 0.027, 95% CI (0.007, 0.105)].

***Conclusion:*** The study identified that most respondents lack adequate knowledge on the method of EC. In addition ever use of EC is very low.

***Recommendations:*** Health professions should give attention in increasing knowledge and uptake of Emergency Contraception.

**Editor:** Kristina Gemzell-Danielsson, Karolinska Institutet, Sweden

**Funding:** Haramaya University supported the study. The study was part of masters thesis. The university has no role in the design and conduct of the study. One of the author is Haramaya University Employee, this does not have any influence on affecting the design, and implementation of the study. The funders had no role in study design, data collection and analysis, decision to publish, or preparation of the manuscript.

**Competing Interests:** The authors have declared that no competing interests exist.

* Email: negaassefa@yahoo.com

## Introduction

Emergency contraceptives (EC) is the only method women can use to prevent pregnancy after they have had unprotected sexual intercourse, have experienced a contraceptive failure, have remembered too late that they have forgotten to take their birth control pills, or have been forced to have sex against their will. EC is sometimes referred to as "morning-after" or "post-coital" contraception. EC is intended for occasional or emergency use only and not as a regular means of contraception. Formerly, EC was thought to be effective only within 72 hours, but recent studies have confirmed it is effective for up to 120 hours [1].The copper-releasing intrauterine device (IUD) can be used safely for EC up to 5 days after unprotected intercourse, reducing the risk of pregnancy by over 99 percent [2].

EC is largely underutilized worldwide and has been referred to as one of the best kept secrets in Reproductive Health [3]. Globally, use of EC is relatively low. In the United States usage has been reported as 9.4%, in South Africa as 4% and in Iran as 5.2% [4,5,6]. In addition, studies have showed that knowledge, and attitude on emergency contraception among women are limited [7].

Each year globally about 250 million pregnancies occur. One-third of these pregnancies are unintended, of which 20% terminated by induced abortion. In low income countries, more than one-third of the 182 million pregnancies are unintended; of which 19% are terminated by induced abortion. Among the induced abortion 11% are unsafe [8].

Due to high unmet need for family planning and its subsequent effect, many women in Ethiopia are experiencing the challenges of abortion and unwanted child birth. As a result, the Federal Ministry of Health of Ethiopia has allowed the distribution of EC in drug stores and the provision of safe abortion services in medical setup for those who demand the service under certain conditions such as rape, incest, sexual violence, etc.

In Dire Dawa, EC pills can be found in any drug retails in a two dose oral pills that should be taken in 12 hours apart. According to the information on the leaflet distributed with the drug, the two doses should be taken within 72 hours after exposure to unprotected sex. In major cities, in Ethiopia, even though EC is easily accessible from drug stores, abortion rate is quite high. For example, the abortion rate in Dire Dawa, is 184 per 1,000 per women of reproductive age, while the national average is 49 per 1,000 [10]. For this, many explain that Dire Dawa is a city, and there are plenty of health facilities, both public and private that render abortion service. Therefore, it is reasonable to have this difference between national average and the city's value.

Abortion, even if performed in safe way, it may be painful, and may have psychological and physical stress. Here, the paradox is while EC service is widely available, why would women prefer to have an abortion in the face of potential problems associated with the procedure. For this, several reasons can be given, yet the dominant one is lack of adequate knowledge on EC among the general public and women in particular.

This study assessed knowledge, attitude and practice (KAP) and determinants of use of emergency contraceptive among women obtaining abortion service in Dire Dawa at selected health institutions. The outcome of this study will be used to put interventions in place in order to increase the use of EC thereby reverse the occurrence of unwanted pregnancy and its sequelae.

## Methods and Materials

Facility based cross-sectional study was conducted from January to February 2014 among women who obtained abortion service in selected health facilities in Dire Dawa city. Dire Dawa city is located in the Eastern part of Ethiopia 505 kms from Addis Ababa, the capital of Ethiopia. Based on the 2007 census conducted by the central statistical agency of Ethiopia, Dire Dawa Administrative council has a total population of 341,834 of whom 171,461 are males and 170,373 are females and the growth rate was 2.5% [11].

The sample size was calculated assuming proportion of EC knowledge of married and unmarried women experienced induced abortion to be 9% and 17.5%, respectively, obtained from previous study in Jimma, Ethiopia [12]. A 5% margin of error, 95% confidence level and adding a non-response rate of 10%. Accordingly, a sample size of 431 was obtained.

A multi-stage sampling technique was used to select 431 study participants. A list of health facilities prepared and the facilities were stratified into government and private for non-profit health facilities. Then they were selected by simple random sampling from the list. The sample size to each selected facility was allocated proportionally using client volume in the facilities served in the year 2013. All women in reproductive age group who came for obtaining abortion service in the selected health facilities during the study period were source of population for the study.

A pre-tested structured questionnaire was used to collect data. The questionnaire was translated into three local languages (Amharic, Oromifa and Somali) and then back to the original English to maintain its consistency. The questionnaire includes socio-demographic variables, knowledge, attitude and practice questions about EC. Seven female diploma nurses collected the data by face-to-face interview. The data collection was supervised by Nurses who have bachelor degree.

Following data collection a unique code was assigned to each questionnaire and checked for completeness then entered into computer on EPI-info software version 3.5.1. Data was cleaned and analyze using Statistical Package for Social Science (SPSS) version 16.1. First, descriptive analysis was done to identify the level knowledge, attitude and practice which is expressed in terms of frequencies and percentages. Knowledge of EC was assessed using questions of awareness about the types, mentioning the time limit for EC use after unprotected sex and responding the dosage of emergency contraceptive. Attitude was assessed using the responses of the way clients were thinking or behaving about EC. Practice was determined based on ever use of EC after exposure to unprotected sexual intercourse to prevent unintended pregnancy.

Seven questions were used to measure knowledge of the respondents on EC. If respondents get the right answer, it was coded as Yes "1" if not it was coded as No "0". The respondent's knowledge scores were aggregated and ranged 0–7. Based on the cumulated score, respondents, who scored above the mean value, were considered as "knowledgeable"; while those who score below the mean were considered as "not knowledgeable".

The respondents' attitude was measured using nine items rated on a five-point Likert scale that was later changed to dichotomous outcome. The scores were aggregated and ranged 0–9. Based on the cumulative score, respondents who scored above the mean of the total were considered as having "positive attitude"; while those scored below the mean of the total were considered as having "negative attitude". Finally, odds ratios with 95% CI were calculated to measure risk and statistical significance of socio-demographic, knowledge and attitude towards use of EC. Logistic regression analysis was used to assess the relative effect of independent variable on the dependent variables.

The study was carried out after obtaining ethical clearance from Institutional Ethical Clearance Board (IRB) of College of Health Sciences, Haramaya University. All participants were informed about the objectives and their right whether to choose to participate or not and their right to leave the study at anytime they wish. A written informed consent was obtained from all participants. Study participants, whose age is less than 18 years, assent was taken from the study participants. For this study group, as the issue is very sensitive, consent was not obtained from the care taker/guardian. All data, consent/assent documents are kept in safe place at the office of the first author. This procedure of taking consent and assent was accepted by the IRB, as the survey took only oral responses. In order to keep confidentiality of respondents' information, only data collector and supervisor were involved in the data collection and supervision process.

## Result

### Socio – Demographic Characteristics of the Respondents

Among women who came for abortions service at the selected health facilities, a total of 390 women were interviewed. The response rate was 90.1%. The minimum and maximum age of the

**Table 1.** Socio-demographic characteristics of women who came for induced abortion in Dire Dawa town, March 2014.

| Variables | Frequency | Percent |
|---|---|---|
| **Age** | | |
| 15–19 | 72 | 18.5 |
| 20–24 | 186 | 47.7 |
| 25–29 | 92 | 23.6 |
| 30+ | 40 | 10.3 |
| Total | 390 | 100 |
| **Living arrangement** | | |
| Parent | 148 | 37.9 |
| Spouse | 139 | 35.6 |
| Friend | 42 | 10.8 |
| Alone | 61 | 15.6 |
| Total | 390 | 100 |
| **Occupation** | | |
| Student | 159 | 40.8 |
| Merchant | 32 | 8.2 |
| House Wife | 70 | 17.9 |
| Commercial Sex Worker | 16 | 4.1 |
| Employee | 113 | 29 |
| Total | 390 | 100 |
| **Education** | | |
| Illiterate | 21 | 5.4 |
| Primary Education | 95 | 24.3 |
| Secondary Education | 149 | 38.2 |
| Diploma and above | 125 | 32.1 |
| Total | 390 | 100 |
| **Marital Status** | | |
| Unmarried | 251 | 64.4 |
| Married | 139 | 35.6 |
| Total | 390 | 100 |
| **Religion** | | |
| Christian | 220 | 69.2 |
| Muslim | 120 | 30.8 |
| Protestant | 53 | 13.6 |
| Catholic | 6 | 1.5 |
| Total | 390 | 100 |

respondents was 16 and 41 respectively. Among the respondents 278 (71.3%) were in the age range of 20–29 years. Regarding educational status, 38.2% had some secondary level education, 32.1% to tertiary level, 24.3% to primary level and 5.4% had no education (Table 1).

## Knowledge on EC among Women who Seek Induced Abortion

Knowledge scores were aggregated and ranged 0–7 with mean 2.04, median 1 and SD 2.96. Based on this result, the summary index for knowledge towards EC showed that 133 (34.1%) women were knowledgeable while 257 (65.9%) were not knowledgeable. When asked about the options available to prevent unintended pregnancy, 249 (63.8%) responded abortion while 114 (29%) reported the use of EC. Regarding EC methods majority 142 (36.4%) respondents mentioned ECP while only one (0.01%) mentioned IUCD. Concerning the appropriate time for taking EC and doses, 72 of them described within 72 hours; 66 women stated two times are the appropriate doses of ECP. Similarly, 74 respondents mentioned 12 hours is the time intervals to take ECP. Regarding the main sources of information about EC, friends and health workers were the main sources (Table 2).

## Attitudes of women attending abortion service towards EC

Attitude scores were aggregated and ranged 0–9 with mean 6.13, median 7 and SD 2.42, Based on this, the overall summary index for attitude assessment towards emergency contraceptive revealed that 51.3% (200) of the respondents had positive attitude towards use of EC (Table 3).

**Table 2.** Knowledge of Emergency Contraceptive among women attending abortion service in Dire Dawa town, March 2014.

| Variables | Frequency | Percent |
|---|---|---|
| **Things to do after unprotected sexual intercourse (correctly replied)** | 114 | 29.2 |
| *Use ECP* | 114 | 29.2 |
| Abortion | 249 | 63.8 |
| No alternative | 6 | 1.5 |
| I don't know | 21 | 5.4 |
| Total | 390 | 100 |
| **Types of EC methods(correctly replied)** | 142 | 36.4 |
| *ECP* | 142 | 36.4 |
| *IUCD* | 1 | 0.3 |
| COC | 0 | 0 |
| Depo | 19 | 4.9 |
| I don't know | 228 | 58.5 |
| Total | 390 | 100 |
| **Time limit to take EC(correctly replied)** | 72 | 18.5 |
| Any time | 8 | 2.1 |
| Before sex | 44 | 11.3 |
| 24 hours after sex | 28 | 7.2 |
| *72 hours after sex* | 72 | 18.5 |
| 120 hours after sex | 5 | 1.3 |
| I don't know | 233 | 59.7 |
| Total | 390 | 100 |
| **Dose of ECP (correctly replied)** | 66 | 14.6 |
| One dose | 57 | 14.6 |
| *Two dose* | *66* | *16.9* |
| Three dose | 9 | 2.3 |
| I don't know | 258 | 66.2 |
| Total | 390 | 100 |
| **Time interval between doses (correctly replied)** | 74 | 19.0 |
| *12 hours* | *74* | *19.0* |
| 24 hours | 31 | 7.9 |
| I don't know | 285 | 73.1 |
| Total | 390 | 100 |
| **Advantage of EC (correctly replied)** | *106* | *27.2* |
| *Prevent pregnancy* | *106* | *27.2* |
| Regular contraceptive | 5 | 1.3 |
| Regulation of menstrual cycle | 54 | 13.8 |
| Abortion | 25 | 6.4 |
| I don't know | 200 | 51.3 |
| Total | 390 | 100 |
| **Situations of requirement EC to prevent unintended pregnancy(correctly replied)** | 101 | 25.9 |
| *Raped* | 13 | 3.3 |
| *Condom breaks* | 27 | 6.9 |
| *Regular pills are missed* | 21 | 5.4 |
| *Use no contraceptives* | 66 | 16.9 |
| ***In all above situations*** | ***101*** | ***25.9*** |
| I don't know | 162 | 41.6 |
| Total | 390 | * |
| **Knowledge of Emergency Contraceptive (summary index)** | | |
| **Not Knowledgeable** | 257 | 65.9 |

**Table 2.** Cont.

| Variables | Frequency | Percent |
|---|---|---|
| **Knowledgeable** | 133 | 34.1 |
| Total | 390 | 100% |

*Percentage could be greater than 100 since multiple responses are possible.
NB: *Italicized fonts are correct responses.*

## Emergency Contraceptive Use

Out of 390 respondents, 38 (9.7%) mentioned that they had ever used ECP at least once. Bad rumour (58), fear of side effect (41), religious prohibition (16) and husband influence (7) were the reasons mentioned by the respondents for not using EC while 228 women never heard of EC and two respondents said that they do not know where EC is available. Among the 38 women who ever used ECP, 24 (63.2%) of them were between the age group of 25–29.

Regarding the living arrangement of those, who ever used EC, 19 live with their parents, 10 live with spouse, three live with friend and six of the respondent live alone. Twenty four of the women were employee while nine of them were students and the remaining six were merchants, housewives, or commercial sex workers. Regarding educational background of the women who ever used ECP, 33 had diploma & above while three had some secondary education and two had some primary education. Of the 38 respondents who ever used EC, 28 women were unmarried; and 35 women were Christian.

## Determinants on the use of Emergency Contraceptives

Socio demographic factors, knowledge and attitude found to be significantly associated on the use of EC. Accordingly, age of respondents was found significantly associated with the use of EC [AOR = 0.2, 95% CI (0.01, 0.8)]. The likelihood of EC usage decreased as the age of the women increased. Women of the age group 20–24 were less likely to use EC compared with the younger age group (15–19) with an AOR 0.18 [CI 0.04, 0.8]. Similarly women who were living with their spouse were less likely to use EC compared to those living alone, AOR 0.001 [0.000, 0.017].

Religion of the respondents was found to be significantly associated with the use EC [p = 0.024]. The study shows that more Christian respondents were using EC than that of Muslim 4.113 [1.205, 14.039]. Marital status significantly associated with the use of EC [p = 0.000]. Married women were less likely to use EC compared to unmarried women. Education is significantly associated with use of EC. The likelihood of using EC increased as the education level of the study subjects increased. Those respondents with diploma & above were more likely to use EC compared to primary and secondary education. Knowledge of respondents towards EC was significantly associated with use of EC [p = 0.000]. The result showed that the likelihood to use EC

**Table 3.** Attitude towards Emergency Contraception among abortion service users in Dire Dawa town, March 2014.

| Variables | S. disagree | Disagree | Neutral | Agree | S. Agree | Total |
|---|---|---|---|---|---|---|
| | % | % | % | % | % | % |
| I would use ECP if I have unprotected sex | 0.0 | 7.7 | 10.8 | 80.0 | 1.5 | 100 |
| EC methods are safe | 1.0 | 20.0 | 17.4 | 60.5 | 1.0 | 100 |
| I would recommend EC methods to a friend | 1.3 | 30.0 | 11.8 | 53.1 | 3.8 | 100 |
| EC methods should be limited because they could have side effect | 5.4 | 62.3 | 11.0 | 18.7 | 2.6 | 100 |
| Increased accessibility of EC brings about irresponsible sexual behavior? | 9.2 | 56.4 | 15.4 | 17.0 | 1.0 | 100 |
| My partner has positive attitude towards EC methods | 0.3 | 23.8 | 12.6 | 62.6 | 0.8 | 100 |
| If male partner knows about EC, he may be less likely to use condoms | 0.8 | 67.9 | 6.7 | 24.1 | 0.5 | 100 |
| Increased accessibility of EC make women stop using other forms of contraceptive | 9.2 | 61.5 | 9.7 | 18.5 | 1.0 | 100 |
| EC methods could have an effect on future fertility | 7.2 | 68.5 | 13.1 | 10.8 | 0.5 | 100 |
| **Attitude towards EC (Summary index)** | **Number** | **%** | | | | |
| **Negative attitude** | 190 | 48.7 | | | | |
| **Positive attitude** | 200 | 51.3 | | | | |

**Table 4.** Determinants of the use Emergency Contraception in Dire Dawa town, March 2014.

| Variables | Practice | | COR (95% CI) | AOR (95% CI) | P-Value |
|---|---|---|---|---|---|
| | Yes | No | | | |
| **Age** | | | | | |
| 15–19 | 3 (0.8) | 69 (17.7) | 1 | 1 | 0.001 |
| 20–24 | 6 (1.5) | 180 (46.2) | **0.226 (0.061, 0.833)** | **0.18 (0.040, 0.821)** | 0.027 |
| 25–29 | 24 (6.2) | 68 (17.4) | 1.727 (0.451, 6.621) | 1.667 (0.331, 8.386) | 0.535 |
| 30+ | 5 (1.3) | 35 (9.0) | 1.607 (0.319, 8.092) | 1.935 (0.256, 14.642) | 0.522 |
| **Living arrangement** | | | | | |
| Alone | 6 (1.5) | 55 (14.1) | 1 | 1 | 0.000 |
| Parent | 19 (4.9) | 129 (33.1) | 3.251 (0.974, 10.857) | 1.974 (0.464, 8.217) | 0.350 |
| Spouse | 10 (2.6) | 129 (33.1) | **0.002 (0.000, 0.021)** | **0.001 (0.000, 0.017)** | 0.000 |
| Friend | 3 (0.8) | 39 (10.0) | 3.509 (0.682, 18.060) | 3.371 (0.494, 23.027) | 0.215 |
| **Occupation** | | | | | |
| Employee | 24 (6.2) | 89 (22.8) | 1 | 1 | 0.005 |
| Student | 9 (2.3) | 150 (38.5) | 0.334 (0.109, 1.021) | 0.427 (0.112, 1.634) | 0.214 |
| Merchant | 2 (0.5) | 30 (7.7) | 3.304 (0.786, 13.893) | 5.014 (0.881, 28.552) | 0.069 |
| House wife | 2 (0.5) | 68 (17.4) | 0.474 (0.124, 1.817) | 0.365 (0.062, 2.147) | 0.265 |
| Commercial sex worker | 1 (0.3) | 15 (3.8) | | *NI | |
| **Education** | | | | | |
| Diploma & above | 33 (8.5) | 92 (23.6) | 1 | 1 | 0.000 |
| Illiterate | 0 | 21 (5.4) | | **NI | |
| Primary Education | 2 (0.5) | 93 (23.8) | **0.056 (0.013, 0.241)** | **0.055 (0.010, 0.293)** | 0.001 |
| Secondary Education | 3 (0.8) | 146 (37.4) | **0.059 (0.017, 0.305)** | **0.059 (0.014, 0.248)** | 0.000 |
| **Marital Status** | | | | | |
| Unmarried | 28 (7.2) | 223 (57.2) | 1 | 1 | |
| Married | 10 (2.6) | 129 (33.1) | **0.002 (0.000, 0.022)** | **0.002 (0.000, 0.020)** | 0.000 |
| **Religion** | | | | | |
| Christian | 35 (9) | 235(60.3) | 1 | 1 | |
| Muslim | 3(0.8) | 117 (30) | 1.853 (0.711, 4.832) | **4.113 (1.205, 14.039)** | 0.024 |
| **Knowledge** | | | | | |
| Knowledgeable | 35 (9) | 98 (25.1) | 1 | 1 | |
| Not Knowledgeable | 3 (0.8) | 254 (65.1 | 0.116 (0.073, 0.183) | **0.027 (0.007, 0.105)** | 0.000 |
| **Attitude** | | | | | |
| Positive attitude | 34 (8.7) | 166 (42.6) | 1 | 1 | |
| Negative attitude | 4 (1) | 186 (47.7) | 0.080 (0.046, 0.137) | 0.605 (0.238, 1.537) | 0.291 |

*NI = Not included as the observations are below 20.
**NI = Not included as the observation group does not use EC.

increased among the knowledgeable respondents. Respondents who had poor knowledge of EC were found less likely to use EC. In the crude analysis, attitude is significant to towards EC [COR = 0.1, 95% CI (0.1, 0.14)]. But it is insignificant after adjusting for possible confounders [p = 0.291] (Table 4).

## Discussion

In this study 34.1% of study participants were knowledgeable on Emergency Contraception. The study also revealed that 51.3% of the respondents had positive attitudes towards EC. Ever use of EC was 38 (9.7%). Knowledge is significantly associated with the use of EC [AOR = 0.027, CI 95% (0.007, 0.105)]. Attitude towards EC found to be insignificant [AOR = 0.605, CI95% (0.238, 1.537)].

Strength of this study is that the respondent's willingness to participate in the study and obtaining the response rate of 90.1%. Some of the limitations are, it is focused on women who were seeking abortion, a specific population with failure in preventing pregnancy; it may not reflect the general condition of women in the city. In addition, the study populations from private health facilities were not included in the study so that this study might not be representing the entire population.

Less than half of the women had heard about EC among which, majority mentioned Emergency Contraception Pill as EC method, while only one woman mentioned Intra Uterine Contraceptive Device. Only 72 women of the respondents correctly identified 72 hours as the time limit for the method use. The study also identified that knowledge of respondents towards EC was significantly associated with the use of EC. Those respondents with poor knowledgeable were less likely to use EC compared to those with good knowledge. The study also indicated that knowledge of unmarried (72.2%) women towards EC was higher than that of married (27.8%). This finding is similar to the study conducted in Jimma (17.5% unmarried and (9%) married [12].

Nearly half of the study participants had a positive attitude towards emergency contraceptives. Although educated women generally have a positive attitudes towards EC, considerable number of women had inappropriate information about EC. Of which only 62 (62%) respondents had appropriate knowledge about EC while 38 (38%) respondents lack adequate information. In a similar study conducted in Kampala, Uganda, 29% of the respondents had inappropriate information [13]. The use of EC among those respondent with negative attitude compared to positive attitude was insignificant [p = 0.291]. The reason could be lack of information on the use and options of EC despite respondents' positive attitude to use of EC. This study also showed that, health care providers were not providing information about the availability and methods of EC to their clients. Out of the 390 respondents, only 34 (8.7%) women mentioned that they were informed by health care providers about EC. This result is almost similar to the study conducted in Nigeria which was 10% [14].

Less than ten percent of the study participants mentioned ever use of EC. This result is slightly higher than the result obtained from Jimma 5.4% [12]. The reason could be associated with the education of the women as most respondents (86%) in this study who ever used ECP had diploma and above. Of the 38 respondents who ever used ECP, majority (35) were Christians while three were Muslim.

Married women were less likely to use EC compared to unmarried women. This finding is different from the study conducted among the college students in Arba Minch town [15]. The result of this study showed that education is significantly associated with the use of EC. The likelihood of EC use increased as the level of education of the study participants increased. Those respondents with diploma & above were more likely to use EC compared to both primary and secondary education level.

Source of information was highly associated to the use EC. In the study, the major source of information was friends. This result is consistent to the study finding in Lusaka, Zambia where majority referred friends as a major source of information for EC. The same study revealed that women who obtained information from friends were less likely to use EC compared to those women who heard from health workers [16].

## Conclusion and Recommendation

In conclusion the great potential of emergency contraceptives to prevent unintended pregnancies and induced abortions was not considered as an option by the study participants. The use of EC is very low. The major reason for this is lack of adequate knowledge on the method and its availability. IUCD as EC is not known at all. This study showed that information on EC is not provided adequately by the health professionals. Hence, there is a need to educate the community, in particular women of reproductive age about ECs. Education on methods available, the correct time limit for use, and accurate message about its effect on health through health professionals and mass media should be given. The health executives should give due attention to design strategies and strengthening the health education in all health facilities as well as high schools and colleges focusing on the availability and options of Emergency contraceptives.

## Acknowledgments

The authors would like to thank women who participated in the study. We are grateful to the health facilities that facilitated data collection. We also would like to thank data collectors and supervisors.

## Author Contributions

Conceived and designed the experiments: MA NA TA. Performed the experiments: MA NA TA. Analyzed the data: MA NA TA. Contributed reagents/materials/analysis tools: MA NA TA. Contributed to the writing of the manuscript: MA NA TA.

## References

1. Schwarz EB, Gerbert B, Gonzales R (2007) Need for emergency contraception in urgent care settings. Contraception 75: 285–288.
2. Cheng L, Gulmenzoglu AM, Piaggio G, Ezcurra E, Van L (2008) Interventions for emergency contraception. Cochrane Database Syst Rev: (2)
3. Wegene T, Fikre E (2007) Knowledge, attitude and practice on emergency contraceptives among female university students in Addis Ababa, Ethiopia, The Ethiopian journal of health development 21: 112–113.
4. Babaee G, Jamali B, Ali M (2003) Investigating the knowledge, attitude and its relationship with the means of using emergency contraception. J Sex Marital Ther. Tehran 29(4): 269–75. Available: http://www.ncbi.nlm.nih.gov/PubMed/5/5/2008.
5. Merchant RC, Casadei K, Gee EM, Bock BC, Becker BM, et al (2007) Patients' emergen-cy contraception comprehension, usage, and view of the emergency department role for emergency contraception. J Emerg Med 33: 367–75.
6. Myer L, Mlobeli R, Cooper D, Smit J, Morroni C (2007) Knowledge and use of emergency contraception among women in the Western Cape province of South Africa: a cross-sectional study. BMC Women's Health: 7: 4. doi:10.1186/1472-6874-7-14. Available: http://www.ncbi.nlm.nih.gov/pubmed/5/5/2008.
7. Seife M, Fikre E (2007) Assessment of level of awareness and utilization of emergency contraception, among college female students in Oromia Regional state, Arsi Zone, Asella. South-East Ethiopia, Mater Thesis Addis Ababa University.
8. WHO, Gutmacher Institute (2007) Facts on induced abortion worldwide. Available: http://www.searo.who.int/LinkFiles/Publications_Facts_on_Induced_Abortion_Worldwide.pdf.
9. Neinstein LS, Gordon MC, Katzman KD, Rosen SD, Woods RE (2008) Adolescent Health Care: a practical guide. 5th Edition, Edited by: Lippincott Williams and Wilkins, Philadelphia; 533–649.
10. Singh S, Fetters T, Gebreselassie H (2010) The estimated incidence of induced abortion in Ethiopia, International Perspectives on Sexual and Reproductive Health. Journal of reproductive health 36(1): 16–25.
11. Dire Dawa City Administration (2010) Dire Dawa profile. Dire Dawa, Ethiopia.
12. Admasu A, Tebeje B (2009) Knowledge, attitudes, practices and barriers to use emergency contraception among women with unsafe abortion in Jimma Marie Stops Clinic, South West Ethiopia. Ethiopian Journal of Reproductive Health, Addis Ababa 3.
13. Stella K (2011) Knowledge, attitudes and practices regarding emergency contraceptive pills among female undergraduate students of Makerere University-Uganda. 2.2.08: Issues in Hormonal Contraceptive Use.
14. Margaret OE, Osarethin AT, EbuchiVictor I (2006) Health Care Providers Knowledge and Attitude towards and Provision of Emergency Contraceptive in Lagos, Nigeria. International Family Planning perspectives 32(2): 89–93.
15. Alemtu W (2011) Knowledge, attitude and practice of emergency contraceptives among female college students in Arba Minch Town, Southern Ethiopia, Ethiopian Journal Health Development, Addis Ababa, Ethiopia 25(3): 176–183.
16. Chavuma N, Chanda DO, Vwalika B (2010) Emergency Contraception Among Women With' Abortion At University Teaching Hospital In Lusaka, Zambia. Medical Journal of Zambia Lusaka, Zamibia 37(4).

# 7

# The Support for Smoke Free Policy and How It Is Influenced by Tolerance to Smoking – Experience of a Developing Country

**Abdul Rashid[1]*, Azizah Ab Manan[2], Noorlia Yahya[2], Lailanor Ibrahim[2]**

1 Department of Public Health Medicine, Penang Medical College, Georgetown, Penang, Malaysia, 2 Penang State Health Department, Georgetown, Penang, Malaysia

## Abstract

This cross sectional survey was conducted to determine the support in making Penang UNESCO World Heritage Site (GTWHS) smoke free and to determine the influence of tolerance towards smoking on this support. This is the first phase in making Penang, Malaysia a smoke free state. A multistage sampling process was done to select a sample of respondents to represent the population of GTWHS. Attitude towards smoking was assessed using tolerance as a proxy. A total of 3,268 members of the community participated in the survey. A big majority (n = 2969; 90.9%) of the respondents supported the initiative. Support was lowest among the owners and residents/tenants, higher age groups, the Chinese, men, respondents who had poor knowledge of the places gazetted as smoke free, and respondents with poor knowledge of the health effects on smokers and on passive smokers. The odds (both adjusted and unadjusted) of not supporting the initiative was high among those tolerant to smoking in public areas. Tolerance towards smoking was associated with 80.3% risk of non-support in the respondents who were tolerant to smoking and a 57.2% risk in the population. Health promotion and education concerning the harm of tobacco smoke in Malaysia, which has mainly targeted smokers, must change. Health education concerning the risks of second hand smoke must also be given to non-smokers and efforts should be made to denormalize smoking.

**Editor:** Qinghua Sun, The Ohio State University, United States of America

**Funding:** The funding for this study was provided by the Malaysian health promotion board (MySihat), Grant number LPKM/04/061/01/321. The funder had no role in the study design, data collection and analysis, decision to publish or preparation of the manuscript.

**Competing Interests:** The authors have declared that no competing interests exist.

* Email: drrashid10@gmail.com

## Introduction

Although smoking prevalence has reduced worldwide, both in men and women, the number of smokers has increased significantly and cigarette smoking is still the chief preventable killer in most countries [1–3]. In Malaysia, according to the Global Adult Tobacco Survey (GATS) 2011, 31% of adults aged 15 years and older were current tobacco smokers, more men (43.9%) than women (1.0%) and highest in the 25 to 44 age group. On the average an adult Malaysian smoked 14 cigarettes a day and among those who had ever smoked on daily basis only 9.5% had quit [4]. The World Health Organization (WHO) recommends a 30% relative reduction in current tobacco use in persons age 15 years and above [5].

Burning of tobacco produces a complex mixture of more than 7000 compounds which are risks for a wide range of diseases and premature deaths [2]. Cigarette smokers have an average 10 years reduced life span and the mortality among cigarette smokers is two to three times the mortality among persons who had never smoked [6]. At present most tobacco related deaths are reported in the developed countries but due to the change in smoking trends it is expected that more tobacco related deaths will occur in underdeveloped and developing countries [2],[6]. In Malaysia, tobacco related diseases accounted for the main causes of deaths in the hospitals operated by the Ministry of Health. Heart and pulmonary circulation diseases ranked first due to tobacco related illnesses followed by malignant neoplasms and cerebrovascular diseases [7]. Smoking not only effects morbidity and mortality but also quality of life, participation in workplace and increased health care costs [2].

Second hand smoke is equally if not more injurious to health [8]. In the United States (US) almost 2.5 million non-smoking Americans died from heart diseases and lung cancer due to exposure to second hand smoke. The loss of productivity due to exposure to second hand smoke is estimated to be about USD5.6 billion per year [2]. In Malaysia, it is estimated that 39.8% of adults who worked indoors have been exposed to second hand smoke and 38.4% adults exposed to second hand smoke at home, 84.9% in cafes/coffee shops/bistros, 78.7% in bars/nightclubs, 71% in restaurants, 28.2% in government buildings, 13.6% in indoor shopping complexes and 8.7% in health care facilities [7].

There are several interventions to combat smoking and the hazards of tobacco smoke. One is to target individual's smoking related attitudes or social influence by implementing anti-smoking policies including laws which discourage smoking [2],[9],[10]. Creation of smoke free areas is an effective intervention because it is easier to discourage people from smoking rather than encourage people to quit smoking once they have started [11],[12]. These smoke free areas not only help educate people on the dangers of second hand smoke but also help denormalize smoking by making smoking less socially acceptable and less convenient [2],[13],[14]. According to MPOWER which is a technical package on evidence based tobacco control interventions to reduce tobacco use to protect people from second hand smoke, all public places should be completely smoke free or at least 90% of the population should be covered by complete subnational smoke free legislation. Forty three countries comprising 1.1 billion people have achieved this level [11].

Malaysia became a signatory of the WHO Framework Convention on Tobacco Control (WHO FCTC) on the 23rd September 2003 and ratified it in 2005 and became an official party to the convention in December 2005. In 2011, as part of an initiative to comply with article 8 of the WHO FCTC, a proposal to create a smoke free zone in Penang, Malaysia was submitted to the Penang State Government with the objective to protect people from second hand smoke. The Ministry of Health had earlier gazetted 21 areas to be smoke free and as a start the Penang State Government had gazetted 6 recreational areas as smoke free zones. The current proposal was to include areas which had commercial and residential units. It was decided that George Town World Heritage Site (GTWHS) would be the first phase in making Penang a smoke free state. Studies conducted elsewhere had shown high level of support towards smoke free policies but different social and cultural values affect smoking habits and attitudes towards second hand smoke differently [15]. Thus before implementing the smoke free policy, a preliminary survey was conducted in this area to assess the level of support of the public to the proposal. The objective of this paper is to show the level of support towards the smoke free policy and the influence of tolerance to smoking on it.

## Materials and Methods

### Study design and Location

This cross sectional survey was conducted in Penang UNESCO World Heritage Site. The survey was commissioned by the Malaysian Health Promotion Board and the Penang State Government to determine the public and the stakeholders' support towards making Penang a smoke free state. The survey commenced from the middle of 2012 and ended in April 2013. Penang is one of the 14 states in Malaysia with a multi-ethnic population. It is one of the most densely populated states in the country with a population of 1,561,853. George Town, the capital of Penang, was inscribed as a UNESCO World Heritage Site on 7th July 2008 under Cultural Heritage Site category. This site features residential, commercial buildings, tourist sites and public open areas.

### Sample

Multistage sampling process was done to select a sample of respondents to represent the population of GTWHS. Samples were taken from eating outlets, accommodation & hotels, places of worship, private and government offices, residences, retail & businesses, hawkers, education facilities, places of tourist attraction and public open spaces. Stata was used to calculate the sample size. Because each premise had a different population size, the sample from each premise was taken with a 5% margin of error. Within each premise/location, the type of respondent ranged from owner or senior management, employee, clients and the general public. This allowed the investigators to capture a wide range of respondents from the different levels. However because of the dynamic population, the study unit from each premise was taken based on the willingness to participate in the study.

### Tool

Data were collected using face to face interviews by trained interviewers. The interviewers were trained comprehensively on accurate methods of data collection to avoid variations and to ensure uniformity. A uniform protocol covering the questionnaire, inclusion and exclusion criteria for each question was set up to minimize error and bias. Besides the baseline demographic information, the questionnaire was used to gather information on the support for making GTWHS a smoke free zone. Other independent variables related to the support including knowledge, attitudes and practices were also included in the questionnaire. Attitude towards smoking was assessed using tolerance as a proxy [16]. There were 16 items in the tolerance scale, the respondents were asked if they would tolerate smoking in 16 different public locations. Respondents were considered not tolerant to smoking if they answered they would not tolerate smoking in all the public places. The smoking tolerance items were examined using Mokken scaling to assess for fit to a single underlying dimension of tolerance. All items on the tolerance scale were selected by the Mokken scaling procedure, and the final scale had an H coefficient of 0·77, indicating that the items met the criteria for a unidimensional scale. The scale had high consistency level (Cronbach alpha reliability 0.97). The scale used to assess the tolerance towards smoking is in Appendix S1.

### Analysis

Data were tabulated and cross tabulated. SPSS version 18 was used to analyse the relationship between the variables using Chi square test. Odds ratio was used to quantify the odds of not supporting the proposal and regression analysis to estimate support for smoke free zone using tolerance as predictor. Stata was used to measure the attributable risk in the exposed and in the population. A probability value of $P<0.05$ was considered to be statistically significant.

### Ethics

The research had received the approval of the Joint Penang independent ethics committee (JPEC 01-13-0014). All respondents were asked to give a written informed consent before starting the interview. The anonymity of the respondents was assured.

## Results

A total of 3,268 members of the community participated in the survey. Most of the participants were interviewed in business premises (n = 771, 23.6%) followed by offices (both government and private) (n = 455, 13.9%) and education premises (n = 404, 12.4%). The majority of the participants were clients/customers/patrons/tourists/general public (44.6%) followed by owners (26.0%), employees (19.9%) and residents/tenants (11.4%). The majority were men (58.8%), age group 25 to 44 (37.6%), Chinese (60.3%), married (61.4%), income group of between RM1001 to 3000 (66.0%) and the highest level of education up to secondary school (51.7%). Most had never smoked (79.4%) and were aware of the national laws prohibiting smoking in certain areas (86.6%)

**Table 1.** Factors associated with non-support to making GTWHS a smoke free zone.

| Variable | N | No support | Support | Chi square/P value |
|---|---|---|---|---|
| **Respondent Type** | | | | 24.76/<0.001 |
| Owner | 851 | 92 (10.8) | 759 (89.2) | |
| Employee | 584 | 38 (6.5) | 546 (93.5) | |
| Clients/customers/patrons/tourists/general public | 1459 | 114 (7.8) | 1345 (92.2) | |
| Residents/tenants | 374 | 55 (14.7) | 319 (85.3) | |
| **Age** | | | | 9.99/0.01 |
| ≤24 | 688 | 61 (8.9) | 627 (91.1) | |
| 25–44 | 1229 | 91 (7.5) | 1125 (92.5) | |
| 45–64 | 1052 | 110 (10.5) | 942 (89.5) | |
| ≥65 | 299 | 37 (12.4) | 262 (87.6) | |
| **Gender** | | | | 16.61/<0.001 |
| Men | 1923 | 209 (10.9) | 1714 (89.1) | |
| Women | 1345 | 90 (6.7) | 1255 (93.3) | |
| **Marital Status** | | | | 0.38/0.95 |
| Married | 2008 | 186 (9.3) | 1822 (90.7) | |
| Divorce | 28 | 3 (10.7) | 25 (89.3) | |
| Widow/widower | 17 | 1 (5.9) | 16 (94.1) | |
| Single | 1215 | 109 (9.0) | 1106 (91.0) | |
| **Race** | | | | 18.74/<0.001 |
| Malay | 634 | 43 (6.8) | 591 (93.2) | |
| Chinese | 1970 | 215 (10.9) | 1755 (89.1) | |
| Indian | 462 | 28 (6.1) | 434 (93.9) | |
| Others | 202 | 13 (6.4) | 189 (93.6) | |
| **Highest Level of Education** | | | | 45.29/<0.001 |
| Illiterate | 61 | 12 (19.7) | 49 (80.3) | |
| Non formal | 29 | 24 (18.6) | 105 (81.4) | |
| Primary | 296 | 46 (15.5) | 250 (84.5) | |
| Secondary | 1691 | 144 (8.5) | 1547 (91.5) | |
| Tertiary | 1091 | 73 (6.7) | 1018 (93.3) | |
| **Income** | | | | 9.71/0.01 |
| ≤RM1000 | 592 | 72 (12.2) | 520 (87.8) | |
| RM1001 to 3000 | 2158 | 191 (8.9) | 1967 (91.1) | |
| ≥RM3001 | 518 | 36 (6.9) | 482 (93.1) | |
| **Smoking status** | | | | 219.89/<0.001 |
| Never smokers | 2596 | 146 (5.6) | 2450 (94.4) | |
| Past smokers | 167 | 20 (12.0) | 147 (88.0) | |
| Current smokers | 505 | 133 (26.3) | 372 (73.7) | |
| **Awareness on the existence of national laws prohibiting smoking in certain areas** | | | | 20.72/<0.001 |
| Yes | 2827 | 236 (8.3) | 2591 (91.7) | |
| No | 129 | 24 (18.6) | 105 (81.4) | |
| Unsure | 312 | 39 (12.5) | 273 (87.5) | |
| **Knowledge of places which are smoke free according to law** | | | | 30.16/<0.001 |
| Poor knowledge | 998 | 133 (13.3) | 865 (86.7) | |
| Good knowledge | 2270 | 166 (7.3) | 2104 (92.7) | |
| **Health effects on smokers** | | | | 122.59/<0.001 |
| Poor knowledge | 2825 | 103 (23.3) | 340 (76.7) | |
| Good knowledge | 443 | 196 (6.9) | 2629 (93.1) | |
| **Health effects on passive smokers** | | | | 83.48/<0.001 |
| Poor knowledge | 1070 | 115 (18.7) | 499 (81.3) | |

**Table 1.** Cont.

| Variable | N | No support | Support | Chi square/P value |
|---|---|---|---|---|
| Good knowledge | 2198 | 184 (6.9) | 2479 (75.6) | |

and had good knowledge of places which were smoke free (69.5%). Most had good knowledge of the health effects of tobacco smoke on smokers (86.4%) as well as on passive smokers (81.2%). Although the majority were not tolerant to tobacco smoke (67.3%), a substantial proportion of the participants were tolerant (32.7%).

A big majority of the respondents supported (n = 2969; 90.9%) the smoke free initiative. As shown in Table 1, more than 10% of the owners and residents/tenants did not support the smoke free zone initiative ($\chi2 = 24.76$; $P<0.001$). The support for the initiative decreased as the age group increased ($\chi2 = 9.99$; $P = 0.01$). Among the races, Chinese had the highest non-support proportion ($\chi2 = 18.74$; $P<0.001$). The support for the initiative increased with increasing education levels ($\chi2 = 45.29$; $P<0.001$), similarly the support increased as the income bracket increased ($\chi2 = 9.71$; $P = 0.01$). Support was highest among those who never smoked followed by past smokers and lowest among current smokers ($\chi2 = 219.89$; $P<0.001$). The support for the initiative was lower among the men ($\chi2 = 16.16$; $P<0.001$), respondents who had poor knowledge of places gazetted as smoke free ($\chi2 = 30.16$; $P<0.001$), poor knowledge of health effects on smokers ($\chi2 = 122.59$; $P<0.001$) and among passive smokers ($\chi2 = 83.48$; $P<0.001$).

The tolerance to smoking among the respondents was 32.7%. As shown in Table 2, there is a six fold odds of not-supporting the smoke free initiative among those tolerant to smoking in public areas. Regression analysis showed that there was a fourfold odds of not supporting the initiative among those tolerant to smoking in public areas. Tolerance towards smoking was associated with 80.3% risk of non-support in the respondents who were tolerant to smoking and a 57.2% risk in the population.

## Discussion

Tobacco control measures have avoided an estimated 8 million premature deaths and extended the mean life span by 19 to 20 years [17]. Although Malaysia is relatively new in actively adopting tobacco control policies, the ministry of health and several Non-Governmental Organizations (NGO) have been actively and consistently disseminating information pertaining to the risks associated with smoking to the public. This could explain the high level of support for the proposed smoke free policy which is comparable with that of developed countries [18–21] and other developing countries like Thailand [22]. The implementation of smoke free legislation has been shown to be effective even in low and middle income countries like Malaysia. In Uruguay the exposure to second hand smoke decreased greatly in indoor public places and workplaces after the implementation of the smoke free legislation [23].

In the present study, a higher proportion of owners and residents/tenants and the Chinese compared to others were non-supportive of the smoke free zone initiative probably because most owners of the premises/businesses in the area are Chinese and they fear that this proposal may affect their businesses. The support for the initiative was higher among women which is similar to the findings of studies conducted elsewhere [10],[16],[19],[24]. This could be because the prevalence of smoking among women is much lower compared to men. The correlation between education and level of support is because of the ability to understand the information on health and the increased self-awareness leading to the decision not to support unhealthy choices [10],[21]. Similarly poor knowledge is associated with lower support of smoke free policies [10],[20],[25],[26]. Better knowledge is associated with improved understanding of the risks associated with smoking and second hand smoke. Hence it is important to create awareness of the smoke free policies which has been shown to be associated with higher intolerance to smoking [27]. Education could also be a reason for the decrease in the support among the older age groups in this study. This finding contradicts the findings of studies conducted elsewhere which showed higher support among older respondents [10],[16],[18–20],[24]. In a relatively young country like Malaysia the younger age groups are more aware of the dangers of smoking and second hand smoke compared to the elderly whose level of education is lower and the knowledge on the adverse effect of smoking on health is limited [25]. The support from adolescents is important because they influence each other's habits though peer influence and social norms [27]. In general, support is high among those who never smoked and lowest among current smokers [18],[21],[26–28]. Although smokers and non-smokers generally believe that there is a harmful effect in passive smoking and both groups support tobacco control measures, non-smokers are usually more in favour of smoking bans than smokers [29]. Furthermore smokers whose social environments condone smoking are even less likely to support tobacco control policies [10].

The authors used tolerance to smoking as an indicator for attitudes towards smoking. Gilpin [16] indicated that a population's belief where smoking should not be allowed can be considered as an indicator of its attitude towards smoking. This study found about one in every third respondents was tolerant

**Table 2.** Tolerance to smoking and its associated risks of non-support to making GTWHS a smoke free zone.

| Variable | Prevalence | Unadjusted Odds ratio | Adjusted odds ratio | Attributable risk exposed | Attributable risk population |
|---|---|---|---|---|---|
| **Tolerance to smoking** | 32.7% | 6.1 (4.7;7.9) | 4.0 (3.0;5.4) | 80.3% | 57.2% |

towards cigarette smoke and the attributable risk of tolerance to non-support was high. The tolerance to tobacco smoke is also high among European Union (EU) citizens where only about half of its citizens (57%) are bothered by the exposure to second hand smoke while 30% are rarely and 27% never bothered and most were concerned about the smell rather than the health consequences [19]. People living in countries with weak smoke free policies are more likely to be exposed to second hand smoke compared with people living in countries with comprehensive smoke free policies [30]. In Thailand where the tobacco control policies are better compared to Malaysia, Thai smokers are more likely to be concerned about harm to others than Malaysian smokers are and they are also more likely to support smoke free policies [22]. In Malaysia, health education and promotion has always mainly targeted smokers in an attempt to get them to quit smoking by primarily educating them on the hazards of smoking. Very little health promotional effort is made to educate the public concerning the harmful effects of second hand smoke. This has resulted in a lower proportion of people believing that breathing other peoples smoke causes serious illness in non-smokers [4]. One of the strategies to change the attitudes towards smoking is by adopting comprehensive smoke free policies which make smoking socially unacceptable. Strong smoke free policies are associated with favourable attitudes [31]. Even with minimal initial support, the adoption of smoke free policy has been shown to increase support over time and the resistance towards such policies diminish once implemented [24],[31–33]. Smoke free policies which are markers for denormalization and social unacceptability of smoking [25],[34] help protect non-smokers from exposure to second hand smoke and reduce tobacco use. Such policies also encourage cessation by providing a supportive environment to quit smoking and these policies reduce tobacco initiation among young people because of the lower visibility of role models, fewer opportunities and diminished social acceptability and social advantages for smoking. These policies eventually result in improved health [2],[12],[16],[29,35–44]. In the US, smoking was acceptable and considered normal prior to the 1964 surgeon general's report on the health effects of smoking. This changed after the report was published, non-smokers rights movement emerged and public policies were introduced to change the attitudes of the public to denormalize smoking by making it socially unacceptable to smoke everywhere. This resulted in reduced smoking rates and the protection of more than half of Americans from second hand smoke [2],[11],[13],[36],[45]. In California the tobacco programme aimed at changing social norms related to smoking by educating the public regarding the dangers of second hand smoke and the setting up of smoke free venues has been shown to be effective in changing population attitudes. Such was its success that smokers have been shown to be more considerate about not smoking in the presence of non-smokers. Furthermore because positive attitudes to smoke free public places stimulate adoption of smoke free homes,[46] more than half of all California smokers' homes were reported smoke free [17]. In most developed countries, as a result of the denormalisation and unacceptance of smoking in public areas, smoking habits now carry a connotation of being a filthy habit [48] and is associated with unemployment, low socioeconomic status and low education [49]. Smokers are ostracised and are obliged to smoke in unpleasant surroundings and in extreme weather conditions and are not eligible for insurance premium reductions as non-smokers [48]. These have helped reduce the prevalence of smoking and reduce the morbidity and mortality related to smoking [50].

## Conclusions

Malaysian health promotion and education on tobacco control has mainly targeted smokers. This must change; education concerning the risks of second hand smoke should also be targeted towards non-smokers. The education provided can increase the knowledge on the adverse effects of tobacco smoke which will help reduce social acceptability of smoking. This will result in the acceptance of policies restricting second hand smoke and the reduction in smoking rates [35–37],[51–54] leading to reduced adverse health consequence [2],[55],[56]. Educating the public on the dangers of second hand smoke using mass media campaigns have been shown to be effective even on people with low levels of education [16],[53]. This would be an effective tool especially among the elderly Malaysians who have lower levels of education compared with the younger population. The information given can empower non-smokers to speak out against smoking habits [34] and win the support of smokers who will better understand the risks associated with second hand smoke which can trigger acceptance of society wide anti-smoking policies [9]. Mass media campaigns aimed at restructuring perception rather than sending pure anti-use messages [57] can also be used to assure hospitality industries that there is no negative economic impact on their businesses and that sales do not decline as a result of smoke free laws [44],[58].

### Limitations

There are several limitations to the study. The main one concerns sampling. Due to the dynamic population in this study the investigators were unable to do probability sampling. However every effort was made to collect data from different levels of the sample units which included the owners or senior management, employees, clients and the general public.

### What This Paper Adds

Denormalization of smoking has been shown to be an effective method of tobacco consumption control in most developed countries. In a developing country like Malaysia the focus of health education and promotion has been towards smokers in an effort to get them to quit smoking. Although this has been shown to be successful to some extent, the high tolerance to smoking is a cause of concern. There is a need to change the tobacco control strategies by focussing the health educational efforts towards non-smokers. The denormalization of smoking will not only help reduce uptake but also increase quit rates.

## Supporting Information

**Appendix S1** Scale used to assess the tolerance towards smoking.

## Acknowledgments

The authors would like to thank the Malaysian Health Promotion Board (MySihat), Ministry of Health Malaysia and the Penang State Government in making this survey a success. The authors would also like to thank Prof Ronan Conroy from the Royal College of Surgeons in Ireland for helping in the data analysis.

## Author Contributions

Conceived and designed the experiments: AR AM NY LI. Performed the experiments: AR AM. Analyzed the data: AR. Wrote the paper: AR AM NY LI.

## References


1. Communication D-Gf (2012) Attitudes of Europeans towards Tobacco. European Union: European Commission. 1–101 p.
2. Department of Health and Human Services US (2014) The Health Consequences of Smoking—50 Years of Progress. A Report of the Surgeon General. Atlanta, GA: Department of Health and Human Services, Centers for Disease Control and Prevention, National Center for Chronic Disease Prevention and Health Promotion, Office on Smoking and Health.
3. Ng M, Freeman MK, Fleming TD, Robinson M, Dwyer-Lindgren L, et al. (2014) Smoking prevalence and cigarette consumption in 187 countries, 1980–2012. JAMA 311: 183–192.
4. Health IfP (2012) Report of the Global Adult Tobacco Survey (GATS) Malaysia, 2011; Health NIo, editor: Ministry of Health Malaysia.
5. Organization WH (2013) Draft action plan for the prevention and control of non-communicable diseases 2013–2020. Geneva: World Health Assembly, World Health Organization.
6. Jha P, Peto R (2014) Global Effects of Smoking, of Quitting, and of Taxing Tobacco. New England Journal of Medicine 370: 60–68.
7. Malaysia MoH (2006) Annual report; System IaD, editor. Kuala Lumpur, Malaysia Ministry of Health Malaysia.
8. Diethelm PA, Rielle JC, McKee M (2005) The whole truth and nothing but the truth? The research that Philip Morris did not want you to see. Lancet 366: 86–92.
9. Zlatev M, Pahl S, White M (2008) Perceived risk and benefit for self and others as predictors of smokers' attitudes towards smoking restrictions. Psychology & Health 25: 167–182.
10. Doucet JM, Velicer WF, Laforge RG (2007) Demographic differences in support for smoking policy interventions. Addict Behav 32: 148–157.
11. Frieden TR (2014) Tobacco control progress and potential. JAMA 311: 133–134.
12. Chapman S, Borland R, Scollo M, Brownson RC, Dominello A, et al. (1999) The impact of smoke-free workplaces on declining cigarette consumption in Australia and the United States. Am J Public Health 89: 1018–1023.
13. Gutman M (2011) Social Norms and Attitudes About Smoking, 1991–2010. Princeton, New Jersey: Robert Wood Johnson Foundation.
14. Malone RE, Grundy Q, Bero LA (2012) Tobacco industry denormalisation as a tobacco control intervention: a review. Tob Control 21: 162–170.
15. Markham WA, Lopez ML, Aveyard P, Herrero P, Bridle C, et al. (2009) Mediated, moderated and direct effects of country of residence, age, and gender on the cognitive and social determinants of adolescent smoking in Spain and the UK: a cross-sectional study. BMC Public Health 9: 1471–2458.
16. Gilpin EA, Lee L, Pierce JP (2004) Changes in population attitudes about where smoking should not be allowed: California versus the rest of the USA. Tob Control 13: 38–44.
17. Holford TR, Meza R, Warner KE, Meernik C, Jeon J, et al. (2014) Tobacco control and the reduction in smoking-related premature deaths in the United States, 1964–2012. JAMA 311: 164–171.
18. Bakhturidze GD, Mittelmark MB, Aaro LE, Peikrishvili NT (2013) Attitudes towards smoking restrictions and tobacco advertisement bans in Georgia. BMJ Open 3: 2013–003461.
19. European Commission (2009) Attitudes of Europeans towards tobacco.
20. Danishevski K, Gilmore A, McKee M (2008) Public attitudes towards smoking and tobacco control policy in Russia. Tob Control 17: 276–283.
21. Maguire RL, Brinkley J, Mansfield C (2010) Custom Attitudes Toward Smoking Restrictions in Work Sites, Restaurants, and Bars Among North Carolinians. N C Med J 71: 511–518.
22. Yong HH, Foong K, Borland R, Omar M, Hamann S, et al. (2010) Support for and reported compliance among smokers with smoke-free policies in air-conditioned hospitality venues in Malaysia and Thailand: findings from the International Tobacco Control Southeast Asia Survey. Asia Pac J Public Health 22: 98–109.
23. Blanco-Marquizo A, Goja B, Peruga A, Jones MR, Yuan J, et al. (2010) Reduction of secondhand tobacco smoke in public places following national smoke-free legislation in Uruguay. Tob Control 19: 231–234.
24. Rosenberg M, Pettigrew S, Wood L, Ferguson R, Houghton S (2012) Public support for tobacco control policy extensions in Western Australia: a cross-sectional study. BMJ Open 2: 2011–000784.
25. Koh HK, Alpert HR, Judge CM, Caughey RW, Elqura LJ, et al. (2011) Understanding worldwide youth attitudes towards smoke-free policies: an analysis of the Global Youth Tobacco Survey. Tob Control 20: 219–225.
26. Ashley MJ, Cohen JE (2003) What the public thinks about the tobacco industry and its products. Tob Control 12: 396–400.
27. Unger JB, Rohrbach LA, Howard KA, Boley Cruz T, Johnson CA, et al. (1999) Attitudes toward anti-tobacco policy among California youth: associations with smoking status, psychosocial variables and advocacy actions. Health Educ Res 14: 751–763.
28. Poland BD, Cohen JE, Ashley MJ, Adlaf E, Ferrence R, et al. (2000) Heterogeneity among smokers and non-smokers in attitudes and behaviour regarding smoking and smoking restrictions. Tob Control 9: 364–371.
29. Thyrian JR, Panagiotakos DB, Polychronopulos E, Willemsen MC, Zatonski W, et al. (2010) The exposure to environmental tobacco smoke and attitudes towards tobacco control measures–a comparison of 5 European countries. Cent Eur J Public Health 18: 87–92.
30. Thrasher JF, Nayeli Abad-Vivero E, Sebrie EM, Barrientos-Gutierrez T, Boado M, et al. (2013) Tobacco smoke exposure in public places and workplaces after smoke-free policy implementation: a longitudinal analysis of smoker cohorts in Mexico and Uruguay. Health Policy Plan 28: 789–798.
31. Hyland A, Higbee C, Borland R, Travers M, Hastings G, et al. (2009) Attitudes and beliefs about secondhand smoke and smoke-free policies in four countries: findings from the International Tobacco Control Four Country Survey. Nicotine Tob Res 11: 642–649.
32. Thrasher JF, Boado M, Sebrie EM, Bianco E (2009) Smoke-free policies and the social acceptability of smoking in Uruguay and Mexico: findings from the International Tobacco Control Policy Evaluation Project. Nicotine Tob Res 11: 591–599.
33. Walsh RA, Paul CL, Tzelepis F, Stojanovski E, Tang A (2008) Is government action out-of-step with public opinion on tobacco control? Results of a New South Wales population survey. Australian and New Zealand Journal of Public Health 32: 482–488.
34. Glantz SA, Jamieson P (2000) Attitudes toward secondhand smoke, smoking, and quitting among young people. Pediatrics 106.
35. Callinan JE, Clarke A, Doherty K, Kelleher C (2010) Legislative smoking bans for reducing secondhand smoke exposure, smoking prevalence and tobacco consumption. Cochrane Database Syst Rev: CD005992.
36. Cummings KM (2002) Programs and policies to discourage the use of tobacco products. Oncogene 21: 7349–7364.
37. Fichtenberg CM, Glantz SA (2002) Effect of smoke-free workplaces on smoking behaviour: systematic review. Bmj 325: 188.
38. Fong GT, Hyland A, Borland R, Hammond D, Hastings G, et al. (2006) Reductions in tobacco smoke pollution and increases in support for smoke-free public places following the implementation of comprehensive smoke-free workplace legislation in the Republic of Ireland: findings from the ITC Ireland/UK Survey. Tob Control 15: iii51–58.
39. Hammond D, Fong GT, Zanna MP, Thrasher JF, Borland R (2006) Tobacco denormalization and industry beliefs among smokers from four countries. Am J Prev Med 31: 225–232.
40. Hublet A, Schmid H, Clays E, Godeau E, Gabhainn SN, et al. (2009) Association between tobacco control policies and smoking behaviour among adolescents in 29 European countries. Addiction 104: 1918–1926.
41. Hyland A, Li Q, Bauer JE, Giovino GA, Steger C, et al. (2004) Predictors of cessation in a cohort of current and former smokers followed over 13 years. Nicotine Tob Res 6: S363–369.
42. Martinez-Sanchez JM, Fernandez E, Fu M, Gallus S, Martinez C, et al. (2010) Smoking behaviour, involuntary smoking, attitudes towards smoke-free legislations, and tobacco control activities in the European Union. PLoS ONE 5: e13881.
43. Thomson G, Wilson N, Edwards R, Woodward A (2008) Should smoking in outside public spaces be banned? Yes. Bmj 337: a2806.
44. Viswanathan B, Plumettaz C, Gedeon J, Bovet P (2011) Impact of a smoking ban in public places: a rapid assessment in the Seychelles. Tob Control 20: 427–430.
45. Borland R, Yong HH, Siahpush M, Hyland A, Campbell S, et al. (2006) Support for and reported compliance with smoke-free restaurants and bars by smokers in four countries: findings from the International Tobacco Control (ITC) Four Country Survey. Tob Control 15: iii34–41.
46. Borland R, Yong HH, Cummings KM, Hyland A, Anderson S, et al. (2006) Determinants and consequences of smoke-free homes: findings from the International Tobacco Control (ITC) Four Country Survey. Tob Control 15: iii42–50.
47. Gilpin EA, Farkas AJ, Emery SL, Ake CF, Pierce JP (2002) Clean indoor air: advances in California, 1990–1999. Am J Public Health 92: 785–791.
48. Chapman S, Freeman B (2008) Markers of the denormalisation of smoking and the tobacco industry. Tob Control 17: 25–31.
49. Siahpush M, Borland R, Yong HH (2007) Sociodemographic and psychosocial correlates of smoking-induced deprivation and its effect on quitting: findings from the International Tobacco Control Policy Evaluation Survey. Tob Control 16.
50. Bayer R (2008) Stigma and the ethics of public health: not can we but should we. Soc Sci Med 67: 463–472.
51. Ashley MJ, Cohen J, Bull S, Ferrence R, Poland B, et al. (2000) Knowledge about tobacco and attitudes toward tobacco control: how different are smokers and nonsmokers? Can J Public Health 91: 376–380.
52. Cohen JE, de Guia NA, Ashley MJ, Ferrence R, Northrup DA, et al. (2002) Predictors of Canadian legislators' support for tobacco control policies. Soc Sci Med 55: 1069–1076.
53. Pierce JP, Macaskill P, Hill D (1990) Long-term effectiveness of mass media led antismoking campaigns in Australia. Am J Public Health 80: 565–569.
54. Rennen E, Nagelhout GE, van den Putte B, Janssen E, Mons U, et al. (2014) Associations between tobacco control policy awareness, social acceptability of smoking and smoking cessation. Findings from the International Tobacco Control (ITC) Europe Surveys. Health Educ Res 29: 72–82.

55. Goodman PG, Haw S, Kabir Z, Clancy L (2009) Are there health benefits associated with comprehensive smoke-free laws. Int J Public Health 54: 367–378.
56. Dinno A, Glantz S (2007) Clean indoor air laws immediately reduce heart attacks. Prev Med 45: 9–11.
57. Totten JW, Cayton BJ (2012) Smokers' Vs. Non-smokers' Attitudes toward Tobacco Usage. Atlantic Marketing Journal 1: 73–74.
58. Scollo M, Lal A, Hyland A, Glantz S (2003) Review of the quality of studies on the economic effects of smoke-free policies on the hospitality industry. Tob Control 12: 13–20.

# 8

# Contribution of Psychosocial Factors to the Association between Socioeconomic Position and Takeaway Food Consumption

**Kyoko Miura[1,2]*, Gavin Turrell[1]**

**1** School of Public Health and Social Work, Faculty of Health, Queensland University of Technology, Kelvin Grove, Queensland, Australia, **2** Cancer and Population Studies Group, QIMR Berghofer Medical Research Institute, Herston, Queensland, Australia

## Abstract

***Objective:*** To examine whether psychosocial factors mediate (explain) the association between socioeconomic position and takeaway food consumption.

***Design:*** A cross-sectional postal survey conducted in 2009.

***Setting:*** Participants reported their usual consumption of 22 takeaway food items, and these were grouped into a "healthy" and "less healthy" index based on each items' nutritional properties. Principal Components Analysis was used to derive three psychosocial scales that measured beliefs about the relationship between diet and health ($\alpha = 0.73$), and perceptions about the value ($\alpha = 0.79$) and pleasure ($\alpha = 0.61$) of takeaway food. A nutrition knowledge index was also used. Socioeconomic position was measured by highest attained education level.

***Subjects:*** Randomly selected adults (n = 1,500) aged between 25–64 years in Brisbane, Australia (response rate = 63.7%, N = 903).

***Results:*** Compared with those with a bachelor degree or higher, participants with a diploma level of education were more likely to consume "healthy" takeaway food ($p = 0.023$) whereas the least educated (high school only) were more likely to consume "less healthy" choices ($p = 0.002$). The least educated were less likely to believe in a relationship between diet and health ($p < 0.001$), and more likely to have lower nutritional knowledge compared with their highly educated counterparts ($p < 0.001$). Education differences in beliefs about the relationship between diet and health partly and significantly mediated the association between education and "healthy" takeaway food consumption. Diet- and health-related beliefs and nutritional knowledge partly and significantly mediated the education differences in "less healthy" takeaway food consumption.

***Conclusions:*** Interventions that target beliefs about the relationship between diet and health, and nutritional knowledge may reduce socioeconomic differences in takeaway food consumption, particularly for "less healthy" options.

**Editor:** Keitaro Matsuo, Kyushu University Faculty of Medical Science, Japan

**Funding:** This research was supported by Queensland University of Technology (operational aspects of the study). GT is supported by the National Health and Medical Research Council of Australia (NHMRC) Senior Research Fellowship (APP1003710). The funders had no role in study design, data collection and analysis, decision to publish, or preparation of the manuscript.

**Competing Interests:** The authors have declared that no competing interests exist.

* Email: Kyoko.Miura@qimrberghofer.edu.au

## Introduction

There are well-established socioeconomic inequalities in health [1,2]. Diet is a major contributing factor to the poor health of socioeconomically disadvantaged groups [3,4], and the dietary patterns of these groups are less likely to be consistent with dietary recommendations [5,6]. In this paper, we examine the relationship between socioeconomic position (SEP) and the consumption of "takeaway food", here defined as foods or meals that are pre-prepared commercially and require no further preparation by the consumer, and can be consumed immediately after purchase. Takeaway foods include "fast-food" and "convenience food", and these types of food are often associated with diets that are high in energy and total fat, and low in essential nutrients (e.g. vitamin A and C); they are also associated with negative health-related outcomes including weight gain [11]. Previous studies have reported that socioeconomically disadvantaged groups are more likely than their advantaged counterparts to consume or purchase takeaway food [7–10] and this might partly explain why disadvantaged groups have a higher prevalence of overweight and obesity [11] and why they experience higher rates of mortality and morbidity for diet-related chronic disease [3,4,12,13]. To date, however, our understanding of why socioeconomic group differ in their consumption of takeaway food is limited. It has been suggested that psychosocial factors might contribute to this association [14–17]; however, no known study has investigated this issue.

We define "psychosocial" as pertaining to the influence of social and structural factors (e.g. SEP) on an individual's psychological disposition (e.g. beliefs, attitudes, perceptions) such that their interrelation shapes and circumscribes behaviour, and ultimately, health. In the context of this study we focus on four individual-level psychological factors—knowledge, beliefs, preferences, and perceptions—and conceptualise these as potentially mediating the effects of SEP on takeaway food consumption.

Nutritional knowledge and health beliefs may partially explain socioeconomic differences in takeaway food consumption. Socio-economically disadvantaged groups are more likely to have low levels of nutritional knowledge and are less likely to believe in the relationship between diet and health compared with advantaged groups [18–20] and these factors have been associated with less healthy dietary intakes [21–23], including frequent fast-food consumption [24].

Taste or food preference is one of the most influential determinants of food choice [25] and is also an important reason for the consumption of fast-food [26]. Hence, taste is also likely to be an important determinant of takeaway food consumption. Food preference may also vary across different socioeconomic groups. Lower income households have been reported to be more likely than their affluent counterparts to dislike foods that were consistent with dietary guideline recommendations [27]. This finding suggests that socioeconomically disadvantaged groups may prefer the taste of takeaway foods more than advantaged groups, and this may contribute to the more frequent takeaway food consumption among disadvantaged groups.

The perception of takeaway food as value for money may be an important factor influencing the decision to consume takeaway food [7,28,29]. Consumers may perceive takeaway food as worth purchasing if they can trade-off the expense for a reduction of time and effort for meal planning, preparation and cleaning up [30]. A previous study found that frequent consumers of takeaway food were more likely to report that convenience food (including takeaway foods) represented value for money compared with those who consumed takeaway food less regularly [28].

In health research, the three most commonly used individual-level measures of SEP are education, occupation, and income [31]. Given that these indicators are only moderately correlated [32], it is likely that they capture different dimensions of the socioeconomic construct and probably reflect distinct aetiological pathways between socioeconomic circumstances and takeaway food consumption [33]. In this paper, we use education as our socioeconomic indicator as it is arguably the most conceptually meaningful socioeconomic determinant of an individual's psychological disposition towards food choice. Education reflects knowledge and skills (cognitive capacities) attained through formal learning (e.g. school, university) and lived experience, and these are likely to be important factors that shape people's dietary beliefs, perceptions and preferences, and influence the acquisition of information and knowledge about healthy dietary behaviours.

While earlier research has investigated psychosocial influences on takeaway or fast-food consumption [7,28,34–37], no known studies have assessed the contribution of psychosocial factors to different types of takeaway food defined as "healthy" or "less healthy": the former may be influenced by different psychosocial factors compared with the latter. For example, consumption of "healthy" takeaway items, such as sushi, may be driven by strong health beliefs or high nutritional knowledge whereas taste may be the dominant reason for the consumption of "less healthy" items such as fried potato chips. The aims of this study are to determine whether psychosocial factors mediate (explain) the association between education and the types of takeaway food consumed among adults.

## Methods

### Study Participants

This cross-sectional study was conducted in the Brisbane metropolitan area (Australia) between July and September 2009. A total of 1,500 adults aged between 25–64 years were randomly selected from the electoral roll of the Brisbane statistical subdivision. Data were collected by a postal survey [38] that asked about usual takeaway food consumption, a range of psychosocial factors that may influence consumption, and socio-demographic characteristics. A total of 903 participants completed the survey (response rate 63.7%). For the purpose of this paper, participants who reported never consuming takeaway food in the previous 12 months (n = 19, 2.1%) were excluded from the analyses. Ethical approval for the study was granted by the Queensland University of Technology Human Research Ethics Committee (ID 0900000445).

### Measures

**Socioeconomic position and covariates.** Education was used as the socioeconomic measure and ascertained by the highest completed qualification. Participant's education was coded as: 1) bachelor degree or higher (latter includes graduate diploma, graduate certificate, and postgraduate degree); 2) diploma (includes associate degree which is generally not a university-level education in Australia); 3) vocational (trade or business certificate); and 4) no post-school qualifications. Covariates used in the multivariable analyses were age (continuous) and sex.

**Psychosocial factors (mediators).** Based on previous research, participants were asked a range of questions about psychosocial factors that may influence takeaway food consumption [8,24,26].

Belief about the diet-health relationship, perceived values of takeaway food, and takeaway food as pleasure: Participants were asked to indicate their level of agreement (1 = strongly disagree, 5 = strongly agree) with the following items: "Eating a diet that is high in fat is a threat to my health", "Being 10 kg or more overweight is a threat to my health" [8], "What you eat can affect your chance of getting cancer or heart disease" [24], "Takeaway foods are value for money", "Takeaway foods are inexpensive", "Takeaway food is fun and entertaining", "Takeaway food is a treat for myself", "Takeaway foods are tasty" [26], and "It is cheaper for me to buy takeaway foods than to cook for myself" [39]. These nine items were included in a Principal Component Analysis to determine if there was an underlying structure to the beliefs and perceptions data. Using Varimax rotation and eigenvalue criteria $\geq 1.0$, three components were identified and subsequently interpreted as "diet-health belief and weight concern", "perceived value of takeaway food" and "takeaway foods as pleasure" (Table 1). These three components had eigenvalues of 2.6, 1.9, and 1.3 respectively, they accounted for 28.9%, 21.1%, and 14.5% of the total variance, and their cumulative contribution was 64.6%. Standardised scoring coefficients were calculated for the items forming the three components and these were used to derive factor scales for each of the constructs.

**Table 1.** Beliefs and perceptions about diet, health, and takeaway food: results of a Principal Components Analysis.

| (N = 801) | Retained components (loadings) | | |
|---|---|---|---|
| | 1 | 2 | 3 |
| **Belief about the diet-health relationship**† | | | |
| Eating a diet that is high in fat is a threat to my health | **0.74** | −0.05 | 0.04 |
| What you eat can affect your chance of getting cancer or heart disease | **0.83** | −0.03 | −0.03 |
| Being 10 kg or more overweight is a threat to my health | **0.84** | −0.10 | 0.00 |
| Cronbach's Alpha | **0.73** | | |
| **Perceived value of takeaway food**† | | | |
| Takeaway foods are value for money | −0.03 | **0.83** | 0.19 |
| Takeaway foods are inexpensive | −0.03 | **0.86** | 0.07 |
| It is cheaper for me to buy takeaway foods than to cook for myself | −0.15 | **0.79** | 0.08 |
| Cronbach's Alpha | | **0.79** | |
| **Takeaway foods as pleasure**† | | | |
| Takeaway food is fun and entertaining | 0.02 | 0.23 | **0.72** |
| Takeaway food is a "treat" for myself | 0.01 | −0.05 | **0.80** |
| Takeaway food is tasty | −0.01 | 0.15 | **0.70** |
| Cronbach's Alpha | | | **0.61** |

†Response options for each item range from 1 = Strongly Disagree to 5 = Strongly Agree.

Nutritional knowledge: A 20-item nutritional knowledge measure was adapted from a previous study [40]. These items cover knowledge about the nutrient content of various foods, the relationship between nutrition and health, and dietary recommendations. Participants had three response options for each statement: "true", "false", or "not sure". A score was calculated to determine each participant's general nutritional knowledge according to their correct answers to the statements: a score of 1 was assigned when the response was correct, and if the response was incorrect or "not sure", the score was 0. A nutritional knowledge index was constructed by summing all items and the index ranged from 0–20 (mean 17.5, SD 2.8; median 18.0). The intra-class correlation coefficient (ICC) of the nutritional knowledge index was 0.91 (95% CI 0.82, 0.95) which is interpreted as "almost perfect" reliability [41].

Takeaway food consumption: As part of the questionnaire, participants were asked *"In the last 12 months, did you eat any takeaway food"?* The response options were "Never", "Rarely", "Less than once a month", "1–3 times per month", "Once per week", "2–4 times per week", "5–6 times per week" and "Once per day". Respondents who indicated "Never" (n = 19) were directed to a section of the questionnaire which explored possible reasons for not consuming takeaway food: these respondents are not included in this present study. Those who reported consuming takeaway food in the last 12 months were then asked to indicate how often they had consumed each of 22 specific takeaway items. The response options for this question were: "Never or rarely", "Less than once a month", "1–3 times per month", "Once per week", "2–4 times per week", "5–6 times per week", "Once per day or more". The 22 takeaway foods were kebab, sandwiches, fried rice, pasta, Asian-style noodles, sushi, salad, diet soft drink, fruit/vegetable juices, fried potato chips, hamburger, pizza, savoury pies, fried fish/seafood, fried chicken, fried dim-sum, curry, cakes, non-diet soft drink, thick/milk shake, flavoured milk, and ice-cream. At the time the questionnaire was administered, these were the most frequently consumed takeaway items in Australia [9].

Each of the 22 items was categorised as either "healthy" or "less healthy" based on the Australian Guide to Healthy Eating (AGHE) [42] which classifies food into five core food groups and an "extra" food group. The "extra" foods (e.g. cakes and deep-fried takeaway foods) are a non-essential part of a diet and are typically high in fat, sodium, or sugar. Most of the "less healthy" takeaway items were consistent with the extra foods. To classify foods not identified in the extra foods list, nutrient composition data were used [43,44]. Specifically, using food classification criteria developed by a number of Australian nutritional authorities [43,44] takeaway items were categorised as "less healthy" if they met one or more of the following criteria:>2500 kJ of energy per serve;> 3 g of saturated fat per 100 g; <2 g of fibre per serve. Beverages classified as "less healthy" were those containing ≥ 300 kJ energy per serve and/or> 3 g of saturated fat per 100 g. Foods or beverages not meeting any of these criteria were considered "healthy" options. This classification resulted in nine "healthy" items and 13 "less healthy" items. "Healthy" takeaway foods comprised the first nine the first nine of the 22 items listed above, and "less healthy" takeaway foods comprised the remaining 13 items on the list. A score was subsequently calculated to characterise each participant's consumption of the 22 takeaway foods as follows: never or rarely = 0, less than once a month = 1, one to three times per month = 2, four times per month = 3, two to four times per week = 4, five to six times per week = 5, and once or more per day = 6 [45]. "Healthy" and "less healthy" takeaway food indices were created by summing the items. Each respondent's score was rescaled to range from 0 to 100 with higher scores being indicative of consuming a wider variety or greater frequency of takeaway food in the last 12 months. The reliability of the "healthy" takeaway food consumption measure was assessed in a separate test-retest sample of 100 individuals in the target age range who completed the same survey twice, four weeks apart. The ICC for the "healthy" takeaway index was 0.72 (95% CI 0.52–0.85) whereas the ICC for the "less healthy" measure was 0.69 (95% CI 0.46–0.83). According to Landis and Koch's scale of strength for reliability coefficients, these ICCs are "substantial" in magnitude [41].

## Statistical analysis

Descriptive statistics were used to describe the participants' demographic and takeaway food consumption patterns. The contribution of psychosocial factors to the association between SEP and the type of takeaway food consumed was examined using a mediation model [46,47]. A series of multiple regression models assessed a number of associations (Figure 1):

Step 1. Association between SEP and takeaway food consumption (Path c)

Step 2. Association between SEP and psychosocial factors (Path a)

Step 3. Association between psychosocial factors and takeaway food consumption (Path b)

Step 4. Association between SEP and takeaway food consumption controlling for each psychosocial factor (Path c'), and the indirect effect of SEP on takeaway food consumption through each psychosocial factor.

The mediated (indirect) effect was formally examined using a non-parametric bootstrapping procedure (n = 5000 samples) that estimated the sampling distribution of the indirect effect and the corresponding bias-corrected and accelerated 95% confidence intervals (95% CI) [46,47]. This procedure is more statistically robust than the Sobel test [46,47]. Indirect effects were considered significant when the 95% CI did not include zero. For all other tests, statistical significance was considered at $p<0.05$ (two-tailed). All models were adjusted for age and sex and the highest education group was the referent category. All analyses were performed in SAS (version 9.2, SAS Institute Inc., Cary, NC, USA).

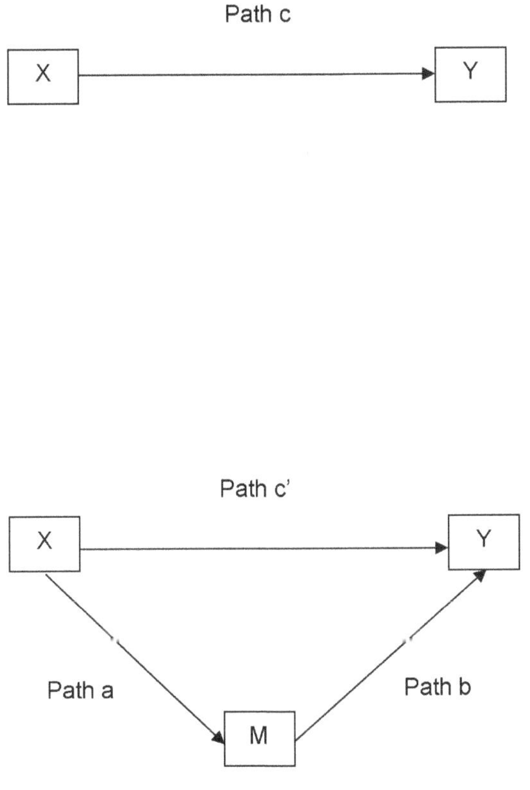


**Figure 1. Conceptual model of the association between socioeconomic position (SEP) and takeaway food consumption and contribution of psychosocial factors to the association (adapted from [39]).** X = the independent variable = SEP (education). Y = the outcome variable = takeaway food consumption ("healthy" and "less healthy", each takeaway food type was examined separately). M = the proposed mediating variable = psychosocial factors (nutritional knowledge, belief about the diet-health relationship, perceived value of takeaway food, and takeaway foods as pleasure), each psychosocial factor was examined separately. Indirect (mediated) effect = a x b = c – c'.

# Results

## Exclusion of participants

Of the 903 questionnaires that were returned, missing or inadequate information was identified for age (n = 16, 1.8%), education (n = 19, 2.1%), and "healthy" and "less healthy" takeaway food indices (n = 10, 1.1%). In total, the number (%) of missing information on the psychosocial factors ranged from 5 (0.6%) to 60 (6.6%) (median n = 13, 1.4%). Participants with missing information on these variables, as well as those who reported never consuming takeaway food, were excluded from all analyses. The resultant final analytical sample was N = 801.

Table 2 shows the socio-demographic characteristics of the included and excluded participants. Over half of the study participants were females (58.8%) and the mean age was 43.8 years (SD 11.6). Compared with those who were excluded from the analyses, retained participants were younger ($p<0.001$) and more educated ($p = 0.002$).

## Association between education and takeaway food consumption (Path c)

Education was associated with type of takeaway food consumed (Figure 2). Compared with participants who had a bachelor degree or higher, those with a diploma level of education were more likely to report that they consumed "healthy" takeaway food ($\beta = 3.02$, $p = 0.023$). The consumption level of participants with no post-school qualifications and vocational education were also higher than that of bachelor degree or higher; however, the difference was not significant (all $p>0.05$). For "less healthy" takeaway food, those with no post-school qualifications scored significantly higher than participants who had a bachelor degree or higher ($\beta = 2.38$, $p = 0.002$). Participants with diploma level of education were also more likely to report that they consumed "less healthy" takeaway food; however, the difference was borderline significant ($\beta = 1.99$, $p = 0.052$).

## Association between education and psychosocial factors (Path a)

There were significant associations between education and diet and health-related beliefs and nutritional knowledge (Table 3). Compared with participants with a bachelor degree or higher, those with a vocational level of education ($\beta = -0.28$, $p = 0.005$) and no post-school qualifications ($\beta = -0.31$, $p<0.001$) were less likely to believe in the diet-health relationship and more likely to have low nutritional knowledge (vocational: $\beta = -0.98$, $p<0.001$; no post school qualifications $\beta = -1.33$, $p<0.001$). There were no education differences in the perceived value of takeaway food and the perception of takeaway food as pleasure.

## Association between psychosocial factors and takeaway food consumption (Path b)

The majority of psychosocial factors were significantly associated with the consumption of takeaway food (Table 4). A high level of "healthy" takeaway food consumption was significantly

**Table 2.** Characteristics of participants and their takeaway food consumption scores.

| | Total (N = 801) | Excluded (n = 102) | Census[†] |
|---|---|---|---|
| **Sex (%)[‡]** | | | |
| Males | 41.2 | 37.3 | 49.2 |
| Females | 58.8 | 62.7 | 50.8 |
| **Age (years) [mean (sd)][§]** | 43.8 (11.0) | 48.2 (11.4)* | 42.7 (11.0) |
| **Education (%)[‡]** | | | |
| Bachelor degree or higher | 36.5 | 21.7* | 28.7 |
| Diploma | 12.4 | 10.8 | 10.0 |
| Vocational | 18.6 | 14.5 | 19.0 |
| No post-school qualifications | 32.6 | 53.0 | 42.3[|] |
| **Healthy takeaway food[¶]** | 13.2 (0.0, 73.3) | 13.2 (0.0, 56.4) | |
| **Less healthy takeaway food[¶]** | 12.8 (0.0, 88.3) | 12.8 (0.0, 42.2) | |

[†]Compared with 2006 Census data (ABS, 2010).
[‡]Chi-square was used to assess the differences between included and excluded participants.
[§]t-test was used to assess the differences between included and excluded participants.
[|]People who answered "not applicable" to non-school qualifications.
[¶]Median (minimum, maximum). Healthy and less healthy takeaway food consumption indices ranged from 0 to 100 with higher scores indicating a wider variety or greater frequency of consumption. Mann-Whitney U-test was used to assess the differences between included and excluded participants.
* $p<0.001$: statistically significant difference in age and education between the analytic sample and excluded participants.

associated with the perception that takeaway food is value for money ($\beta = 1.46$, $p<0.001$) or lower nutritional knowledge ($\beta = -0.55$, $p<0.001$). Belief in the diet-health relationship and the perception of takeaway food as pleasure was not associated with "healthy" takeaway food consumption. A high "less healthy" takeaway food score was observed among those who had a weaker belief in the diet-health relationship ($\beta = -1.10$, $p<0.001$), and those who perceived that takeaway food was value for money ($\beta = 1.52$, $p<0.001$). Participants who perceived takeaway food a pleasure ($\beta = 1.39$, $p<0.001$) and those who had lower nutritional knowledge ($\beta = -0.45$, $p<0.001$) were also significantly more likely to consume "less healthy" takeaway food.

### Psychosocial contributions to the association between education and takeaway food consumption (Path c′)

Table 5 presents the association between education and takeaway food consumption (Path c), and the mediating effects of this association (Path c′). Lower educated groups consumed a high level of "healthy" takeaway food compared with those with a bachelor degree or higher.

After the inclusion of nutritional knowledge in the Path c model, the magnitude of the association was attenuated. However, differences between participants with a bachelor degree or higher and those with a diploma level of education remained significant ($\beta = 2.80$, $p = 0.035$). In general, these non-significant associations (except those with diploma level of education) were slightly reduced after the inclusion of other psychosocial factors. The indirect (mediated) effects of nutritional knowledge were significant among those with no post-school qualifications and vocational

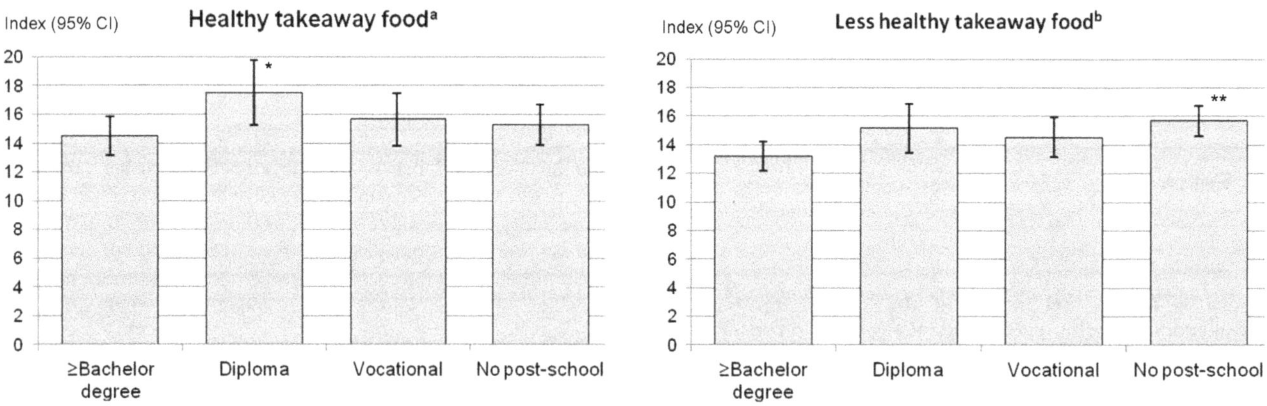


**Figure 2. The average "healthy" and "less healthy" takeaway food consumption indices by education.** The mean consumption values with their 95% confidence intervals. * $p<0.05$, ** $p<0.01$ compared with participants with a bachelor degree or higher. All analyses adjusted for age and sex. [a] The "healthy" takeaway food consumption index (ranged from 0 to 100; mean 15.3, SD 11.7), with high score indicating a wide variety or greater frequency of consumption. *P*-for trend = 0.512. [b] The "less healthy" takeaway food consumption index (ranged from 0 to 100; mean 14.0, SD 9.3), with high score indicating a wide variety or greater frequency of consumption. *P*-for trend = 0.004.

**Table 3.** Associations between education level and beliefs, perceptions and knowledge about diet, health, and takeaway food[†].

| (N = 801) | β (SE)[‡] | *p*-value |
|---|---|---|
| **Belief about the diet-health relationship** | | |
| Bachelor degree or higher | Reference[§] | – |
| Diploma | −0.09 (0.11) | 0.435 |
| Vocational | −0.28 (0.10) | 0.005 |
| No post-school qualifications | −0.31 (0.08) | <0.001 |
| **Perceived values of takeaway food** | | |
| Bachelor degree or higher | Reference[§] | – |
| Diploma | −0.04 (0.12) | 0.735 |
| Vocational | −0.12 (0.10) | 0.222 |
| No post-school qualifications | 0.05 (0.09) | 0.550 |
| **Takeaway food as pleasure** | | |
| Bachelor degree or higher | Reference[§] | – |
| Diploma | 0.07 (0.12) | 0.554 |
| Vocational | −0.06 (0.10) | 0.538 |
| No post-school qualifications | −0.01 (0.09) | 0.903 |
| **Nutritional knowledge** | | |
| Bachelor degree or higher | Reference[§] | – |
| Diploma | −0.42 (0.31) | 0.178 |
| Vocational | −0.98 (0.27) | <0.001 |
| No post-school qualifications | −1.33 (0.23) | <0.001 |

[†]These analyses examine the association between the independent variable (education) and each mediating variable (psychosocial factor): see Figure 1, Path a.
[‡]All analyses are adjusted for age and sex.
[§]The regression coefficients quantify the absolute difference between the reference category and the other education categories in their mean scores on each of the psychosocial measures.

education as the 95% CI did not include zero. The largest absolute indirect effect was observed among participants with no post-school qualifications (indirect effect 0.72; 95% CI 0.30, 1.30) compared with other education groups. None of other psychosocial factors showed significant indirect effects in the consumption of "healthy" takeaway food.

Lower educated groups also scored higher for "less healthy" takeaway food (Path c). The magnitude of this baseline education difference was attenuated when diet and health-related beliefs were included in the Path c model. Among participants with no post-school education, however, the association remained significant with adjustment for the diet and health-related relationship ($\beta = 2.04$, $p = 0.007$). Likewise, the magnitude of the association was attenuated when nutritional knowledge was included in the Path c model. Nonetheless, differences in consumption between participants with a bachelor degree or higher and those with no post-school qualifications remained significant ($\beta = 1.78$, $p = 0.020$). When the variables perceived value of takeaway food and takeaway food as pleasure were included in the Path c model, the magnitude of the associations changed only slightly all levels. Significant indirect effects were observed for both diet and health-related beliefs and nutritional knowledge among those with no

**Table 4.** Associations between psychosocial factors and takeaway food consumption[†,‡].

| (N = 801) | Healthy takeaway food[§] | p-value | Less healthy takeaway food[|] | p-value |
|---|---|---|---|---|
| **Belief about the diet-health relationship** | −0.61 | 0.139 | 1.10 | <0.001 |
| **Perceived value of takeaway food** | 1.46 | <0.001 | 1.52 | <0.001 |
| **Takeaway food as pleasure** | 0.12 | 0.765 | 1.39 | <0.001 |
| **Nutritional knowledge** | −0.55 | <0.001 | −0.45 | <0.001 |

[†]These analyses examine the association between the mediating variables (psychosocial factors) and the outcome variables (takeaway consumption): see Figure 1, Path b.
[‡]All analyses adjusted for age, sex, and education.
[§]The healthy takeaway food consumption index ranged from 0 to 100 (median 13.2), with higher scores indicating a wider variety or greater frequency of consumption.
[|]The less healthy takeaway food consumption index ranged from 0 to 100 (median 12.8) with higher scores indicating a wider variety or greater frequency of consumption.

**Table 5.** Contribution of psychosocial factors to the association between education and takeaway food consumption.

| (N = 801) | Education[†] | | | | | | | | |
|---|---|---|---|---|---|---|---|---|---|
| | Diploma | | | Vocational | | | No post-school qualifications | | |
| | β (SE)[‡] | *p*-value[§] | Indirect effects (95% CI) | β (SE)[‡] | *p*-value[§] | Indirect effects (95% CI) | β (SE)[‡] | *p*-value[§] | Indirect effects (95% CI) |
| **"Healthy" takeaway food[‡]** | | | | | | | | | |
| Path c | 3.02 (1.33) | 0.023 | — | 1.16 (1.15) | 0.313 | — | 0.83 (0.98) | 0.402 | — |
| *Potential mediator* | | | | | | | | | |
| Belief about the diet-health relationship | 2.97 (1.33) | 0.026 | 0.05 (−0.04, 0.31) | 0.99 (1.16) | 0.392 | 0.17 (−0.02, 0.57) | 0.63 (0.99) | 0.523 | 0.19 (−0.04, 0.54) |
| Perceived value of takeaway food | 3.08 (1.32) | 0.020 | −0.06 (−0.44, 0.29) | 1.34 (1.15) | 0.242 | −0.18 (−0.53, 0.07) | 0.75 (0.98) | 0.443 | 0.07 (−0.18, 0.35) |
| Takeaway food as pleasure | 3.02 (1.33) | 0.024 | 0.01 (−0.07, 0.20) | 1.17 (1.15) | 0.310 | −0.01 (−0.19, 0.07) | 0.82 (0.99) | 0.403 | 0.01 (−0.06, 0.11) |
| Nutritional knowledge | 2.80 (1.32) | 0.035 | 0.23 (0.00, 0.73) | 0.63 (1.15) | 0.586 | 0.53 (0.22, 1.05)* | 0.10 (0.99) | 0.920 | 0.72 (0.30, 1.30)* |
| **"Less healthy" takeaway food[‖]** | | | | | | | | | |
| Path c | 1.99 (1.02) | 0.052 | — | 1.11 (0.88) | 0.209 | — | 2.38 (0.76) | 0.002 | — |
| *Potential mediators* | | | | | | | | | |
| Belief about the diet-health relationship | 1.90 (1.02) | 0.062 | 0.10 (−0.10, 0.39) | 0.81 (0.88) | 0.362 | 0.31 (0.08, 0.70)* | 2.04 (0.76) | 0.007 | 0.34 (0.12, 0.70)* |
| Perceived value of takeaway food | 2.05 (1.01) | 0.042 | −0.06 (−0.44, 0.30) | 1.30 (0.87) | 0.137 | −0.19 (−0.50, 0.06) | 2.30 (0.75) | 0.002 | 0.08 (−0.19, 0.38) |
| Takeaway food as pleasure | 1.90 (1.01) | 0.061 | 0.09 (−0.19, 0.44) | 1.20 (0.87) | 0.171 | −0.09 (−0.42, 0.17) | 2.36 (0.75) | 0.002 | 0.01 (−0.24, 0.26) |
| Nutritional knowledge | 1.80 (1.01) | 0.076 | 0.19 (−0.01, 0.56) | 0.67 (0.88) | 0.448 | 0.44 (0.17, 0.91)* | 1.78 (0.76) | 0.020 | 0.60 (0.21, 1.08)* |

[†]Reference category: Bachelor degree or higher.
[‡]The regression coefficients quantify the absolute difference between the reference category (Bachelor degree or higher) and the other education categories in their mean scores on the "healthy" and "less healthy" takeaway consumption indexes before (Path c, Figure 1) and after adjusting for each psychosocial mediator.
[§]All analyses adjusted for age and sex.
* Statistically significant indirect (mediated) effect.

post-school qualifications and vocational education. The largest absolute indirect effect was observed among participants with no post-school qualifications when the mediation effect of nutritional knowledge was assessed (indirect effect 0.60; 95% CI 0.21, 1.08).

## Discussion

This study examined whether psychosocial factors contributed to the association between education and the type of takeaway food consumed. The study found that lower educated groups were more likely to consume takeaway food, especially "less healthy" options, which was similar to previous research [7,8,10]. The observed association between education and "healthy" takeaway food consumption was partly mediated by nutritional knowledge. Similarly, beliefs about the diet and health relationship and nutritional knowledge partly explained the education differences in "less healthy" takeaway food consumption.

Similar to this current study, previous research indicates that less educated groups have lower health considerations [48], are less likely to believe in diet-health relationships [18–20], and have lower nutritional knowledge [40,49] than their more educated counterparts. Findings from this present study were also similar to studies which have shown that low nutritional knowledge and weak diet and health-related beliefs were associated with less healthy dietary patterns such as frequent fast-food consumption [20,24,50]. These findings suggest that intervention programs focusing on cognitive factors, especially nutritional knowledge, are likely to be important in reducing socioeconomic differences in takeaway food consumption, particularly "less healthy" options.

While nutritional knowledge and/or belief in the diet-health relationship significantly mediated the association between education and takeaway food consumption, these psychosocial factors did not completely explain the relationship. An individual's food choice is complex and is influenced by numerous factors [51] such as where the foods are to be consumed (work, leisure or home), other contexts (e.g. alone or in the presence of others) [52], culture, marketing [53] and cost [7]. Perception about the accessibility and availability of food has also been reported as influencing food choice [53]. It is possible that lower socioeconomic groups may have easier access to takeaway food outlets (i.e. greater number in their neighbourhood, more proximal) which may be one contributing factor to the high consumption of takeaway foods among these groups [54,55]. Additionally, the availability of "healthy" and "less healthy" choices may also determine the type of takeaway food consumed, and may be a reason for the observed associations. For example, US and New Zealand studies have found that "less healthy" takeaway options are more readily available than "healthy" options at major fast-food outlets in these countries [56,57]. Increasing and promoting the availability of healthier takeaway options, as well as facilitating the within-store purchase of healthy options, are likely to be important future directions of interventions. However, since takeaway foods are generally less nutritious than food prepared at home [58], efforts are also needed to improve the nutrient content of takeaway foods.

In this study, nutritional knowledge and the perception that takeaway foods are value for money were important determinants of both "healthy" and "less healthy" takeaway food consumption. However, there were some differences in the association between psychosocial factors and the type of takeaway food. Diet and health-related beliefs, and the perception that takeaway food is pleasure, influenced the consumption of "less healthy" takeaway food whereas these factors were not associated with "healthy" takeaway food consumption. It is unknown why diet and health-related beliefs were associated with the consumption of "less healthy" but not "healthy" takeaway food. The perception of takeaway food as pleasure was associated only with the consumption of "less healthy" takeaway food. This finding may be a reflection of the notion that, in general, eating situations (e.g. eating with others) changes an individuals' emotional state which may influence their decision to choose more "indulgent" or "less healthy" food types [59] rather than continuing to eat healthily. Likewise, the decision to consume "less healthy" takeaway food may also be driven by taste preference, which has been shown to be a strongly influential predictor of food consumption [7,60].

Some limitations of this study need to be acknowledged. First, due to the cross-sectional design of this study, temporal direction of causal order (i.e. exposure variable precedes mediator, and the mediator precedes outcome) cannot be determined. Second, all data were collected by self-report and hence are prone to bias such as social desirability bias. These biases may be different according to participants' education level. Third, the classification of "healthy" and "less healthy" takeaway choices was made based on the AGHE [42] and nutrient composition criteria used in the Australian State Hospitals and schools [43,44]. However, not all items in the "healthy" and "less healthy" takeaway food categories were necessarily healthy or unhealthy respectively as nutrient contents vary considerably within each food group [57,61]. Fourth, the current study employed only one socioeconomic indicator: this is likely to have underestimated the total socioeconomic effect of takeaway food consumption. Further, the current study achieved a moderately high response rate; however, 36.7% of those approached did not respond. Typically, the most disadvantaged groups are more likely to be non-responders in a postal survey, and in general these groups are more likely to exhibit less healthy behaviours [62,63]. In this present study, the lower educated groups were underrepresented compared with the Brisbane population hence the magnitude of the association between education and takeaway food consumption may have been underestimated.

In conclusion, intervention programs addressing nutrition and health-related beliefs and knowledge may contribute to a reduction in socioeconomic differences in takeaway food consumption. Nevertheless, the increasing popularity of takeaway food is likely to continue [64] regardless of a person's SEP, and this has implications for dietary quality, overweight/obesity and diet-related chronic disease for the whole population. Policies aimed at promoting healthy eating may need to be focused on improving the nutritional value of takeaway food and ensuring that healthy options are available. Future research should consider a wider array of psychosocial concepts (e.g. values, perceptions, and motivations) to identify and assess whether these contribute to our understanding of socioeconomic differences in takeaway food consumption.

## Author Contributions

Conceived and designed the experiments: KM. Performed the experiments: KM. Analyzed the data: KM. Contributed reagents/materials/analysis tools: GT. Wrote the paper: KM GT. Aided the interpretation of the data: GT.

## References


1. Kawachi I, Kennedy BP (1999) Income inequality and health: pathways and mechanisms. Health Serv Res 34: 215–227.
2. Mackenbach JP, Kunst AE (1997) Measuring the magnitude of socio-economic inequalities in health: An overview of available measures illustrated with two examples from Europe. Soc Sci Med 44: 757–771.
3. Davey Smith G, Brunner E (1997) Socio-economic differentials in health: the role of nutrition. Proc Nutr Soc 56: 75–90.
4. James WPT, Nelson M, Ralph A, Leather S (1997) The contribution of nutrition to inequalities in health. Br Med J 314: 1545–1549.
5. Giskes K, Turrell G, van Lenthe FJ, Brug J, Mackenbach JP (2006) A multilevel study of socio-economic inequalities in food choice behaviour and dietary intake among the Dutch population: the GLOBE study. Public Health Nutr 9: 75–83.
6. Turrell G, Hewitt B, Patterson C, Oldenburg B, Gould T (2002) Socioeconomic differences in food purchasing behaviour and suggested implications for diet-related health promotion. J Hum Nutr Diet 15: 355–364.
7. Blanck HM, Yaroch AL, Atienza AA, Yi SL, Jian Zhang, et al. (2009) Factors influencing lunchtime food choices among working Americans. Health Educ Behav 36: 289–301.
8. Glanz K, Basil M, Maibach E, Goldberg J, Snyder D (1998) Why Americans eat what they do: taste, nutrition, cost, convenience, and weight control concerns as influences on food consumption. J Am Diet Assoc 98: 1118–1126.
9. Miura K, Giskes K, Turrell G (2012) Socio-economic differences in takeaway food consumption among adults. Public Health Nutr 15: 218–226.
10. Thornton LE, Bentley RJ, Kavanagh AM (2011) Individual and area-level socioeconomic associations with fast food purchasing. J Epidemiol Community Health 65: 873–880.
11. Miura K, Turrell G (2014) Reported consumption of takeaway food and its contribution to socioeconomic inequalities in body mass index. Appetite 74: 116–124.
12. Agardh E, Allebeck P, Hallqvist J, Moradi T, Sidorchuk A (2011) Type 2 diabetes incidence and socio-economic position: a systematic review and meta-analysis. Int J Epidemiol 40: 804–818.
13. Pujades-Rodriguez M, Timmis A, Stogiannis D, Rapsomaniki E, Denaxas S, et al. (2014) Socioeconomic deprivation and the incidence of 12 cardiovascular diseases in 1.9 million women and men: implications for risk prediction and prevention. PLoS One 9: e104671.
14. Kearney M, Kearney JM, Dunne A, Gibney MJ (2000) Sociodemographic determinants of perceived influences on food choice in a nationally representative sample of Irish adults. Public Health Nutr 3: 219–226.
15. Lynch JW, Kaplan GA, Salonen JT (1997) Why do poor people behave poorly? Variation in adult health behaviours and psychosocial characteristics by stages of the socioeconomic lifecourse. Soc Sci Med 44: 809–819.
16. Lê J, Dallongeville J, Wagner A, Arveiler D, Haas B, et al. (2013) Attitudes toward healthy eating: a mediator of the educational level-diet relationship. Eur J Clin Nutr 67: 808–814.
17. Wang Y, Chen X (2011) How much of racial/ethnic disparities in dietary intakes, exercise, and weight status can be explained by nutrition- and health-related psychosocial factors and socioeconomic status among US adults? J Am Diet Assoc 111: 1904–1911.
18. Girois S, Kumanyika S, Morabia A, Mauger E (2001) A comparison of knowledge and attitudes about diet and health among 35- to 75-year-old adults in the United States and Geneva, Switzerland. Am J Public Health 91: 418–424.
19. Kearney M, Kelly A, Gibney MJ (1998) Attitudes toward and beliefs about nutrition and health among a nationally representative sample of Irish adults: Application of logistic regression modelling. J Nutr Educ 30: 139–148.
20. Wardle J, Steptoe A (2003) Socioeconomic differences in attitudes and beliefs about healthy lifestyles. J Epidemiol Community Health 57: 440–443.
21. Beydoun MA, Wang Y (2008) Do nutrition knowledge and beliefs modify the association of socio-economic factors and diet quality among US adults? Prev Med 46: 145–153.
22. Guillaumie L, Godin G, Vezina-Im LA (2010) Psychosocial determinants of fruit and vegetable intake in adult population: a systematic review. International Journal of Behavioral Nutrition and Physical Activity 7: 12.
23. Wardle J, Parmenter K, Waller J (2000) Nutrition knowledge and food intake. Appetite 34: 269–275.
24. Satia JA, Galanko JA, Siega-Riz AM (2004) Eating at fast-food restaurants is associated with dietary intake, demographic, psychosocial and behavioural factors among African Americans in North Carolina. Public Health Nutr 7: 1089–1096.
25. Aikman SN, Min KE, Graham D (2006) Food attitudes, eating behavior, and the information underlying food attitudes. Appetite 47: 111–114.
26. Rydell SA, Harnack LJ, Oakes JM, Story M, Jeffery RW, et al. (2008) Why eat at fast-food restaurants: reported reasons among frequent consumers. J Am Diet Assoc 108: 2066–2070.
27. Turrell G (1998) Socioeconomic differences in food preference and their influence on healthy food purchasing choices. J Hum Nutr Diet 11: 135–149.
28. de Boer M, McCarthy M, Cowan C, Ryan I (2004) The influence of lifestyle characteristics and beliefs about convenience food on the demand for convenience foods in the Irish market. Food Qual Prefer 15: 155–165.
29. Mahon D, Cowan C, McCarthy M (2006) The role of attitudes, subjective norm, perceived control and habit in the consumption of ready meals and takeaways in Great Britain. Food Qual Prefer 17: 474–481.
30. Beck ME (2007) Dinner preparation in the modern United States. Br Food J 109: 531–547.
31. Dutton T, Turrell G, Oldenburg B (2005) Measuring socioeconomic position in population health monitoring and health research. Brisbane: Queensland University of Technology, School of Public Health.
32. Turrell G, Hewitt B, Patterson C, Oldenburg B (2003) Measuring socio-economic position in dietary research: is choice of socio-economic indicator important? Public Health Nutr 6: 191–200.
33. Galobardes B, Morabia A, Bernstein MS (2001) Diet and socioeconomic position: does the use of different indicators matter? Int J Epidemiol 30: 334–340.
34. Dunn KI, Mohr P, Wilson CJ, Wittert GA (2011) Determinants of fast-food consumption. An application of the Theory of Planned Behaviour. Appetite 57: 349–357.
35. Dunn KI, Mohr PB, Wilson CJ, Wittert GA (2008) Beliefs about fast food in Australia: A qualitative analysis. Appetite 51: 331–334.
36. Dave JM, An LC, Jeffery RW, Ahluwalia JS (2009) Relationship of attitudes toward fast food and frequency of fast-food Intake in adults. Obesity 17: 1164–1170.
37. van der Horst K, Brunner TA, Siegrist M (2011) Fast food and take-away food consumption are associated with different lifestyle characteristics. J Hum Nutr Diet 24: 596–602.
38. Dillman DA (2000) Mail and Internet Surveys: The Tailored Design Method. New York: John Wiley & Sons, Inc.
39. Lea EJ, Crawford D, Worsley A (2006) Public views of the benefits and barriers to the consumption of a plant-based diet. Eur J Clin Nutr 60: 828–837.
40. Turrell G, Kavanagh AM (2006) Socio-economic pathways to diet: modelling the association between socio-economic position and food purchasing behaviour. Public Health Nutr 9: 375–383.
41. Landis JR, Koch GG (1977) The measurement of observer agreement for categorical data. Biometrics 33: 159–174.
42. The Commonwealth Department of Health and Family Services (1998) The Australian Guide to Healthy Eating: Background Information for Nutrition Educators: Department of Health and Family Services.
43. New South Wales Health and New South Wales Department of Education and Training (2006) Fresh Tastes at School: NSW Healthy School Canteen Strategy Canteen Menu Planning Guide. 2nd ed: New South Wales Health and New South Wales Department of Education and Training.
44. Queensland Health (2007) A Better Choice Healthy Food and Drink Supply Strategy for Queensland Health Facilities. Queensland Health.
45. Miura K, Giskes K, Turrell G (2011) Contribution of take-out food consumption to socioeconomic differences in fruit and vegetable Intake: a mediation analysis. J Am Diet Assoc 111: 1556–1562.
46. Preacher KJ, Hayes A (2004) SPSS and SAS procedures for estimating indirect effects in simple mediation models. Behav Res Methods Instrum Comput 36: 717–731.
47. Hayes AF (2013) Introduction to Mediation, Moderation, and Conditional Process Analysis: A Regression-Based Approach. New York: Guilford Press.
48. Ball K, Crawford D, Mishra G (2006) Socio-economic inequalities in women's fruit and vegetable intakes: a multilevel study of individual, social and environmental mediators. Public Health Nutr 9: 623–630.
49. Parmenter K, Waller J, Wardle J (2000) Demographic variation in nutrition knowledge in England. Health Educ Res 15: 163–174.
50. Beydoun MA, Powell LM, Wang Y (2008) Reduced away-from-home food expenditure and better nutrition knowledge and belief can improve quality of dietary intake among US adults. Public Health Nutr 12: 369–381.
51. Conner M, Armitage CJ (2006) Social Psychological Models of Food Choice. In: Shepherd R, Raats M, editors. The Psychology of Food Choice. Wallingford, Oxfordshire, UK: CABI Press.
52. Devine CM (2005) A life course perspective: understanding food choices in time, social location, and history. J Nutr Educ Behav 37: 121–128.
53. Shepherd R (1999) Social determinants of food choice. Proc Nutr Soc 58: 807–812.
54. Burns CM, Inglis AD (2007) Measuring food access in Melbourne: access to healthy and fast foods by car, bus and foot in an urban municipality in Melbourne. Health Place 13: 877–885.
55. Reidpath DD, Burns C, Garrard J, Mahoney M, Townsend M (2002) An ecological study of the relationship between social and environmental determinants of obesity. Health Place 8: 141–145.
56. Saelens BE, Glanz K, Sallis JF, Frank LD (2007) Nutrition Environment Measures Study in Restaurants (NEMS-R): development and evaluation. Am J Prev Med 32: 273–281.
57. Chand A, Eyles H, Ni Mhurchu C (2012) Availability and accessibility of healthier options and nutrition information at New Zealand fast food restaurants. Appetite 58: 227–233.
58. Guthrie JF, Lin B-H, Frazao E (2002) Role of food prepared away from home in the American diet, 1977-78 versus 1994-96: changes and consequences. J Nutr Educ Behav 34: 140–150.

59. Vue H, Degeneffe D, Reicks M (2008) Need states based on eating occasions experienced by midlife women. J Nutr Educ Behav 40: 378–384.
60. Tuorila H, Pangborn RM (1988) Prediction of reported consumption of selected fat-containing foods. Appetite 11: 81–95.
61. Dunford E, Webster J, Barzi F, Neal B (2010) Nutrient content of products served by leading Australian fast food chains. Appetite 55: 484–489.
62. Batty G, Gale C (2009) Impact of resurvey non-response on the associations between baseline risk factors and cardiovascular disease mortality: prospective cohort study. J Epidemiol Community Health 63: 952–955.
63. Tolonen H, Dobson A, Kulathinal S, the WHO MONICA Project (2005) Effect on trend estimates of the difference between survey respondents and non-respondents: results from 27 populations in the WHO MONICA Project. Eur J Epidemiol 20: 887–898.
64. Jaworowska A, Blackham T, Davies IG, Stevenson L (2013) Nutritional challenges and health implications of takeaway and fast food. Nutr Rev 71: 310–318.

# Comparison of Diabetes Management Status between Cancer Survivors and the General Population: Results from a Korean Population-Based Survey

**Ji-Yeon Shin[1], Hye Young Shim[2], Jae Kwan Jun[2]***

1 Department of Preventive Medicine, School of Medicine, Eulji University, Daejeon, Republic of Korea, 2 National Cancer Control Institute, National Cancer Center, Goyang, Republic of Korea

## Abstract

***Purpose:*** This study aimed to determine and compare the prevalences of diabetes awareness, treatment, and adequate glycemic control among cancer survivors in a Korean population and two non-cancer control groups, comprising individuals without a history of cancer but with other chronic diseases (non-cancer, chronic disease controls) and individuals without a history of cancer or any other chronic disease (non-cancer, non-chronic disease controls).

***Methods:*** We analyzed data from 2,660 subjects with prevalent diabetes (aged ≥30 years), who had participated in the 2007–2011 Korea National Health and Nutrition Examination Survey. Awareness was defined as a subject having been diagnosed with diabetes by a clinician. Treatment was defined as a subject who was taking anti-diabetic medicine. Adequate glycemic control was defined as a hemoglobin $A1_c$ level of <7%. Multivariable logistic regression and predictive margins were used to evaluate whether awareness, treatment, or adequate glycemic control differed among cancer survivors and the two non-cancer control groups.

***Results:*** Cancer survivors had greater awareness compared with the non-cancer, chronic disease and non-cancer, non-chronic disease control groups (85.1%, 80.4%, and 60.4%, respectively). Although the prevalences of treatment and adequate glycemic control were higher for survivors compared with the non-cancer, non-chronic disease controls, they were lower compared with the non-cancer, chronic disease controls. The prevalence of diabetes treatment was 67.5% for cancer survivors, 69.5% for non-cancer, chronic disease controls, and 46.7% for non-cancer, non-chronic disease controls; the prevalences of adequate glycemic control in these three groups were 31.7%, 34.6%, and 17.8%, respectively.

***Conclusions:*** Cancer survivors were less likely than the non-cancer chronic disease subjects to receive diabetes management and to achieve adequate glycemic targets. Special attention and education are required to ensure that this population receives optimal diabetes care, and the systematic roles for primary care and specialist physicians need to be determined.

**Editor:** Andrea Icks, Heinrich-Heine University, Faculty of Medicine, Germany

**Funding:** This work was supported by a grant from the National R&D Program for Cancer Control, No. 1310231 (http://ncc.re.kr/english/index.jsp). The funders had no role in study design, data collection and analysis, decision to publish, or preparation of the manuscript.

**Competing Interests:** The authors have declared that no competing interests exist.

* Email: jkjun@ncc.re.kr

## Introduction

Due to advances in early detection and improvement in the treatment of cancer, cancer survivors represent a growing population. There are currently more than 13 million cancer survivors in the U.S., and the long-term cancer survivor population continues to grow [1]. In Korea, the 5-year relative survival rate from 2006–2011 was 64.1%, which represents a 22.9% increase from the 1993–1995 survival rate [2]. In 2011, there were approximately one million cancer survivors estimated in Korea [2].

As the number and survival time of cancer survivors increase, the comorbid conditions and resulting non-cancer mortality of this population have become an important focus of attention. Diabetes is one chronic disease that can strongly influence the prognosis of cancer survivors [3–7]. Cancer patients with diabetes showed a 41% higher all-cause mortality compared with individuals without diabetes, according to a pooled-analysis comprising 23 studies on different cancer types [7]. The association of diabetes with cardiovascular mortality is well known [8], and cardiovascular disease is the most important cause of non-cancer deaths in cancer survivors, accounting for 50% of those in the U.S. [9] and for 31.4% in South Korea [10]. Furthermore, diabetes has been reported to increase cancer-specific mortality [3,4]. Patients with a fasting serum glucose level above 140 mg/dL had a 29% higher death rate from all cancers combined compared with those with <90 mg/dL, [4] and significant associations were found for cancer mortalities of the colon, pancreas, and liver [3,4]. Diabetes can affect the quality of life (QOL) of cancer survivors. Individuals with both diabetes and cancer had a clinically important and significantly lower health-related QOL (HRQL) than did those with either condition alone [11]. Moreover, second primary cancers are more likely to develop in cancer survivors with diabetes, since hyperglycemia and/or diabetes is associated with an increased risk of cancer [4,12,13].

Some cancer survivors, especially those with former childhood, testicular, and hematological cancers, were reported to have an increased risk of developing diabetes or metabolic syndrome, especially considering that chemotherapy and hormonal therapy are known to affect endocrine function [14,15]. Therefore, continued diabetes monitoring and management are important issues for cancer survivors. However, diabetes management status, such as adherence to treatment or the glycemic control rate, in cancer survivors has not been investigated extensively. Previous studies showed that cancer survivors were less likely to receive recommended care, such as diabetic and preventive care and appropriate follow-ups for heart failure, compared with general population [16,17]. Thus, overall diabetes management in these individuals is likely to be suboptimal. In this study, we investigated overall diabetes management status, including diabetes awareness, treatment, and adequate glycemic control rates, in cancer survivors compared with two non-cancer control groups; i.e., subjects with no history of cancer but with other chronic diseases, and subjects with no history of cancer or other chronic diseases.

## Materials and Methods

The data were derived from the 2007–2011 Korea National Health and Nutrition Examination Survey (KNHANES). The KNHANES is an ongoing, multicomponent, nationally representative survey of the non-institutionalized Korean population, administered by the Korea Centers for Disease Control and Prevention (KCDC). The survey uses a stratified, multistage probability sampling design, with selections made from sampling units, using household registries, based on geographical area, sex, and age-group. The target population of the survey consisted of non-institutionalized South Korean civilians aged 1 year or older. In 2007 the KNHANES became a year-round investigation employing a rolling sample design. For the KNHANES IV (2007–2009) dataset, 200 sampling units were selected randomly from the primary sampling units encompassing the target population in South Korea. Subsequently, 23 households per sampling unit were subsequently selected (total = 4600 households) in each year. For the KNHANES 2010–2011 dataset, 192 sampling units were selected randomly from the primary sampling units; 20 households per sampling unit were selected (total = 3840 households) in each year [18,19]. KNHANES consists of a health interview, health examination, and nutritional survey. We used data from the health interview and health examination to obtain information regarding sociodemographic characteristics, medical history, and anthropometric and laboratory measurements. The KNHANES was approved by the KCDC Institutional Review Board, and all subjects signed written informed consent forms. Details of the survey have been described elsewhere [18].

We combined data from the 2007–2011 surveys into a large cross-sectional dataset. A total of 4,594 of 6,455 subjects (71.2%) in 2007, 9,744 of 12,528 subjects (77.8%) in 2008, 10,533 of 12,722 subjects (82.8%) in 2009, 8,958 of 10,938 subjects (81.9%) in 2010, and 8,518 of 10,589 subjects (80.4%) in 2011 participated in each survey. Among the 42,347 total subjects, our study sample consisted of the 2,726 subjects with prevalent diabetes. "Prevalent diabetes" was applicable to individuals with a fasting plasma glucose level of ≥126 mg/dL or to subjects responding "yes" to any of the following questions: "Have you ever been told by a doctor that you have diabetes?"; "Are you now taking insulin?"; and "Are you currently taking oral hypoglycemic agents?" To limit the analysis to adults with type 2 diabetes, we excluded subjects whose age at diagnosis was <30 years [20] or whose age at the time of the survey was <30 years. After applying the exclusions, 2,660 subjects remained for analysis (Figure 1).

Among the prevalent diabetes subjects, those who had been diagnosed with diabetes by a clinician were considered to be aware of their diabetes status. Subjects who were on pharmacological treatment (either insulin, oral anti-diabetic drugs, or both) for diabetes were considered as "treated". Subjects were characterized as displaying adequate glucose control when their hemoglobin $A1_c$ (HbA1c) levels were <7% [21]. We classified the subjects as cancer survivors if they answered "yes" to the interview question, "Have you ever been told by a doctor that you have cancer or a malignancy of any kind?" The type of cancer and the age at diagnosis were also noted. Since we assumed that frequent contacts with health professionals were associated with the quality of care the patient received, we separated the remaining subjects into two non-cancer control groups: those without cancer but with chronic disease and those without cancer or any other chronic disease. In accordance with a previous study, we operationally defined chronic disease as incurable and usually associated with a life-time increase of medical encounters [22]. Participants who had been diagnosed by a physician, with hypertension, arthritis, heart disease, stroke, asthma, or chronic obstructive pulmonary disease, comprised the chronic disease group [22].

Blood samples were obtained from subjects after a minimum 8-h fast. The serum fasting glucose levels were measured enzymatically at a central laboratory, using Advia 1650/2400 (Siemens, New York, USA) during the 2007 KNHANES and using an automatic analyzer 7600 (Hitachi, Tokyo, Japan) during the 2008–2011 KNHANES. In the 2007–2010 KNHANES, HbA1c was measured in the subjects with fasting plasma glucose levels ≥126 mg/dL or in those who were taking insulin or oral anti-diabetic medication, while in the 2011 KNHANES, HbA1c was measured in all subjects 10 years of age or older. HbA1c levels were measured using a high-performance liquid chromatography Varian II assay (Bio-Rad, Carlsbad, CA, USA) in the 2007 KNHANES and using a high-performance liquid chromatography-723G7 (Tosoh, Japan) in the 2008 KNHANES. Rigorous quality-control (QC) programs were employed in both surveys, and HbA1c measurements were reportedly comparable [23]. The detailed methods for comparing and assessing the validity and reliability of each survey are described elsewhere [23,24].

All statistical analyses were performed using the software package SAS (ver. 9.2, SAS Institute, Cary, NC, USA), with a survey procedure that adjusted for the complex survey design and included appropriate sampling weights to obtain accurate estimates representative of the non-institutionalized Korean population (according to KCDC guidelines) [18]. A descriptive analysis was used to assess the characteristics of the cancer survivors and control subjects with diabetes. A chi-square analysis was used to compare the categorical variables among the three groups. Next, we compared the prevalence of diabetes awareness, treatment, and adequate glycemic control among the three groups. We used multivariable logistic regression analyses to compute adjusted prevalence estimates (*i.e.*, predicted population margins) as well as adjusted odds ratios (ORs) and confidence intervals (CIs) [25,26]. We considered age (30–49, 50–59, 60–69, and ≥70 years), sex, education (elementary school or less, middle or high school graduates, and college or higher graduates), and body mass index (BMI) as potential confounders when calculating the adjusted prevalence, according to previous studies [20,27,28].

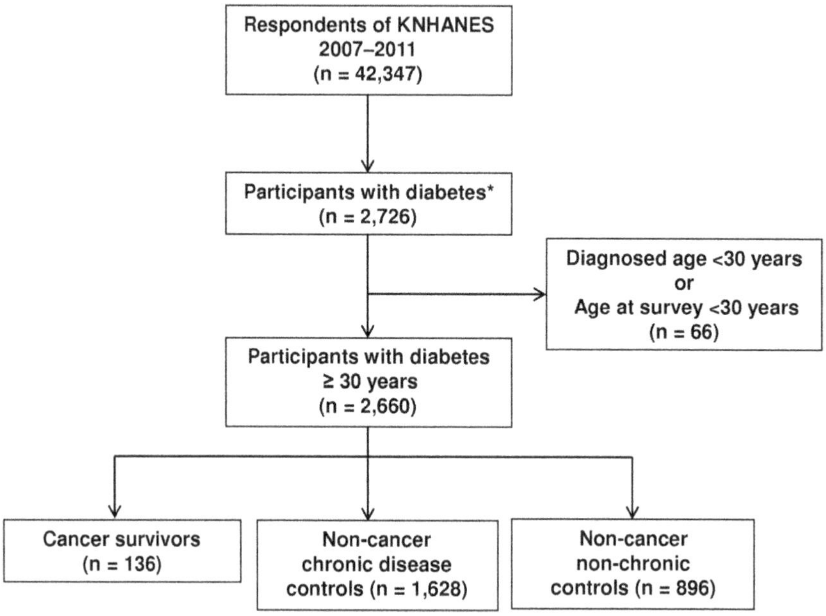


**Figure 1. The process used to select the study population.** KNHANES, Korea National Health and Nutrition Examination Survey. *Subjects with fasting plasma glucose levels of ≥126 mg/dL, or with a previous clinical diagnosis of diabetes made by a physician, or taking insulin or oral anti-diabetic medication.

BMI was calculated as weight in kilograms divided by height in meters squared. The statistical significance of the differences in prevalence was determined using the $t$ statistic derived from the general linear contrast procedure. We adjusted for multiple tests by applying the Bonferroni correction [26]. Since glycemic control is associated with diabetes duration [29], we conducted additional subgroup analyses, for treatment and adequate glycemic control, according to diabetes duration (*i.e.*, ≤5 years and >5 years). This procedure is in line with previous studies [30,31]. In the HbA1c-based analyses of glycemic control, we excluded subjects whose HbA1c levels had not been measured; therefore, a total of 2,556 subjects were included in the analyses. We considered a two-tailed $p$ value<0.05 as statistically significant.

## Results

Our study population comprised 136 cancer survivors, 1,628 non-cancer chronic disease controls, and 896 non-cancer non-chronic disease controls, all with diabetes, and their mean ages were 65.2, 62.6, and 52.8 years, respectively. Of the 136 cancer survivors, 58.8% reported having one of the following four types of cancer: stomach (n = 26), colorectal (n = 21), cervical (n = 20), or breast cancer (n = 13).

Table 1 presents the descriptive analyses for the cancer survivors and the two control groups. Cancer survivors had somewhat different sociodemographic characteristics compared with the non-cancer non-chronic disease controls. The cancer survivors were more likely to be older, female, unmarried, to have a lower level of education and a lower monthly income. Moreover, they were more likely to have had a longer diabetes duration. In contrast, cancer survivors and non-cancer chronic disease controls had similar sociodemographic characteristics, with the exceptions that the former were more likely to be older, non-obese, and to have-longer-term diabetes than the latter.

Table 2 lists the prevalences, odds ratios (ORs), and 95% confidence intervals (CIs) for the diabetes awareness, treatment, and adequate glycemic control variables of each group. Cancer survivors had a higher awareness than did both the non-cancer chronic disease controls and non-cancer non-chronic disease controls (85.1%, 80.4%, and 60.4%, respectively). Following adjustment for other covariates, awareness remained higher in cancer survivors compared with the control groups. Diabetes awareness ORs (which cannot be interpreted as relative risks) in the non-cancer chronic disease and cancer survivor groups, were 2.0 (95% CI: 1.6, 2.7) and 2.5 (95% CI: 1.4, 4.4), respectively, when the non-cancer, non-chronic disease group was used as the reference (Table 2, Model 2).

The prevalence of diabetes treatment in the cancer survivors (67.5%) was significantly higher compared with the non-cancer, non-chronic disease controls (46.7%), but lower compared with the non-cancer, chronic disease controls (69.5%). The prevalence of diabetes treatment in the cancer survivor group was lower compared with the non-cancer, chronic disease controls following adjustment for other covariates, but this difference was not statistically significant.

The prevalence of adequate glycemic control was also lower, but not significantly so, in the cancer survivors compared with the non-cancer chronic disease controls (31.7% and 34.6%, respectively). However, the prevalences in both groups were significantly higher compared with the rate of the non-cancer, non-chronic disease control group (17.8%). The non-cancer chronic disease control group had the highest prevalence of adequate glycemic control, followed by the cancer survivor and non-cancer, non-chronic disease control groups, although group differences decreased following adjustment for age, sex, education, and BMI (29.5%, 25.2%, and 18.7%, respectively; Table 2, Model 2).

Figure 2 illustrates the prevalences of diabetes treatment and adequate glycemic control, following stratification according to diabetes duration (≤5 years and >5 years). Cancer survivors showed the lowest prevalence of treatment among the three groups, regardless of duration. For subjects with a diabetes duration of ≤5 years, the prevalences of adequate glycemic

**Table 1.** Characteristics of cancer survivors and controls with prevalent diabetes among the pooled subjects from the 2007–2011 Korea National Health and Nutrition Examination Survey.

| | All | | Cancer survivors (n = 136) | Non-cancer chronic disease controls (n = 1,628) | Non-cancer non-chronic disease controls (n = 896) | |
|---|---|---|---|---|---|---|
| **Variable** | **Unweighted No.** | **% (SE)** | **% (SE)** | **% (SE)** | **% (SE)** | ***P* value** |
| Age (years) | | | | | | |
| 30–49 | 425 | 24.4(1.2) | 12.4(3.5) | 12.0(1.2) | 43.2(2.1) | <0.001 |
| 50–59 | 593 | 28.2(1.1) | 11.9(3.1) | 27.7(1.4) | 30.5(1.8) | |
| 60–69 | 881 | 25.9(0.9) | 41.4(4.5) | 31.4(1.3) | 16.7(1.3) | |
| ≥70 | 761 | 21.5(0.9) | 34.2(3.8) | 29.0(1.3) | 9.7 (0.9) | |
| Gender | | | | | | |
| Male | 1333 | 55.6(1.1) | 43.5(4.5) | 49.1(1.5) | 66.1(1.9) | <0.001 |
| Female | 1327 | 44.4(1.1) | 56.5(4.5) | 50.9(1.5) | 33.9(1.9) | |
| Education[a] | | | | | | |
| Middle school and under | 1306 | 42(1.2) | 53.7(4.5) | 52.9(1.5) | 25.2(1.6) | <0.001 |
| Middle-high school | 1018 | 42.9(1.2) | 36.3(4.4) | 37.7(1.4) | 51.0(1.9) | |
| College and above | 324 | 15.1(1) | 10.0(3.6) | 9.4 (1.0) | 23.7(1.8) | |
| Marital status | | | | | | |
| Married | 2026 | 77.7(1.0) | 69.0(4.5) | 72.9(1.4) | 85.4(1.3) | <0.001 |
| Unmarried (Single, divorced, widowed) | 634 | 22.3(1.0) | 31.0(4.5) | 27.1(1.4) | 14.6(1.3) | |
| Monthly household income | | | | | | |
| <1000 USD | 925 | 27.8(1.1) | 34.4(4.5) | 34.6(1.5) | 17.4(1.4) | <0.001 |
| 1000–3000 USD | 944 | 36.9(1.2) | 28.8(4.2) | 35.1(1.5) | 40.2(2.1) | |
| ≥3000 USD | 791 | 35.3(1.3) | 36.8(4.2) | 30.2(1.6) | 42.4(2.1) | |
| Health insurance type | | | | | | |
| National Health Insurance | 2469 | 93.5(0.6) | 92.1(2.6) | 92.6(0.8) | 94.9(0.9) | 0.11 |
| Medicaid/none/others | 191 | 6.5(0.6) | 7.9 (2.6) | 7.4 (0.8) | 5.1 (0.9) | |
| Residential area | | | | | | |
| City | 1901 | 76.8(1.8) | 74.0(3.7) | 76.0(1.9) | 78.2(2.2) | 0.43 |
| Rural | 759 | 23.2(1.8) | 26.0(3.7) | 24.0(1.9) | 21.8(2.2) | |
| Duration of diabetes[a] (years) | | | | | | |
| ≤1 | 312 | 16.9(1.1) | 16.4(3.7) | 15.3(1.3) | 20.0(2.1) | <0.001 |
| 2–5 | 667 | 34.6(1.3) | 21.0(4.4) | 34.6(1.6) | 36.4(2.5) | |
| >5 | 1053 | 48.5(1.4) | 62.6(4.8) | 50.1(1.7) | 43.6(2.6) | |
| Body mass index (kg/m$^2$) | | | | | | |
| <25.0 | 1387 | 50.8(1.2) | 58.4(4.5) | 45.1(1.6) | 58.2(1.9) | <0.001 |
| 25.0–29.9 | 1091 | 41.7(1.2) | 36.3(4.3) | 46.6(1.6) | 35.1(1.8) | |

**Table 1.** Cont.

| Variable | All | | Cancer survivors (n = 136) | Non-cancer chronic disease controls (n = 1,628) | Non-cancer non-chronic disease controls (n = 896) | |
|---|---|---|---|---|---|---|
| | Unweighted No. | % (SE) | % (SE) | % (SE) | % (SE) | *P* value |
| ≥30 | 182 | 7.5(0.7) | 5.3 (1.8) | 8.3 (0.9) | 6.7 (1.1) | |

[a]The total number of subjects among these categories does not equal 2,660 due to missing data.

control in the cancer survivors, non-cancer chronic disease controls, and non-cancer, non-chronic disease controls were 66.5%, 81.0%, and 68.5%, respectively: the cancer survivor and non-cancer, chronic disease control group difference was marginally significant. Even though the overall prevalence of treatment in subjects with a diabetes duration of >5 years was higher compared with subjects with a duration of ≤5 years, the trends observed in each model did not differ (Figure 2a).

Moreover, and following stratification according to diabetes duration, the prevalence of adequate glycemic control of the cancer survivor group was lower compared with the non-cancer, chronic disease group, but higher compared with the non-cancer, non-chronic disease control group. However, the differences among the survivors and control groups were not statistically significant. For the ≤5-year diabetes duration subjects, the prevalence of adequate glycemic control was 45.0% in the cancer survivor group, 49.1% in the non-cancer chronic disease control group, and 35.5% in the non-cancer non-chronic disease control group. These values were higher than those of the >5-year diabetes duration subjects (33.3%, 37.1%, and 23.9%, respectively). This trend did not change after adjusting for other covariates (Figure 2b).

## Discussion

To our knowledge, this is the first study to compare the diabetes management status of cancer survivors with the general population based on a nationally representative population. According to the results, diabetes awareness in cancer survivors was significantly higher than in both non-cancer control groups. However, the prevalences of diabetes treatment and adequate glycemic control of cancer survivors were lower compared with that of the non-cancer, chronic disease controls. Even after adjusting for or stratifying by covariates that could affect diabetes management, the results remained the same.

Our finding that cancer survivors demonstrated higher levels of awareness of diabetes and a higher prevalence of adequate glycemic control, compared with non-cancer, non-chronic disease control subjects, appears to be associated with the typically greater number of medical contacts made by the former group. Non-cancer, non-chronic disease subjects might predominately comprise individuals who do not visit their physicians, such that the frequency of undiagnosed diabetes could be higher in this population compared with the other groups. The frequency of medical encounters has been suggested to be an important determinant of the quality of care that patients receive [32]. A previous study reported that breast cancer survivors were more likely to receive routine preventive services than individuals without a history of cancer [32]. In a Korean multicenter study, cancer survivors with hypertension were more likely to regularly take antihypertensive medication than the general population [33]. In addition, cancer survivors were more likely to undergo cancer screening in accordance with guidelines than those without a history of cancer [22,32,34]. We found that the non-cancer chronic disease control subjects, who were generally considered to have more frequent contacts with physicians than the non-cancer non-chronic disease controls, also displayed higher awareness than did the non-cancer non-chronic disease subjects; this finding demonstrates the potential impact of frequent medical contact on diabetes awareness.

Interestingly, even though the subjects of both groups were considered to have frequent contact with physicians, the cancer survivors showed lower treatment and control than those in non-cancer chronic disease controls. There are several possibilities for

**Table 2.** Prevalence, odds ratios (ORs), and 95% confidence intervals (CIs) for diabetes awareness, treatment, and adequate glycemic control in the cancer survivor and control groups with prevalent diabetes.

| | Cancer survivors | | Non-cancer chronic disease controls | | Non-cancer non-chronic disease controls | |
|---|---|---|---|---|---|---|
| | % | OR | % | OR | % | OR |
| **Variables** | **(95% CI)** | **(95% CI)** | **(95% CI)** | **(95% CI)** | **(95% CI)** | **(95% CI)** |
| Awareness | | | | | | |
| Crude | 85.1 | 3.7 | 80.4[b] | 2.7 | 60.4[a] | Reference |
| | (76.[illegible]–91.0) | (2.0–6.9) | (77.8–82.8) | (2.2–3.4) | (56.4–64.2) | |
| Model 1 | 83.0 | 2.4 | 78.8[b] | 1.8 | 67.1[a] | Reference |
| | (73.[illegible]–89.5) | (1.3–4.4) | (75.9–81.4) | (1.4–2.4) | (62.8–71.1) | |
| Model 2 | 81.4 | 2.5 | 78.4[b] | 2.0 | 64.0[a] | Reference |
| | (72.0–88.2) | (1.4–4.4) | (74.6–81.8) | (1.6–2.7) | (58.8–68.9) | |
| Treatment | | | | | | |
| Crude | 67.5 | 2.4 | 69.5[b] | 2.6 | 46.7[a] | Reference |
| | (57.1–76.4) | (1.5–3.8) | (66.7–72.1) | (2.1–3.2) | (42.8–50.6) | |
| Model 1 | 62.8 | 1.5 | 66.6[b] | 1.8 | 53.2[c] | Reference |
| | (52.2–72.2) | (0.9–2.4) | (63.6–69.4) | (1.4–2.2) | (49.0–57.3) | |
| Model 2 | 60.5 | 1.5 | 65.0[b] | 1.8 | 51.1[c] | Reference |
| | (49.4–70.5) | (0.9–2.3) | (60.9–68.9) | (1.4–2.2) | (46.0–56.2) | |
| Adequate glycemic control | | | | | | |
| Crude | 31.7 | 2.1 | 34.6[b] | 2.4 | 17.8[a] | Reference |
| | (23.2–41.6) | (1.3–3.5) | (31.9–37.3) | (1.9–3.1) | (15.0–21.1) | |
| Model 1 | 27.1 | 1.5 | 31.3[b] | 1.8 | 20.0[c] | Reference |
| | (19.1–36.8) | (0.9–2.4) | (28.4–34.4) | (1.4–2.3) | (16.9–23.5) | |
| Model 2 | 25.2 | 1.5 | 29.5[b] | 1.8 | 18.7[c] | Reference |
| | (17.5–34.8) | (0.9–2.4) | (25.6–33.6) | (1.4–2.3) | (15.1–22.8) | |

Model 1 was adjusted for age and sex; Model 2 was also adjusted for education and body mass index.
We adjusted for multiple tests by applying the Bonferroni method.
Awareness: proportion of prevalent diabetes subjects who had been diagnosed with diabetes by a clinician.
Treatment: proportion of prevalent diabetes subjects who were receiving pharmacological treatment (either insulin, oral anti-diabetic drugs, or both).
Adequate glycemic control: proportion of prevalent diabetes subjects displaying hemoglobin A1c (HbA1c) levels of <7%.
[a] $p$-value $<0.05$ when compared with cancer survivors.
[b] $p$-value $<0.05$ when compared with non-cancer non-chronic disease controls.
[c] $p$-value $<0.15$ when compared with cancer survivors.

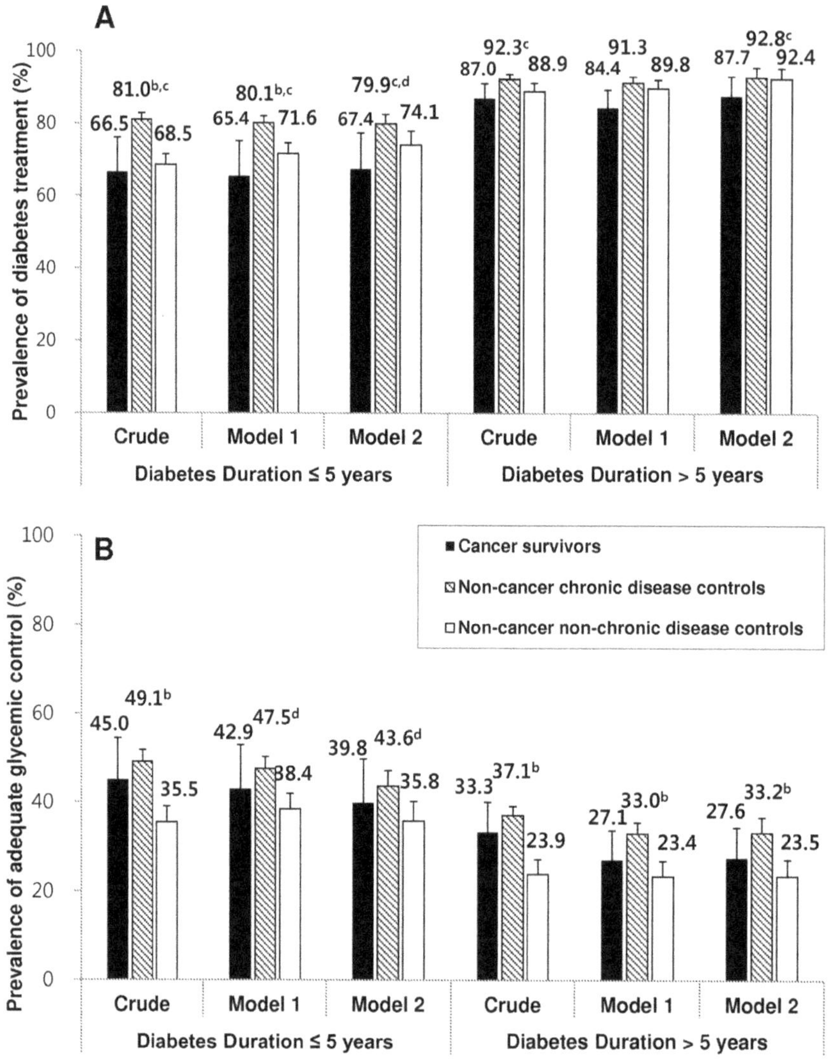


**Figure 2. Prevalence of: (A) diabetes treatment; and (B) adequate glycemic control, among the cancer survivor and control groups with prevalent diabetes, according to diabetes duration.** Model 1 was adjusted for age and sex; Model 2 was additionally adjusted for education and BMI. We adjusted for multiple tests by applying the Bonferroni method. [a]*p*-value<0.05 when compared with cancer survivors. [b]*p*-value<0.05 when compared with non-cancer non-chronic disease controls. [c]*p*-value<0.15 when compared with cancer survivors. [d]*p*-value<0.15 when compared with non-cancer non-chronic disease controls.

this. First, cancer survivors tend to have greater difficulty maintaining general medical check-ups and receiving comprehensive health management for other diseases than non-cancer chronic disease controls. Even though cancer survivors visit oncology specialists at tertiary hospitals for cancer-related follow-up, it is difficult for the oncology specialist to provide comprehensive care. In fact, oncologists do not always assume the primary care role that cancer patients expect of them [17], and to some extent, they are not willing or equipped to deal with such problems [35]. In addition, cancer patients often expect their oncologist to be their sole care provider [36], potentially losing contact with non-cancer providers who are critical for overall health care [17]. In Korea, there is neither a family doctor referral system, designated physician, nor an organized care system for long-term follow-up of cancer survivors. Thus, the difficulties in management of chronic comorbid disease for cancer survivors appear to be exacerbated in Korea.

Second, cancer survivors might frequently be unaware of the effects of diabetes and poor glycemic control on their disease prognosis, or of the risk that it confers regarding the development of other cancers. Previous studies suggest that cancer survivors are characterized by a knowledge deficit regarding the late effects of treatment and individual health risks [37,38]. In contrast, patients with non-cancer-related chronic diseases, such as hypertension and cardiovascular disease, are relatively more likely to be aware of the risk that diabetes imposes upon their disease. According to the Health Belief Model, perceived susceptibility is critical for healthy behaviors [39]. In addition, perceived benefits (related to treatment efficacy) and perceived severity contribute to sick-role behavior after diagnosis [39]. If cancer patients realize the impact of diabetes on disease prognosis and take the risk of diabetes more seriously, then their health behaviors are more likely to change.

Third, diabetes treatment and management are not likely major priorities for cancer patients, regardless of whether they recognize the risk of diabetes. The work by Earle and Neville indicated that having a prior cancer diagnosis can shift attention away from other important health issues [17], and Shin *et al.* argued that some cancer survivors are relatively ignorant of their health needs outside of cancer, tending to only focus on cancer treatment [40]. In many cases, diabetes management is a lower priority than cancer care, causing cancer survivors to be negligent in diabetes management.

In regards to the second and third possibilities, educating cancer survivors about the importance of diabetes management may be beneficial. If the patients recognize the impacts of uncontrolled blood sugar on cancer-related prognoses and/or cancer-unrelated health, diabetes care may increase enough in priority to improve their self-glycemic control.

The question as to who is responsible for patient education in our current healthcare system is connected to the question of which system should be applied to the long-term care of cancer survivors. During the last few years, there has been intense discussion in regards to follow-up care of cancer survivors [35]. The American Society of Clinical Oncology recommends promoting successful models of survivor care and tools that optimize the transition process between oncologist and primary care providers to achieve high-quality cancer survivor care [36]. Studies have shown that survivors who visited both primary care physicians (PCP) and oncologists received better comorbidity management and care than did cancer patients who only visited oncologists [16,17]. Since an oncologist alone cannot be responsible for all areas of care, it is desirable that PCPs take partial responsibility for care of cancer survivors. Yet, this creates ambiguity in several areas; e.g., screening for specific cancers, screening for other cancers, and ongoing comorbidity management [35]. Further studies and discussions are needed to ensure that the roles of oncology specialists and PCPs are systematically coordinated in the future.

This study had a number of limitations. The KNHANES was not designed to investigate cancer survivorship. For this reason, the number of cancer survivors included in the study was relatively small. The limited sample size of the cancer survivor group caused the predictions derived from the subgroup analyses less stable and more difficult to conduct further analyses based on factors such as cancer type and age. Moreover, KNHANES classified cancer into only the six-most prevalent types in Korea (gastric, liver, colorectal, breast, cervical, and lung cancers), and consequently data for the other types were absent, creating several missing values for the "cancer type" variable. In addition, because additional information, such as the cancer stage and treatment method (*i.e.*, the use of chemotherapy or radiotherapy), was not collected in KNHANES, we could not assess the associations of these variables with diabetes management. Second, cancer and other chronic disease diagnoses and the use of diabetes medication were self-reported, which could lead to misclassification bias. Third, we were unable to consider the effects of order. Due to the numerous missing values among the dates of diagnosis, we could not confirm whether cancer, or other chronic diseases, manifested before or after the diabetes diagnosis. Fourth, we could not rule out the possibility of survival bias, because the KNHANES uses a cross-sectional design. Therefore, our finding that the prevalences of treatment and adequate glycemic control of the cancer survivors and non-cancer chronic disease patients were higher, compared with the non-cancer, non-chronic disease group, could be due to the poor health status of the former subjects, which had either already resulted in death or prevented their participation in the investigation.

Despite these limitations, our finding that cancer survivors had a suboptimal diabetes management status compared to that of the non-cancer chronic disease group suggests there is room for improvement in the management of diabetes in cancer survivors. Taking this into consideration, the additional finding that the prevalences of treatment and adequate glycemic control were lower in cancer survivors compared with the non-cancer, chronic disease group, despite greater awareness of diabetes in the cancer survivors, strongly indicates that there are certain barriers to adequate diabetes management in cancer survivors. Our findings illustrate the issues with the health care system for cancer survivors in Korea, in terms of the ambiguity in care responsibility between oncologists and PCPs. Inadequate glycemic control in cancer survivors could lead to severe cardiovascular or oncogenic consequences, and special attention to diabetes management and proactive education is needed to ensure that survivors receive optimal diabetes care. Regardless of who is responsible, general primary care issues, including glycemic control in cancer survivors, should be addressed with greater priority. Further studies in this area are warranted to determine the optimum roles of primary care and specialist physicians.

## Author Contributions

Conceived and designed the experiments: JYS HYS JKJ. Analyzed the data: JYS. Contributed reagents/materials/analysis tools: JYS HYS JKJ. Wrote the paper: JYS JKJ.

## References

1. Siegel R, DeSantis C, Virgo K, Stein K, Mariotto A, et al. (2012) Cancer treatment and survivorship statistics, 2012. CA Cancer J Clin 62: 220–241.
2. Jung KW, Won YJ, Kong HJ, Oh CM, Seo HG, et al. (2013) Cancer statistics in Korea: incidence, mortality, survival and prevalence in 2010. Cancer Res Treat 45: 1–14.
3. Coughlin SS, Calle EE, Teras LR, Petrelli J, Thun MJ (2004) Diabetes Mellitus as a Predictor of Cancer Mortality in a Large Cohort of US Adults. Am J Epidemiol 159: 1160–1167.
4. Jee S, Ohrr H, Sull J, Yun J, Ji M, et al. (2005) Fasting serum glucose level and cancer risk in korean men and women. JAMA 293: 194–202.
5. Lipscombe L, Goodwin P, Zinman B, McLaughlin J, Hux J (2008) The impact of diabetes on survival following breast cancer. Breast Cancer Res Treat 109: 389–395.
6. Park SM, Lim MK, Shin SA, Yun YH (2006) Impact of prediagnosis smoking, alcohol, obesity, and insulin resistance on survival in male cancer patients: National Health Insurance Corporation Study. J Clin Oncol 24: 5017–5024.
7. Barone BB, Yeh H, Snyder CF (2008) Long-term all-cause mortality in cancer patients with preexisting diabetes mellitus: A systematic review and meta-analysis. JAMA 300: 2754–2764.
8. Bjørnholt JV, Erikssen G, Aaser E, Sandvik L, Nitter-Hauge S, et al. (1999) Fasting blood glucose: an underestimated risk factor for cardiovascular death. Results from a 22-year follow-up of healthy nondiabetic men. Diabetes Care 22: 45–49.
9. Brown BW, Brauner C, Minnotte MC (1993) Noncancer deaths in white adult cancer patients. J Natl Cancer Inst 85: 979–987.
10. Shin D, Ahn E, Kim H, Park S, Kim Y, et al. (2010) Non-cancer mortality among long-term survivors of adult cancer in Korea: national cancer registry study. Cancer Causes Control 21: 919–929.
11. Bowker S, Pohar S, Johnson J (2006) A cross-sectional study of health-related quality of life deficits in individuals with comorbid diabetes and cancer. Health Qual Life Outcomes 4: 17.
12. Hu FB, Manson JE, Liu S, Hunter D, Colditz GA, et al. (1999) Prospective study of adult onset diabetes mellitus (type 2) and risk of colorectal cancer in women. J Natl Cancer Inst 91: 542–547.
13. Stattin P, Björ O, Ferrari P, Lukanova A, Lenner P, et al. (2007) Prospective study of hyperglycemia and cancer risk. Diabetes Care 30: 561–567.
14. De Haas EC, Oosting SF, Lefrandt JD, Wolffenbuttel BHR, Sleijfer DT, et al. (2010) The metabolic syndrome in cancer survivors. Lancet Oncol 11: 193–203.
15. Nuver J, Smit AJ, Postma A, Sleijfer DT, Gietema JA (2002) The metabolic syndrome in long-term cancer survivors, and important target for secondary preventive measures. Cancer Treat Rev 28: 195–214.
16. Snyder CF, Frick KD, Kantsiper ME, Peairs KS, Herbert RJ, et al. (2009) Prevention, screening, and surveillance care for breast cancer survivors

compared with controls: changes from 1998 to 2002. J Clin Oncol 27: 1054–1061.
17. Earle CC, Neville BA (2004) Under use of necessary care among cancer survivors. Cancer 101: 1712–1719.
18. The Ministry of Health and Welfare (2012) The guideline for the usage of Korean National Health and Nutrition Survey raw data. Seoul: Korea Centers for Disease Control and Prevention.
19. Sim CS, Kim Y, Lee H, Park CY, Ham JO, et al. (2014) Iron deficiency increases blood lead levels in boys and pre-menarche girls surveyed in KNHANES 2010–2011. Environ Res 130: 1–6.
20. Koro CE, Bowlin SJ, Bourgeois N, Fedder DO (2004) Glycemic control from 1988 to 2000 among U.S. adults diagnosed with type 2 diabetes: a preliminary report. Diabetes Care 27: 17–20.
21. American Diabetes Association (2010) Standards of Medical Care in Diabetes—2010. Diabetes Care 33: S11–S61.
22. Cho J, Guallar E, Hsu YJ, Shin D, Lee WC (2010) A comparison of cancer screening practices in cancer survivors and in the general population: the Korean national health and nutrition examination survey (KNHANES) 2001–2007. Cancer Causes Control 21: 2203–2212.
23. Korea Centers for Disease Control and Prevention (2009) Quality control and development of standardization manual for the medical laboratory tests in the nation-wide health survey of 2008 year. Seoul: Korea Centers for Disease Control and Prevention.
24. Korea Centers for Disease Control and Prevention (2013) Korea National Health and Nutrition Examination Survey. Available: https://knhanes.cdc.go.kr/knhanes/sub02/sub02_05.jsp. Accessed 9 May 2014.
25. Graubard BI, Korn EL (1999) Predictive margins with survey data. Biometrics 55: 652–659.
26. SAS Institute (2014) SAS SAS/STAT(R) 9.22 User's Guide. Available: http://support.sas.com/documentation/cdl/en/statug/63347/HTML/default/viewer.htm#statug_logistic_sect074.htm. Assessed 6 july 2014.
27. Ong KL, Cheung BMY, Wong LYF, Wat NMS, Tan KCB, et al. (2008) Prevalence, treatment, and control of diagnosed diabetes in the U.S. National Health and Nutrition Examination Survey 1999–2004. Ann Epidemiol 18: 222–229.
28. Shaya FT, Yan X, Lin P-J, Simoni-Wastila L, Bron M, et al. (2010) US trends in glycemic control, treatment, and comorbidity burden in patients with diabetes. J Clin Hypertens 12: 826–832.
29. Clauson P, Linnarsson R, Gottsäter A, Sundkvist G, Grill V (1994) Relationships between diabetes duration, metabolic control and β-cell function in a representative population of type 2 diabetic patients in Sweden. Diabet Med 11: 794–801.
30. Byun SH, Ma SH, Jun JK, Jung KW, Park B (2013) Screening for Diabetic Retinopathy and Nephropathy in Patients with Diabetes: A Nationwide Survey in Korea. PLoS One 8: e62991.
31. Hoerger TJ, Segel JE, Gregg EW, Saaddine JB (2008) Is glycemic control improving in US adults? Diabetes Care 31: 81–86.
32. Earle CC, Burstein HJ, Winer EP, Weeks JC (2003) Quality of non–breast cancer health maintenance among elderly breast cancer survivors. J Clin Oncol 21: 1447–1451.
33. Shin D, Kim S, Cho J, Yang HK, Cho B, et al. (2012) Comparison of hypertension management between cancer survivors and the general public. Hypertens Res 35: 935–939.
34. Trask PC, Rabin C, Rogers ML, Whiteley J, Nash J, et al. (2005) Cancer screening practices among cancer survivors. Am J Prev Med 28: 351–356.
35. Jacobs LA, Palmer SC, Schwartz LA, DeMichele A, Mao JJ, et al. (2009) Adult cancer survivorship: evolution, research, and planning care. CA Cancer J Clin 59: 391–410.
36. McCabe MS, Bhatia S, Oeffinger KC, Reaman GH, Tyne C, et al. (2013) American Society of Clinical Oncology Statement: Achieving high-quality cancer survivorship care. J Clin Oncol 31: 631–640.
37. Landier W, Wallace WHB, Hudson MM (2006) Long-term follow-up of pediatric cancer survivors: Education, surveillance, and screening. Pediatr Blood Cancer 46: 149–158.
38. Hudson MM, Tyc V, Srivastava D, Gattuso J, Quargnenti A, et al. (2002) Multi-component behavioral intervention to promote health protective behaviors in childhood cancer survivors: The Protect Study. Med Pediatr Oncol 39: 2–11.
39. Harvey JN, Lawson VL (2009) The importance of health belief models in determining self-care behaviour in diabetes. Diabet Med 26: 5–13.
40. Shin D, Park J, Park J, Park E, Kim S, et al. (2011) Antihypertensive medication adherence in cancer survivors and its affecting factors: results of a Korean population-based study. Support Care Cancer 19: 211–220.

# 10

# Development and Validation of the Pre-Hospital Stroke Symptoms Coping Test

**Qiuli Zhao[1*¶], Li Yang[1¶], Xiao Zhang[1¶], Xuemei Zhu[1], Qingqing Zuo[1], Yanni Wu[2], Liu Yang[1], Wei Gao[1], Minghui Li[1], Shanshan Cheng[1]**

**1** School of Nursing, The 2nd Affiliated Hospital of Harbin Medical University, Harbin Medical University, Harbin, China, **2** Department of Nursing department, The 2nd Affiliated Hospital of Harbin Medical University, Harbin Medical University, Harbin, China

## Abstract

***Background and Purpose:*** Measures of specific knowledge of coping with pre-hospital stroke symptoms can help educate high-risk patients and family caregivers. This study aimed to develop and validate the Pre-hospital Stroke Symptoms Coping Test (PSSCT).

***Materials and Methods:*** Reliability and validity were analyzed using multiple data sources. The Delphi expert consultation method was applied to assess the test's surface validity and content validity index. The final edition of the 19-item PSSCT contained 3 sections assessing coping with typical symptoms and symptoms associated with vomiting and twitching. Its psychometric properties were investigated in a community sample of 300 high-risk patients and family members.

***Results:*** The PSSCT was readily accepted by participants. It demonstrated adequate surface validity and content validity, and good internal consistency ($KR_{20} = 0.822$) and test-retest reliability (0.769), with difficulty (P) and degree of differentiation (D) ranges of 0.28–0.83 and 0.15–0.66, respectively. It was also able to distinguish between individuals who had/had not experienced a stroke. Experienced individuals scored significantly higher overall and on coping with typical symptoms and twitching ($P<0.01$).

***Conclusions:*** The PSSCT can practically and directly assess critical knowledge regarding coping with pre-hospital stroke symptoms and has good reliability and validity.

**Editor:** Chiara Lazzeri, Azienda Ospedaliero-Universitaria Careggi, Italy

**Funding:** The development and evaluation of the PSSCT was supported by a grant from the China National Natural Science Foundation (Grant No: 81273194). The funders had no role in study design, data collection and analysis, decision to publish, or preparation of the manuscript.

**Competing Interests:** The authors have declared that no competing interests exist.

* Email: zhaoqiuli1957@163.com

¶ These authors contributed equally to this work.

## Introduction

The global burden of stroke is rapidly increasing. Worldwide, someone is thought to suffer a stroke every other second, with a stroke-related death occurring every six seconds [1]. Thus, strokes are a major cause of death and long-term disability globally, including in developing countries [2]. In China, strokes are also the leading cause of morbidity and mortality [3], with prevalence rates having risen sharply over the past decade. More specifically, approximately 1,500,000 to 2,000,000 new stroke cases are anticipated each year. Its prevalence and mortality rates are estimated to be around 116–219/100,000/year and 58–142/100,000/year, respectively [4], after corrections for age. In order to obtain more satisfactory treatment effects, it is important for patients to find warning signs in a timely manner, adopt the correct pre-hospital coping strategies, and detect and correct inefficient coping methods early; in other words, patients can improve outcomes if they are able to arrive at a specialist or general hospital ward for treatment early on. Several studies have shown that the capacity to identify stroke signs, knowledge of coping with stroke symptoms, and emergency coping abilities during the pre-hospital period are major determinants of successful stroke prevention and treatment [5–7]. It is particularly important for family members to have proper knowledge on how to cope with strokes, including their occurrence, prevention, and prognosis [8,9]. Several studies have demonstrated that the level of knowledge about strokes in the general population is low, which can be improved with the implementation of appropriate health education interventions [10–12]. Thus, there is a need for valid assessment tools or evaluations of the effectiveness of stroke education and rehabilitation programs.

A number of tests have been developed to assess specific stroke knowledge, including the Stroke Symptom Questionnaire [13], Stroke Action Test [14], and Stroke Awareness Questionnaire (SAQ) [15], in which residents learn how to dial 911, etc., for general directions when a stroke has occurred. However, there are presently no references to methods assessing community resident knowledge regarding ways to cope with pre-hospital stroke symptoms in the scientific literature. Thus, having an instrument which would allow evaluations of such knowledge among high-risk populations and family members would be a valuable asset to healthcare providers, as it would enable them to more effectively tailor stroke education interventions to help overcome patient concerns. In order to meet the need for a suitable assessment tool, the present study aimed to develop and validate a Chinese test assessing specific knowledge of coping with pre-hospital stroke symptoms among high-risk populations and their family members, known as the Pre-hospital Stroke Symptoms Coping Test (PSSCT). Specifically, our research objectives were to (1) develop the PSSCT and assess its acceptability and feasibility as a tool for evaluating knowledge on coping with pre-hospital stroke symptoms among high-risk populations and their family members, and (2) assess the psychometric properties of the PSSCT.

## Materials and Methods

This experiment was conducted in accordance with the Declaration of Helsinki (1964). All study participants provided informed consent, and the study design was approved by the appropriate ethics review boards.

We used a methodological research design to develop and psychometrically evaluate the PSSCT in this study. The study consisted of two phases, namely (1) the instrument development phase and (2) the evaluation of psychometric properties phase.

### Research Procedure

**Phase I.** Instrument development A total of 25 potential items were originally identified. Of these, twenty were derived from a review of the literature, monographs on stroke knowledge, and the cerebrovascular guidelines for Chinese public health education programs on strokes [4], [16–19]. Furthermore, we conducted semi-structured interviews with stroke patients and recorded their answers to these questions. We then extracted a total of five items from the contents of patients' answers (see **Table 1** for an outline of the interviews).

An expert panel of 11 health care providers, including 6 doctors and 5 nurses from the emergency, brain surgery, and neurology departments, was invited to review the items for content, breadth, and applicability, and rate each item on its validity and relevance. The experts were selected according to whether they satisfied the following criteria: (1) possess a high level of training or relevant academic qualifications in the area of cerebral apoplexy (e.g., an associate professor or deputy director of both junior and senior personnel); (2) have a profound interest in and rich clinical knowledge of stroke symptoms, especially with regard to coping with them; (3) have a master's degree or at least 10 years of clinical experience; and (4) demonstrate a rigorous practical scientific attitude.

The content validity index (CVI) of each item was calculated, and 6 items with indexes $<0.70$ were subsequently deleted. The 19 items of the PSSCT were finalized after a Delphi expert consultation was conducted. The test was composed of three main parts focusing on coping with typical stroke symptoms and symptoms associated with vomiting and twitching. Dichotomous response options were used. The accuracy of responses, according to guidelines on cerebrovascular care and a review of the literature, was ascertained. A correct answer was given 1 point, and an incorrect one was given 0 points. The total score on the PSSCT reflected the individual's mastery (i.e., the community resident's level of knowledge) with regard to coping with pre-hospital stroke symptoms.

**Table 1.** Outline of semi-structured interviews.

| Interview questions |
|---|
| - How do you cope when stroke symptoms occur? |
| - Can you talk about how you coped with specific symptoms? |

**Phase II.** Pilot psychometric testing of the PSSCT The 19-item PSSCT was pilot-tested with 150 individuals at high risk of stroke and 150 of their relatives. Eligible participants were recruited from 3 different communities consecutively across Harbin, China, through posters placed in community publicity columns until the required sample size was reached. The appropriate sample size was determined by the number of participants needed to perform the factor analysis for psychometric assessment of the instrument. As there were 19 potential items, the sample size was calculated based on the subject-to-item ratio of 10–20:1 [20].

We performed a project analysis of the test (i.e., of item difficulty and degree of differentiation) based on the results of the evaluation in order to validate the effectiveness of the final version of the PSSCT. Its reliability and validity were also assessed. Kuder-Richardson ($KR_{20}$) and test-retest reliability coefficients were used as measures of test reliability, and both content and discriminant validity were evaluated.

### Selection of Research Participants

A sample size of 300 participants was required for this study. The inclusion criteria for 150 high-risk patients coincided with criteria for ascertaining whether individuals were susceptible to stroke: (1) being over 40 years of age; (2) having more than one of several risk factors, including high blood pressure, dyslipidemia (or unknown), diabetes mellitus, atrial fibrillation, and heart valve disease; and (3) clinically diagnosed with cerebral apoplexy (in the past or present).

Meanwhile, the inclusion criterion for 150 of their family members was being a family member of the participant who had close contact with the high-risk population. They could include patients' children, other family members, friends, or a domestic helper. Exclusion criteria were having mental disabilities or a medical background/education.

### Ethical Considerations

The protocol for this study complies with the Declaration of Helsinki and was approved by the Institutional Review Board of the second affiliated hospital of Harbin Medical University, China. The study was briefly explained to potential participants, who were informed that involvement was completely voluntary and that they could refuse to participate or withdraw from the study at any time without losing benefits or being penalized.

### Statistical Analysis

Descriptive statistics (means and standard deviations) were calculated for the continuous variables, such as descriptions of participants' clinical-demographic characteristics. The $KR_{20}$ coefficient was used to assess the reliability of the PSSCT. A CVI of $\geq 0.70$ was used as the cut-off to indicate sufficient content validity. We also compared the scores of participants who had and had not experienced a stroke to determine the discriminant validity. A significance level of 0.01 was used for all statistical analyses. All data entry and analyses were performed with the SPSS version 17.0 (SPSS Inc., Chicago, IL, USA), and Epidata 3.0

software, where significance levels were set at a two-tailed p-value of <0.01.

## Results

### Demographic Characteristics of Participants

Three hundred community residents, including patients at high risk of stroke and their family members, were recruited from three local communities to participate in this study. Five pairs of high-risk patients and their family members ($n = 10$) were excluded, because their knowledge of coping with pre-hospital stroke symptoms could not be evaluated due to logistical reasons. Therefore, 290 (96.7%) valid questionnaires were obtained. The remaining 290 participants (135 males, 155 females; mean age = 62.03 years, SD = 12.69 years) were included in the internal reliability and validity assessments. Most participants ($n = 220$) had not experienced a stroke, and the remaining 70 had personal experiences with stroke.

The average time taken to complete the original version of the 19-item PSSCT was approximately 5 minutes (no more than 10). The results suggested that the PSSCT had adequate surface validity and was readily accepted by participants. Scores on the test's 19 items are presented in **Table 2**, according to participants' characteristics. Total mean scores differed significantly by level of family income per capita, physical condition, living arrangement, health insurance coverage, and smoking habits.

### Analysis of items

Difficulty (P): The difficulty level of a question is typically defined as the proportion of respondents who answer it correctly. Possible values range from 0.0 to 1.0. Items on which more than 90% of respondents answer correctly (i.e., items with a value >0.9) are generally considered to be too easy, while items on which less than 10% of respondents answer correctly (i.e., items with a value <0.1) are considered to be too difficult [21]. In the present study, the analysis revealed that the difficulty (P) of items on the PSSCT ranged from 0.28 to 0.83, as shown in **Table 3**. This range indicated that individual items were answered correctly by 28% to 83% of respondents.

Degree of differentiation (D): An item's discriminative value indicates how well it distinguishes between high and low scorers. In order to calculate the discriminative value of each item, respondents were first divided into groups of high and low scorers, comprised of the 27% of highest scorers and 27% of lowest scorers. Then, the following formula was used:

$$\frac{\text{Number of correct answers in high group} - \text{number of correct answers in low group}}{\text{Total number in both groups}}$$

Values of 0.3 or higher commonly indicate (very) good differentiation. Values ranging from 0.15 to 0.3 are indicative of satisfactory to good differentiation, whereas values less than 0.15 are considered poor to mediocre [21]. Our analysis showed that the degree of differentiation (**D**) of items on the PSSCT ranged from 0.15 to 0.66, as shown in **Table 3**.

### PSSCT readability and content validity

To maximize the likelihood that PSSCT items would be easily comprehended by participants, items were written in plain language, and expert reviewers were asked specifically to comment on clarity and assess comprehensibility. The PSSCT was then subjected to participants' examination; it was administered to the 290 participants with instructions to comment on any difficulties experienced with the items. No difficulties were reported. Thus, the PSSCT showed good readability.

The PSSCT's $KR_{20}$ was calculated to evaluate its internal consistency, which, according to accepted standards of reliability, was good ($KR_{20} = 0.822$). The test-retest reliability was also good at 0.769. Through the Delphi expert enquiry method, data on the PSSCT's content validity were obtained. More specifically, to determine the CVI of each item, the experts were asked to evaluate the relevance of the initial test items with regard to coping with pre-hospital stroke symptoms by using a scale of 1 to 4, where 1 = "absolutely relevant," 2 = "relevant, but not necessary," 3 = "a little relevant," and 4 = "not relevant." A CVI was then calculated for each item, which reflected the proportion of consulted experts who agreed on the content validity of the item. The results showed that the CVI of test items were all ≥0.7, as shown in **Table 3**.

### Discriminate validity

Significant differences in scores on coping with typical stroke symptoms and coping with twitching were observed between the group of participants who had experienced a stroke and the group who had not. This difference was also evident in participants' total coping scores ($P<0.01$). As expected, participants without personal experiences of strokes scored lower than did those with such experience (see **Table 4**), indicating that the PSSCT has good discriminant validity.

## Discussion

This is the first report to describe the development and psychometric validation of a Chinese test assessing specific knowledge of coping with pre-hospital stroke symptoms among patients at high risk for stroke and their families. The PSSCT demonstrated good readability and was easily understood by participants, as a majority of them completed the test in 5 minutes. The results indicated that the PSSCT scores of individuals who did not smoke and who underwent annual physical examinations were higher than the scores of those who smoked and did not undergo annual physical examinations. These findings paralleled Yoon and Hickey's findings [22,23]. They also found that smoking was the most common risk factor for stroke, and observed that participants who did not smoke and who underwent annual physical examinations scored higher for recognition of stroke risk factors and warning signs. In addition, the highest scores in this study were found among participants who lived with their families and friends. This was consistent with previous reports [15] in which individuals with family support scored noticeably higher than did those with poor family support on knowledge of risk factors for stroke. It is possible that increased levels of social support (including informational support) contributed to higher levels of knowledge in participants; familial responsibilities have also been found to influence the use of health services [24,25]. In our study, the PSSCT scores of individuals whose family incomes per capita were high and who had free medical insurance were higher than were those of other participants. This has also verified in previous stroke-related knowledge-based surveys [26,27]. In other words, our study, as well as previous research on identification of stroke risk factors and warning signals, indicates that a greater concern for one's health (e.g., not smoking and going for regular physical examinations) and stronger support (e.g., greater family support and income, good health insurance coverage) lead to better stroke-related knowledge.

Item analyses allow revisions of tests on the basis of their scores, and are an essential part of improving instructions for respondents [28]. Thus, the difficulty level and discriminative value (degree of

**Table 2.** Scores on 19 items according to participants' characteristics (n = 290).

| Characteristic | N | Participants (%) | Mean Score ± SD | P |
|---|---|---|---|---|
| **Gender** | | | | P = 0.318 |
| Male | 135 | 46.55 | 11.25±3.47 | |
| Female | 155 | 53.45 | 11.65±3.33 | |
| **Age** | | | | |
| <60 | 88 | 30.34 | 10.90±3.44 | P = 0.06 |
| ≥60 | 202 | 69.66 | 11.71±3. 36 | |
| **Home address** | | | | |
| Urban | 206 | 71.03 | 11.71±3.25 | P = 0.15 |
| Suburban | 28 | 9.66 | 10.79±3.50 | |
| Rural | 56 | 19.31 | 10.89±3.80 | |
| **Have the disease now** | | | | P = 0.56 |
| Yes | 218 | 75.17 | 11.53±3.34 | |
| No | 72 | 24.83 | 11.26±3.58 | |
| **Living arrangement** | | | | *P = 0.04 |
| Living alone | 25 | 8.62 | 11.68±3.35 | |
| With family | 248 | 85.52 | 11.31±3.41 | |
| With friends | 17 | 5.86 | 13.41±2.76 | |
| **Average family income** | | | | *P = 0.00 |
| <1000 RMB | 46 | 15.86 | 10.02±3.53 | |
| 1000–2000 RMB | 102 | 35.17 | 11.05±3.55 | |
| >2000 RMB | 142 | 48.97 | 12.23±3.04 | |
| **Medical insurance** | | | | *P = 0.03 |
| Social medical insurance | 175 | 60.34 | 11.49±3.20 | |
| Free medical insurance | 17 | 5.86 | 13. 41±2.70 | |
| Rural cooperative insurance | 65 | 22.41 | 10.71±3. 76 | |
| At one's own expense | 20 | 6.90 | 12.35±3.33 | |
| Others | 13 | 4.49 | 11.00±4.04 | |
| **Physical examination** | | | | |
| Many times in a year | 26 | 8.97 | 11.77±3.15 | *P = 0.00 |
| Once a year | 83 | 28.62 | 11.77±3.14 | |
| Once every few years | 80 | 27.59 | 12.38±3.08 | |
| Never | 101 | 34.82 | 10.42±3.66 | |
| **Smoking** | | | | *P = 0.00 |
| Yes | 160 | 55.17 | 10.55±3.34 | |
| No | 130 | 44.83 | 12.58±3.13 | |

SD = standard deviation; *P<0.05.

differentiation) of each item on the test were analyzed and found to be appropriate. In intervention studies, the validity of measurement/evaluation tools is an important measure of performance [29], as is the difficulty level of a question, often defined in terms of the proportion of respondents who answer it correctly. The PSSCT, a test containing 19 items of varying difficulty levels, was used to evaluate individuals' cognitions regarding the correct coping responses to stroke symptoms in this study. However, when respondents were tested on their knowledge regarding the onset of stroke symptoms with the items "I lack the proper medical knowledge, so I do not give any help to the patient" and "We should give the patient nitroglycerin or antihypertensive drugs for lower blood pressure, etc.," only about 28% and 29% of them (i.e., item difficulty levels = 0.28 and 0.29, respectively) were able to recognize the correct coping responses. This worrying result suggests the urgent need to improve the level of coping knowledge with regard to stroke symptoms among high-risk stroke patients and their family members in order to reduce the harm caused by strokes. Thus, designing and implementing comprehensive, professionally organized stroke health education programs aimed at community residents should be a priority.

The primary aim of this study was to develop the PSSCT as an evaluation tool with sound psychometric properties. The $KR_{20}$ coefficient was used in this study to estimate the reliability of the test as a whole and of each of its dimensions through all the stages of its development. The PSSCT yielded an overall $KR_{20}$ coefficient of 0.822. Prior research has indicated that content validity is the most important type of validity because it ensures

**Table 3.** The CVI, P, and D of each item on the test.

| Part | Please judge the appropriateness of the following coping responses in a situation where someone appears to be dizzy and falls suddenly to the ground, showing weakness on one side of the body, numbness, difficulty walking or speaking clearly, or is unconscious or has severe dizziness/headache: | CVI | P | D |
|---|---|---|---|---|
| Part I (coping with typical symptoms) | 1. I will call the patient and shake his/her body, checking whether the patient is conscious. | 0.85 | 0.66 | 0.54 |
| | 2. I will place the patient prostrate on the bed, with his/her head raised (on a pillow). | 0.90 | 0.64 | 0.16 |
| | 3. I will pick the patient up from the ground immediately, and check whether he/she is injured. | 0.80 | 0.72 | 0.62 |
| | 4. We should place the patient on our backs, and bring him/her to the ambulance. | 0.80 | 0.79 | 0.56 |
| | 5. We can support the patient with our hands, and bring him/her to the ambulance. | 0.85 | 0.66 | 0.60 |
| | 6. We can observe the patient for a moment; maybe after a moment, he/she will recover. | 0.70 | 0.60 | 0.50 |
| | 7. If the patient has suffered a head injury and is bleeding after falling, we can bandage his/her head to stop the bleeding. | 0.90 | 0.83 | 0.18 |
| | 8. I lack the proper medical knowledge, so I do not give any help to the patient. | 0.85 | 0.28 | 0.15 |
| | 9. We should prevent compression of the patient's numbness or paralysis of limbs. | 0.70 | 0.87 | 0.19 |
| | 10. We should give the patient nitroglycerin or antihypertensive drugs for lower blood pressure, etc. | 0.75 | 0.29 | 0.30 |
| | 11. We can drop the patient on the bed, and wait for the arrival of emergency personnel. | 0.78 | 0.70 | 0.66 |
| **Part II (coping with vomiting)** | **Please judge the appropriateness of the following coping responses in a situation where someone appears to have the abovementioned symptoms accompanied by nausea and vomiting:** | **CVI** | **P** | **D** |
| | 12. We should let the patient lie on the bed, with his/her head to one side. | 0.90 | 0.75 | 0.33 |
| | 13. We can flop the patient onto his/her back immediately. | 0.75 | 0.63 | 0.55 |
| | 14. We can give the patient water to eliminate food residues in his\her mouth cavity. | 0.85 | 0.39 | 0.49 |
| | 15. When the patient experiences shortness of breath and has phlegm in his/her throat, we can instruct him/her to cough. | 0.70 | 0.39 | 0.37 |
| | 16. When the patient is vomiting, we can thump the patient's back, so that we can get the vomit out. | 0.72 | 0.31 | 0.33 |
| **Part III (coping with twitching)** | **Please judge the appropriateness of the following coping responses in a situation where someone appears to have the abovementioned symptoms accompanied by twitching:** | **CVI** | **P** | **D** |
| | 17. If the patient is lying on the ground, we should pick the patient up and bring him/her to the hospital quickly. | 0.90 | 0.56 | 0.65 |
| | 18. When the patient twitches, we should turn his/her head to one side, in order to prevent asphyxia. | 0.90 | 0.83 | 0.25 |
| | 19. When the patient twitches and symptoms appear to have disappeared, there is no need to go to the hospital; the patient can have a good rest at home. | 0.70 | 0.70 | 0.44 |

CVI = content validity index; P = difficulty (of a test item); D = degree of differentiation (of a test item).

congruence between the research target and data collection tool [20]. Evidence for the PSSCT's content validity was based on both a review of the literature and the evaluation of eleven experts through the Delphi expert consultation method. The results demonstrated that all of the instrument's 19 items met acceptable CVI values of 0.70 or greater [30].

In this study, the PSSCT scores of individuals who had experienced a stroke were higher than were those of individuals who had not, which coincided with previous findings [31–33]. Our analysis revealed that those with experience had significantly higher total coping scores than did those without experience. Individuals who had experienced a stroke also scored significantly higher on coping with typical stroke symptoms and coping with twitching. This was likely the result of various factors. First, participants with such experience had been at the scene of the onset of a stroke or had personally encountered a stroke. They also tended to remember the stories of others they had met who had also experienced a stroke. Second, the caregivers of individuals

**Table 4.** The PSSCT scores of individuals who had experienced a stroke versus those who had not.

| PSSCT part | Score (mean ± SD) | | P |
|---|---|---|---|
| | With experience n = 70 | Without experience n = 220 | |
| Coping with typical stroke symptoms | 7.14±2.01 | 6.19±2.30 | *P = 0.001 |
| Coping with vomiting | 2.54±1.29 | 2.26±1.26 | P = 0.109 |
| Coping with twitching | 2.18±0.83 | 1.79±0.85 | *P = 0.001 |
| Total coping score | 11.86±3.27 | 10.23±3.51 | *P = 0.000 |

SD = standard deviation; *P<0.01.

who had experienced a stroke were usually long term. These caregivers were also typically responsible for managing not only the patients' daily lives but also their disease-related issues [34,35]. For example, caregivers were often very active in gathering information/knowledge about strokes. However, no significant differences in mean scores for coping with vomiting were observed between the two groups of participants in this study. Furthermore, when they were assessed on their knowledge pertaining to coping with the onset of symptoms associated with vomiting (e.g., "We can give the patient water to eliminate food residues in his\her mouth cavity;" "When the patient experiences shortness of breath and has phlegm in his/her throat, we can instruct him/her to cough;" and "When the patient is vomiting, we can thump the patient's back so that we can get the vomit out"), only about 30% to 40% of the residents knew how to respond correctly. A possible explanation for this discrepancy is that the occurrence of vomiting is relatively common and one that people tend to ignore. On the other hand, it might be an indication of the lack of knowledge residents have on how to cope with symptoms.

In addition to the abovementioned robust psychometric evidence, data and information presented in the section 3 provided support for the ability of PSSCT scores to reflect individuals' knowledge pertaining to coping with pre-hospital stroke symptoms. Several studies have shown that community residents lack stroke-related knowledge [12,19,22], including knowledge regarding risk factors for stroke and stroke warning signs, and awareness of strokes and transient ischemic attacks. What remains less clear is the extent of their knowledge regarding coping with stroke symptoms. Thus, the present study was conducted to fill this gap in understanding.

As with other instruments, there were several limitations to the PSSCT. The PSSCT can replicate only a part of what would actually be experienced by community residents in a real stroke situation. Therefore, continued efforts to portray symptoms in a more realistic manner are necessary. For example, multimedia technology (e.g., animation technology or vivid pictures) might be utilized to further increase the predictive value of test scores. Second, the purpose of this study was to develop and validate the PSSCT and not to conduct an epidemiological investigation. The participants recruited into the study might not have been representative of China's population at large. Therefore, caution is needed when generalizing the results of this study to other situations. Finally, a factor analysis was not performed in this study. Further examinations of the instrument's construct validity are thus required. Recommendations for future research include conducting further evaluations of the instrument in a greater number and wider range of groups, and developing and validating a culturally sensitive English language version of the PSSCT.

## Conclusion

This study aimed to develop a practical 19-item instrument to evaluate knowledge of coping with pre-hospital stroke symptoms among community residents. The PSSCT demonstrated robust internal consistency reliability and validity. Our findings also highlighted the importance of or necessity for community-oriented public education programs on the subject, as many residents lacked essential coping knowledge with regard to pre-hospital stroke symptoms. The insufficient coping knowledge of high-risk populations susceptible to stroke and their family members observed in this study presents a critical problem, but also vital clues into future directions for community health education on stroke. Furthermore, use of a standardized instrument, such as the PSSCT, would greatly facilitate cross-study comparisons.

## Acknowledgments

The authors would like to thank all community service personnel who helped with the research, and the participants of this study.

## Author Contributions

Conceived and designed the experiments: Q. Zhao Li Yang X. Zhang. Performed the experiments: Q. Zhao Li Yang X. Zhang X. Zhu Q. Zuo YW Liu Yang WG ML SC. Analyzed the data: Q. Zhao Li Yang X. Zhang. Contributed reagents/materials/analysis tools: X. Zhang YW. Contributed to the writing of the manuscript: Q. Zhao Li Yang X. Zhang.

## References

1. Kaste M, Norrving B (2010) From the World Stroke Day to the World Stroke Campaign: one in six: act now! Int J Stroke 5: 342–343.
2. Donnan GA (2011) Stroke in developing countries: the looming epidemic. Int J Stroke 6: 97.
3. Ministry of Health of the People's Republic of China (2008) The third national retrospect spot-check of death-cause. Neurol Res 17(5): 344–345.
4. Wang YJ, Zhang SM, Zhang L, Wang CX, Dong Q, et al. (2012) Chinese guidelines for the secondary prevention of ischemic stroke and transient ischemic attack 2010. CNS Neurosci Ther 18: 93–101.
5. Baldereschi M, Piccardi B, Di Carlo A, Lucente G, Guidetti D, et al. (2012) Relevance of prehospital stroke code activation for acute treatment measures in stroke care: a review. Cerebrovasc Dis 34: 182–190.
6. Bouckaert M, Lemmens R, Thijs V (2009) Reducing prehospital delay in acute stroke. Nat Rev Neurol 5: 477–483.
7. Ebinger M, Rozanski M, Waldschmidt C, Weber J, Wendt M, et al. (2012) PHANTOM-S: the prehospital acute neurological therapy and optimization of medical care in stroke patients - study. Int J Stroke 7: 348–353.
8. Weltermann BM, Homann J, Rogalewski A, Brach S, Voss S, et al. (2000) Stroke Knowledge Among Stroke Support Group Members. Stroke 31: 1230–1233.
9. Teuschl Y, Brainin M (2010) Stroke education: discrepancies among factors influencing prehospital delay and stroke knowledge. Int J Stroke 5: 187–208.
10. Lecouturier J, Rodgers H, Murtagh MJ, White M, Ford GA, et al. (2010) Systematic review of mass.

11. Fogle CC, Oser CS, Troutman TP, McNamara M, Williamson AP, et al. (2008) Public education strategies to increase awareness of stroke warning signs and the need to call 911. J Public Health Manage Pract 14: E17–E22.
12. Neau JP, Ingrand P, Godeneche G (2009) Awareness within the French population concerning stroke signs, symptoms, and risk factors. Clin Neurol Neurosurg 111: 659–664.
13. Abe IM, Lotufo PA, Goulart AC, Bensenor IM (2011) Stroke prevalence in a poor neighbourhood of Sao Paulo, Brazil: applying a stroke symptom questionnaire. Int J Stroke 6: 33–39.
14. Billings-Gagliardi S, Mazor KM (2005) Development and validation of the stroke action test. Stroke 36: 1035–1039.
15. Hickey A, Holly D, McGee H, Conroy R, Shelley E (2012) Knowledge of stroke risk factors and warning signs in Ireland: development and application of the Stroke Awareness Questionnaire (SAQ). Int J Stroke 7: 298–306.
16. Long A, Hesketh A, Bowen A (2009) Communication outcome after stroke: a new measure of the carer'perspective. Clinical Rehabilitation 23: 846–856.
17. Ferris A, Robertson RM, Fabunmi R, Mosca L (2005) American Heart Association and American Stroke Association national survey of stroke risk awareness among women. Circulation 111: 1321–1326.
18. The European Stroke Organisation (ESO) Executive Committee and the ESO Writing Committee (2008) Guidelines for management of ischaemic stroke and transient ischaemic attack 2008. Cerebrovasc Dis 25: 457–507.
19. Weltermann BM, Berger K, Rogalewski A, Homann J, Schulte H, et al. (1999) Knowledge about stroke in a German occupational cohort [in German]. Aktuelle Neurol 26: V87.
20. Nunnally JC (1994) Psychometric theory. New York: McGraw-Hill.
21. Labeau SO, Witdouck SS, Vandijck DM, Claes B, Rello J, et al (2010) Nurses' Knowledge of Evidence-Based Guidelines for the Prevention of Surgical Site Infection. Worldviews on Evidence-Based Nursing 7: 16–24.
22. Sug Yoon S, Heller RF, Levi C, Wiggers J, Fitzgerald PE (2001) Knowledge of Stroke Risk Factors, Warning Symptoms, and Treatment Among an Australian Urban Population. Stroke 32: 1926–1930.
23. Hickey A, O'Hanlon A, McGee H, Donnellan C, Shelley E, et al. (2009) Stroke awareness in the general population: knowledge of stroke risk factors and warning signs in older adults. BMC Geriatr 9: 35.
24. Umberson D (1987) Family status and health behaviors: social control as a dimension of social integration. Health Soc Behav 28: 306–319.
25. Dubois S, Loiselle CG (2009) Cancer informational support and health care service use among individuals newly diagnosed: a mixed methods approach. J Eval Clin Pract 15: 346–359.
26. Yusuf S, Islam S, Chow CK, Rangarajan S, Dagenais G, et al. (2011) Use of secondary prevention drugs for cardiovascular disease in the community in high-income, middle-income, and low-income countries (the PURE Study): a prospective epidemiological survey. 378: 1231–43.
27. Braig S, Peter R, Nagel G, Hermann S, Rohrmann S, et al. (2011) The impact of social status inconsistency on cardiovascular risk factors, myocardial infarction and stroke in the EPIC-Heidelberg cohort. BMC Public Health 11: 104.
28. Haladyna TM (1999) Developing and validating multiple-choice test items. Hillsdale. NJ: Lawrence Erlbaum Asso-ciates.
29. van der Meulen I, van de Sandt-Koenderman WM, Duivenvoorden HJ, Ribbers GM (2010) Measuring verbal and non-verbal communication in aphasia: reliability, validity, and sensitivity to change of the Scenario Test. Int J Lang Commun Disord 45: 424–435.
30. Polit DF, Beck CT, Owen SV (2007) Is the CVI an acceptable indicator of content validity? Appraisal and recommendations. Res Nurs Health 30: 459–467.
31. Góngora-Rivera F, Gutiérrez-Jiménez E, Zenteno MA, GEPEVC Investigators (2009) Knowledge of ischemic stroke among a Mexico City population. J Stroke Cerebrovasc Dis 18: 208–213.
32. Kim YS, Park SS, Bae HJ, Cho AH, Cho YJ, et al. (2011) Stroke awareness decreases prehospital delay after acute ischemic stroke in Korea. BMC Neurol 11: 2.
33. White JH, Bynon BL, Marquez J, Sweetapple A, Pollack M (2013)' Masterstroke: a pilot group stroke prevention program for community dwelling stroke survivors'. Disabil Rehabil 35: 931–938.
34. Robinson-Smith G, Mahoney C (1995) Coping and marital equilibrium after stroke J Neurosci Nurs 27: 83–89.
35. Exall K, Johnston H (1999) Caring for carers coping with stroke Nurs Times 95: 50–51.

# 11

# Understanding of Factors that Enable Health Promoters in Implementing Health-Promoting Schools: A Systematic Review and Narrative Synthesis of Qualitative Evidence

**Tommy Tsz Man Hung[1]*, Vico Chung Lim Chiang[1], Angela Dawson[2], Regina Lai Tong Lee[1]**

**1** School of Nursing, The Hong Kong Polytechnic University, Hung Hom, Kowloon, HKSAR, **2** Health Services and Practice, Faculty of Health, University of Technology, Sydney, Australia

## Abstract

Health-promoting schools have been regarded as an important initiative in promoting child and adolescent health in school settings using the whole-school approach. Quantitative research has proved its effectiveness in various school-based programmes. However, few qualitative studies have been conducted to investigate the strategies used by health promoters to implement such initiatives. In this study, the researchers conducted a systematic review and narrative synthesis of the qualitative literature to identify important enablers assisting the implementation of health-promoting schools from the perspectives of health promoters. Five enablers have been identified from the review: (a) Following a framework/guideline to implement health-promoting schools; (b) Obtaining committed support and contributions from the school staff, school board management, government authorities, health agencies and other stakeholders; (c) Adopting a multidisciplinary, collaborative approach to implementing HPS; (d) Establishing professional networks and relationships; and (e) Continuing training and education in school health promotion. This highlights the importance of developing school health policies that meet local health needs, and socio-cultural characteristics that can foster mutual understanding between the health and education sectors so as to foster health promotion in children and adolescents.

**Editor:** Yoshihiro Kokubo, National Cardiovascular Center Hospital, Japan

**Funding:** The authors have no support or funding to report.

**Competing Interests:** The authors have declared that no competing interests exist.

* Email: tommy.hung@connect.polyu.hk

## Introduction

The concept of Health-Promoting Schools (HPS) evolved in the 1980s and has been regularly advocated as an effective approach to promoting health in schools [1,2]. The concept of HPS embodies a whole-school approach to community health promotion, in which a broad health education curriculum is supported by the ethos and the environment of the school [3–5]. The World Health Organization [WHO] [6] states that "a health-promoting school is one that constantly strengthens its capacity as a healthy setting for living, learning and working". It is effective in encouraging children to adopt health-enhancing behaviours and in reducing health-compromising behaviours [2,7]. The HPS approach has been widely accepted by the education sector as an effective and important method of implementing a school health programme [8–10]. However, collaboration between the health and education sectors is not always optimal to achieve the common goal of improving students' health, due their traditionally-rooted role expectations [11], such as the fact that teachers are expected to ensure students' academic achievement while school nurses aim for behavioural changes among the students [11]. Although the health and education sectors may share the same goal of improving students' health, their different approaches to the issue and the outcome measures developed are based on different assumptions [11]. Traditionally, educators assume that students are able to make relevant health-related behavioural changes if they have acquired the appropriate knowledge, thus the outcomes are based on cognitive skills such as remembering, understanding, applying, analysing, evaluating and creating [11]. On the other hand, training in the health sector requires healthcare professionals to assess biometric outcomes and the prevalence of diseases, such as body mass index and the prevalence of substance use in the school setting [11]. This fundamental difference between the health and education sectors has led to different understandings of the terms "health education" and "health promotion", which are often applied differently or interchangeably [12], as well as different theoretical bases used in conducting school-based health interventions [1].

The WHO Ottawa Charter for Health Promotion [13] has inspired healthcare professionals to re-define suitable strategies for health promotion. The Ottawa Charter identified five key action strategies: *building healthy public policy, creating supportive environments, strengthening community action, developing personal skills* and *reorienting health services*. These key strategies have advanced the traditional way of school-based health intervention from focusing on biometrics outcome-based evaluation (which is usually from the health sector perspective) to the multifaceted whole-school approach, which also emphasizes collaboration within and outside schools. However, Croghan, Johnson and Aveyard [14] suggested that historical, political, cultural and contextual sphere influence the health promoters' potential in practising school health promotion. This means that even in schools that have "explicitly" adopted the HPS initiative, variations occur in the implementation process as well as the outcomes, in addition to the fact that evaluation of the HPS is challenging in itself due to the complexity of school settings and the ambiguity of definitions and understandings of "health education" and "health promotion" by different staff in schools [1,5,12]. Therefore, in order to understand how schools successfully implement HPS, process evaluation has been widely suggested by different authors after they have performed intervention studies or systematic reviews [1,2,15]. However, they also comment that process evaluation is difficult due to the lack of detailed descriptions of every single step of the health intervention programmes, as well as the fact that it is frequently necessary for implementers to modify the programmes in the complex, ever-changing school settings [1,2,15].

As a result, the authors here attempted to use qualitative methods to explore factors that facilitate collaborative action in order to deliver effective HPS from the perspectives of both health and education providers. This review sought to identify:

(a) The factors that facilitate the delivery of HPS (the enablers), and

(b) Strategies to better support health promoters in delivering the HPS intervention.

In this paper, we refer to both health and education professionals who contribute to school health education or health promotion as health promoters.

## Methodology

We employed a narrative synthesis methodology in this integrative review of peer-reviewed literature due to the variety of study methodologies, interventions, settings and influencing factors [14]. Narrative synthesis is suitable for synthesizing findings from a range of studies that are insufficiently similar to use specialist synthesis approaches such as statistical meta-analysis and meta-ethnography [16]. A number of systematic reviews have been done that aimed at finding evidence of the effectiveness of the HPS approach [1,2,15]. The inclusion criteria in these reviews varied, yet all of the articles included were solely experimental studies. In addition, these reviews discussed and questioned the appropriateness of adopting RCTs to study school health promotion interventions or programmes. For example, the flexible and whole-school approach of HPS, which involves the participation and interaction of the health promoters, makes it too complex to perform a RCT [17]. RCTs involve statistical assumptions that yield large sample sizes, making the interventions expensive and difficult to implement [1,15]. The heterogeneity of different interventions make the combination of results (e.g. meta-analysis) impossible, and even process evaluations are difficult as the interventions are likely to be implemented poorly [15]. Further, in some cases these intervention- or curriculum-based approaches might not necessarily reflect the whole-school philosophy of HPS [18]. Therefore, incorporating qualitative approaches in research on HPS has been suggested [1,15,17,18], and this systematic review adopts a narrative synthesis approach which targets studies that focus on the whole-school approach of HPS. This review was undertaken according to Popay et al.'s guidance on conducting narrative synthesis in systematic reviews [16].

### Search methods

The search aimed to identify the textual and narrative evidence from the literature on health promoters' experiences in implementing HPS. Four electronic databases, CINAHL, Ovid, Medline and Web of Knowledge, were searched, as well as The Journal of School Nursing and the Journal of School Health. The databases were searched for the period from 2002 to December 2012, so that the selected articles would be relevant to the current societal and educational climate [19]. The date of the last search was 31 December 2013. A combination of keywords and thesaurus terms was used in the databases: health promoters (or health promotion actors, principals, teachers, school nurses, stakeholders), AND school (or school-based), AND health promotion (or promoting school, comprehensive school health, and coordinated school health), AND qualitative research (or focus groups, grounded theory, semi-structured interviews and framework). The results obtained were then combined with experience, strategy, programme and/or implementation. Reference lists of related articles were reviewed, and experts in the areas were approached to suggest relevant studies. In order to achieve a broad scope of literature, there were no restrictions on language, publication type or study design. Non-English articles were only excluded for eligibility at the full-text assessment stage. Studies were included if (a) the research included health promoters (principals, teachers, school nurses and/or other staff involved in school health promotion), and (b) the study aimed to explore the views of the process of implementing health-promoting schools.

The review employed the PRISMA (Preferred Reporting Items for Systematic Reviews and Meta-Analysis) statement [20]. The PRISMA flow diagram (Figure S1 and Checklist S1) illustrates the process followed in this review.

### Quality appraisal

The Critical Appraisal Skills Programme (CASP) Qualitative Checklist was used to assess the quality of the six included studies [21]. It contains 10 questions (items) which guide researchers in reviewing qualitative studies. Each item was checked "Yes", "Can't tell" or "No". Under each item, there were hints (guiding questions) for consideration. For items that were checked "Can't tell" or "No" in the appraisal, comments were given independently and discussed between the first and last authors (TTMH & RLTL) in case of disagreement (Table 1). All the six included articles were checked "Yes" for items 1, 2, 3, 7, 8, and 9. The comments are discussed in the following paragraphs.

Inchley et al. [27] did not fully explain how and why they selected the "key stakeholders" for in-depth interviews, or the criteria for student and teacher selection in the focus group interviews (item 4). Pryjmachuk et al. [31] conducted focus group interviews in which all of the participants were female. However, they did not explain why or the potential bias in their results due to the absence of young males (item 4). Keshavarz et al. [28] did not report how they interviewed the staff (item 5). Inchley et al. [27], Keshavarz et al. [28], Morberg et al. [29], and Gugglberger [32] inadequately considered the relationship between researcher and participants in the data collection, discussion and limitations sections of their articles (item 6).

However, all six studies were considered as having passed the quality appraisal after being scrutinized and evaluated by the four authors, as they were important in contributing qualitative

**Table 1.** Summary of characteristics of the six included articles (part 1/3).

| Article | Total sample size | Participants involved | Number of participants contributing qualitative evidence | Study methods | Methods yielding qualitative evidence | Number of interviews/ questions, duration, group size | Main results | Quality appraisal CASP Qualitative Checklist (items 1–9 only) |
|---|---|---|---|---|---|---|---|---|
| [27] | 25 | Health promotion specialists, education officers/advisers, client services officers, catering manager, kitchen supervisor, community dietician, school project coordinator, and other school staff | 25 | Evaluation of the process of a 4-year project within the European Network of Health Promoting Schools in Scotland by multiple case studies | Analysed thematically; in-depth individual interviews; focus group interviews | Forty interviews (baseline and follow-up); duration not mentioned | *Four themes highlighted factors that facilitate translation of HPS principles into practice:*Ownership and empowerment, leadership and management, collaboration, Integration. | 1. Yes; 2. Yes; 3. Yes; 4. Can't tell; 5. Yes; 6. No; 7. Yes; 8. Yes; 9. Yes |
| [28] | 26 | Principals and teachers | 26 | Examining the educational perspectives on implementation of a health-promoting school programme in Sydney | Analysing process drew upon the framework of *complex adaptive systems;* semi-structured individual interviews | Not mentioned | In light of the *complex adaptive systems*: Diversity of component parts and sub-systems of the schools was acknowledged; diversity in and between schools led to diversity of opinion; reaching an agreement on "rules" became difficult; operating context is unique for each school. Failure to recognize the contextual differences led to unrealistic expectations of what schools might achieve; various interaction patterns identified; interactions between schools and the health sector were limited; lots of health-related information which needed prioritization in its flow. | 1. Yes; 2. Yes; 3. Yes; 4. Yes; 5. No; 6. No; 7. Yes; 8. Yes; 9. Yes |

evidence relating to health promoters' experiences in implementing HPS (item 10).

## Data abstraction

All articles were read and the data extracted by two reviewers (TTMH & RLTL) who made decisions regarding inclusion or exclusion. Where possible, consensus was obtained by meeting to compare decisions. In the event of disagreement, a third reviewer (VCLC or AD) read the articles and contributed to decisions and consensus.

## Synthesis

According to [16], one of the purposes of narrative synthesis is to organize findings from included studies in order to identify and list the enablers and the strategies supporting implementation, as well as exploring the relationship between the reported enablers and the supportive strategies. The descriptions may point to a linear process, yet it is a back and forth process in which the synthesis begins as early as in the line-by-line coding [22]. The synthesis was done by data extraction from all of the text labelled as "results" or "findings" in the included studies [22]. Coding was done with the focus on the aim of the present study, at the same time being open-minded to allow for the possibility of different or better fit of codes emerging [22,23]. Each reviewer did the coding and synthesis independently, and through discussion more abstract or analytical themes began to emerge.

# Results

The study characteristics for the six included articles are summarized in Table 1–3. The full text of articles was included when they met the inclusion criteria and passed the quality appraisal. All other included studies mentioned adopting the WHO HPS. The WHO's definition of a HPS is 'one that constantly strengthens its capacity as a healthy setting for living, learning and working'. All included articles are considered to have adopted the whole-school approach, with health promotion supported by the ethos and the environment of the school, rather than just from a narrow perspective reflecting the current health issues of the country or region [2,11]. Most of the studies were conducted in European countries that possess a long history of implementation of HPS [24,25]. Three studies drew upon the HPS concept [26–28]. Three articles, although not stating explicitly whether they were adopting the HPS concept, were conducted in Sweden [29,30] and the UK [31], which have joined the HPS-driven SHE Network. All of them were qualitative research studies that identified and reported themes as findings. Two studies [29,32] used the grounded theory approach in analysing data, but did not aim to generate theory. One study [31] used the framework approach in analysing data. One study [28] presented theory-based qualitative analysis by drawing upon the concept of complex adaptive systems. Five articles have been suggested by experts in the field [14,19,33–35], but they were excluded due to being in non-school settings, focusing on school nurses' role only, solely quantitative design, or beyond the time span covered (Figure S1).

Five key themes were identified in the narrative synthesis that provided insights into the enablers of the delivery of HPS, including supportive strategies to assist health promoters. The findings extracted from the original articles, the examples of codes and the five themes synthesised from the narrative synthesis are outlined in Table 4–9. The themes (enablers) are described below and the synthesised strategies to better support health promoters in implementing HPS are addressed in the discussion.

## Enabler 1: Following a framework/guideline to implement HPS

Keshavarz et al. [28] and Morberg et al. [29] mentioned that a clear, well-defined and systematic framework of HPS is needed in order to carry out specific programmes successfully. Even policies that were "evidence-informed" might not yield similar outcomes due to the diversity in and between schools, which should be addressed by health promoters and external stakeholders so as to formulate realistic health goals for different schools [28]. Keshavarz et al. [28] also reported that there were not many guidelines that might direct schools to become HPS, nor would the schools follow externally imposed ones. Echoing Keshavarz et al.'s notion of setting up realistic health goals for different schools, Gugglberger suggested that school health promotion should be "precisely structured with certain phases, aims and milestones", and that "systematic proceedings are necessary for a mutually successful project" ([32], p. 452). Thus, the schools following the HPS framework should consider tailoring their efforts to the individual local context [28]. As reported in the included studies, some health promoters viewed HPS as "add-ons" [27] and "taking extra time" [28], often competing with other programmes or basic routines [30]. As a result, the health promoters, particularly teachers and school nurses as reported, had to prioritise their work, although health promotion was usually given lower priority than "educational achievement" [27,28,30].

The staff might lose their enthusiasm for carrying on the school health promotion work, regardless of the apparent immediate results, because a sense of ownership by the individual school was insufficient [27]. In order to develop this sense of ownership, the HPS framework should enable "each member to play a much fuller role in strategic planning and professional decision-making" [27]. The health promoters should also be empowered with the autonomy to set health promotion as the priority [29], with the framework/guideline being flexible in its interpretation, assessment of school needs, developing aims and objectives of school health promotion, allocation of budgets, implementation and evaluation of outcomes [27,28].

## Enabler 2: Obtaining committed support and contributions from the school staff, school board management, government authorities, health agencies and other stakeholders

A number of studies in this review identified the critical role of the school board management in supporting the implementation of HPS in terms of finance, coordination, policy and commitment [27–30,32]. "[The support] is the duty of the school administration, it's a very important function... otherwise the school [will] get lost" ([32], p. 452). "It's scary how crucial [senior management] are because it can be frustrating... because there is no support" ([27], p. 68). The principal's individual motivation played a key role in establishing relationships and fostering interactions between schools and the health sector, and also between the health-promoting schools [28,32], which in turn facilitated the exchanges of health-related knowledge, experiences, and resources [28]. As also mentioned in Enabler 1, the sense of ownership and empowerment was related to financial support, especially if the health promoters "could spend that money how they felt it should spent" ([27], p.68). Another request for financial support from the school board management is to pay for the overtime work and extra contributions of the health promoters, particularly the teachers. One of the researchers commented that "[the lack of] financial incentives for teachers was therefore

**Table 2.** Summary of characteristics of the six included articles (part 2/3).

| Article | Total sample size | Participants involved | Number of participants contributing qualitative evidence | Study methods | Methods yielding qualitative evidence | Number of interviews/ questions, duration, group size | Main results | Quality appraisal CASP Qualitative Checklist (items 1–9 only) |
|---|---|---|---|---|---|---|---|---|
| [28] (continued) | | | | | | | Quality and quantity of the information was not always productive; formal and informal feedback loops identified among teachers, students and their parent; formal organization "rules" vs perceived and internalized "rules"; limited sections of curriculum or rules/policies to guide schools in becoming HPS; various attributes of credit and blame to the schools, including award schemes and media coverage; various changes required learning and adaptation, which may not lead to positive change from a health perspective; school behaviour was emergent in nature | |
| [29] | 9 | Head school nurses | 9 | To gain a deeper understanding of how head school nurses in Sweden perceive their leadership in developing school health care | Constructivist grounded theory approach; individual interviews (informal conversation) | Twelve interviews lasting 90 minutes each | *Core category* – Balancing between vague formal goals and strong informal goals. Vague formal goals (subcategory): vague political/state directives for school health care; vague organizational delegation for school health care. Strong informal goals (subcategory): Protecting professional boundaries; protecting traditional routines. Creating local goals (subcategory): Construction, negotiation and implementation of local goals; meeting school nurses' expectations of supportive leadership | 1. Yes; 2. Yes; 3. Yes; 4. Yes; 5. Yes; 6. Can't tell; 7. Yes; 8. Yes; 9. Yes |

**Table 3.** Summary of characteristics of the six included articles (part 3/3).

| Article | Total sample size | Participants involved | Number of participants contributing qualitative evidence | Study methods | Methods yielding qualitative evidence | Number of interviews/ questions, duration, group size | Main results | Quality appraisal CASP Qualitative Checklist (items 1–9 only) |
|---|---|---|---|---|---|---|---|---|
| [30] | 8 | School nurses | 8 | Description of school health nurses' experiences of the conditions for health promotion work and the aspects that they found important for the success of school health promotion. | Data analysed by content analysis; semi-structured individual interviews | Eight interviews lasting about one hour each | *Three themes that school nurses considered to be important for school health promotion:* Organization, support, and knowledge. | All Yes for item 1–9 |
| [31] | 33 | School nurses | 33 | Exploring school nurses' perspective on managing mental health problems in children and young people. | Data analysed using the framework approach; focus group interviews | Four focus group interviews each involving six to twelve participants and lasting around one hour | *Four main themes on the views of school nurses regarding mental health work in young people:* The mental health of children and young people, organizational issues, barriers to doing mental health work, and facilitators of doing mental health work. | All "Yes" except item 4 ("Can't tell") |
| [32] | 23 | HP actors | 23 | Developing a typology of supporting strategies for schools in Austria. | Grounded theory approach; in-depth face-to-face semi-structured interviews; documents | Eighteen interviews lasting between thirty to one hundred and twenty four minutes | *Five types of support for HPS:* Organise exchanges among schools, establish certification and quality control of school health promotion efforts, offer consultation and information concerning health promotion, carry out specific health promotion programmes, and coordinate health promotion actors and information. | All "Yes" except item 6 ("Can't tell") |

**Table 4.** Enabler 1 and supportive strategies through narrative synthesis.

| Synthesized theme | Examples of codes | Examples identified in original texts (author, year, page) | Possible supportive strategies |
|---|---|---|---|
| Enabler 1: Following a framework/ guideline to implement HPS | Lack of rules/ policies | [The] formal rules sometimes were not very simple or were not followed by all agents of the schools. There were not many rules/policies that might guide schools in becoming health-promoting schools" [28]. | Simplify rules/policies that guide schools in becoming HPS |
| | Lack of guidelines | "When I [the school nurse] started five years ago, there was nothing, absolutely nothing. There was no handbook, no common guidelines' " [29]. | Establish a health-related framework/guideline for school health promoters |
| | Rules/policies are flexible to be interpreted; tailored implementation of rules/policies | "We [the school] have to say that we fit into the Department of Education... so our core has to be the parameters that they set. How we interpret [the parameters] has to reflect the needs of the children that we have in our school" [28]. | Adopt the framework/ guideline in a flexible manner to meet individual schools' needs |
| | Huge workload; prioritising work; competing tasks | "Demands usually come that way and it just keeps raining and we [teachers] just can't keep up with them all, which is why we have to prioritise" [28]. "I [school nurse] think I can set the priorities on my own but I have to stick to the basic programme, which stipulates what I have to do during the school year" [30]. "...Many of the staff said, 'I haven't got time to give (to health), apart from the normal sports time' " [28]. | Prioritise health in school policies |
| | Time-consuming; HPS as an extracurricular activity | "One of the difficulties of the health-promoting schools is that it takes away from something else... So if you are going to have one of those, something else has to give a little, because it takes extra time, it takes extra lessons often, to cover the curriculum fully" [28]. | Incorporate HPS into the curriculum |

identified as the biggest hindering factor for HP [health promotion] intervention by the actors" [32].

Besides the support from the school board management, the attitudes and the commitment of the school staff played a vital part in the success. A positive attitude such as not seeing the HPS as an "add-on" [27], and the willingness to commit time [28] determined the contribution of the health promoters. For example, huge workloads and time constraints were commonly reported in most of the selected studies [27,28,30,32]. "Many of the staff have said, 'I haven't got any time to give [to health], apart from the normal sport time' " ([28], p. 1471). Some health promoters were motivated by appreciation for their efforts from external parties

**Table 5.** Enabler 2 and supportive strategies through narrative synthesis (part 1/2).

| Synthesized theme | Examples of codes | Examples identified in original texts (author, year, page) | Possible supportive strategies |
|---|---|---|---|
| Enabler 2: Obtaining committed support and contributions from the school staff, school board management, government authorities, health agencies and other stakeholders | School management's support; worked over-time; financial support; government's help; empowering | "School boards financed additional teachers' hours with the help of the provincial governments" [32]. "I think [the money] was really important for the school... It gave them a sense of empowerment surrounding their part in the project, that they could spend that money how they felt it should be spent..." [27]. | To compensate teachers for extra hours spent on school health promotion |
| | School management's support | "One condition of health promotion activities is that there is a [head teacher] and other people in managerial positions who believe that activities to promote health are important" [30]. | To obtain the committed support of school management |
| | Appreciation; media/ marketing; politics/ politicians; recognising efforts; under-recognising the importance of health | "At my [HP actor] visits to schools I see that they are terribly glad when someone says that they're doing a great job. That's very important, also in the media, also from politics, a big recognition" [32]. The 'Healthy School' seal of approval is an outwardly visible sign that concepts and measures of school health promotion are applied in a school [32]. [The] certificate was a way to show appreciation for the school. [The health promotion actors] also stressed that: "It's important to make schools' achievements visible" [32]. School nurses' availability was reported as a factor for school security, as well as an advantage in marketing local schools [29]. | To recognise health promoters'/schools' efforts through certification, marketing and political means |
| | Cultures in society; emphasising academic achievement over children's health | "[Health] gets pushed to the side. Because then the media comes at you and says why aren't you teaching kids to read properly and we get the blame. It's better to let the child get fat than to let the child get low marks. Why? Because that's what society thinks is more important, a lot of people anyway." [28]. | To cultivate a health-oriented culture in society |

**Table 6.** Enabler 2 and supportive strategies through narrative synthesis (part 2/2).

| Synthesized theme | Examples of codes | Examples identified in original texts (author, year, page) | Possible supportive strategies |
|---|---|---|---|
| Enabler 2 (continued): Obtaining committed support and contributions from the school staff, school board management, government authorities, health agencies and other stakeholders | Banning the selling of unhealthy food and its advertisement (school management support); choosing of food suppliers and the food provided (food suppliers' cooperation) | The banning of advertising or selling 'unhealthy food' in canteens in many schools had led to changes in the food suppliers' practices towards providing more healthy options [28]. | To ban the sale and advertisement of unhealthy food in schools; to choose appropriate food suppliers that provide healthy food options |
| | Coordinating; school administration | "It's the duty of the school administration, it's a very important function, the task of coordination and to repeatedly suggest what's new, what you can do, how to develop. Otherwise the schools get lost." [32]. | To coordinate the implementation of health-promoting schools |
| | Lack of communication between schools and between school and health sectors limited the exchange of knowledge, experiences and resources | "...[The] limitations on interactions between schools and the health sector, and also between the health-promoting schools, there were relatively few exchanges of health-related knowledge, experiences, and resources" [28]. | To communicate between schools and between the school and health sectors to facilitate exchanges of knowledge, experiences and resources |
| | School management's support; enthusiastic teachers; school management's motivation; low level of commitment | "It's scary how crucial [senior management] are because it can be quite frustrating, particularly if you have enthusiastic teachers but they don't get anything moving forward because there's no support..." [27]. "It appears that the principal's individual motivation played a key role in establishing this relationship where it existed" [28]. | To assimilate the teachers and the school management's attitude to school health promotion |

**Table 7.** Enabler 3 and supportive strategies through narrative synthesis.

| Synthesized theme | Examples of codes | Examples identified in original texts (author, year, page) | Possible supportive strategies |
|---|---|---|---|
| Enabler 3: Adopting a multidisciplinary, collaborative approach to implementing HPS | Organisational linkages; networking; regular meetings | "What I think is missing is to link up the organizations. Cooperation and collaboration across the provinces and with national [health promoters] was rare ... Only the social security institutions have a supra-provincial structure and meet regularly" [32]. | To organise regular sessions for mutual support, exchanging health-related information and school health promotion experiences between health promoters, between schools, and between schools and parents |
| | Exchanging information and experiences | "[Schools] exchange experiences and see how the others are doing, with the aim of getting new input" [32]. | |
| | Exchanging information between schools and parents | "A member of the catering staff attended a parents' evening, providing information about school meals service and the quality of the food [that] they had started to supply" [27]. | |
| | Preserving resources; Working together | [Exchange] encourage[s] reflection in schools, so that schools might be able to save resources by working together on [health promotion] issues, and [so] that they can discuss problems and solutions [32]. | |
| | Exchanging information | Exchang[ing] [information and experiences] can have long-term and sustainable effects that last even if the supporting structure is no longer provided [32]. | |
| | Multidisciplinary; assigning roles/ responsibilities collaboration | "If you are going to have a multi-agency, multi-disciplinary group... people do need to have a clear and distinct role within it. And if that's kind of thrashed out beforehand then I think it makes things easier in terms of the action plan and who's going to play what part" [27]. "What we are doing now seems to be more of an integral part of the school, but in a much wider sense because [the Catering Manager] and [Deputy Head Teacher] see a lot of each other and we discuss things..." [27]. | To adopt a multidisciplinary collaborative approach with clear assignment of roles/ responsibilities |
| | Clear organisational structure; assigning roles/responsibilities; unclear assignment of roles/ responsibilities | When there was a clear organisational structure with a clear division of responsibilities, this was good for health promotion activities in school, according to the school health nurses [30]. "I'm [the head school nurse] responsible for the activity manager's tasks, but again I'm not, I don't know... they're not formally delegated to me but I still do the task. Developing healthcare quality, for example, I think the activity manager is also responsible for developing quality" [29]. | To establish a clear organisational structure with clear assignment of roles/responsibilities |
| | Involving students | "The student council has a suggestion box... for new things in the school or something to be improved..." [27]. | Incorporate students' opinions |

**Table 8.** Enabler 4 and supportive strategies through narrative synthesis.

| Synthesized theme | Examples of codes | Examples identified in original texts (author, year, page) | Possible supportive strategies |
|---|---|---|---|
| Enabler 4: Establishing networks and relationships with stakeholders | Collaborating with specialists | "I'd like to work with a school doctor who's specialized in children and young people. That would be really good" [30]. "Cooperation between the SHS in my school and the ear specialist in the municipality functions very well, so we send referrals to him and then he comes here and informs us what he and we can do in the school… it's the same with the skin specialist, she comes here and gives presentations and we discuss pupils' problems" [30]. | To establish professional networks |
| | Maintaining relationships within and outside schools | [School nurses] described how space and legitimacy for the work of school nurses depended on trust and a good relationship between the head school nurse and the head teachers, as well as local politicians and organisational leaders [29]. Good relationships [between the school nurses and CAMHS] tended to be a facilitator of school nurses… [31]. | To maintain a positive relationship with school health promotion stakeholders |
| | Acting as a coordinator | "[Health promotion specialists play] a crucial role in being "the glue", in keeping everything together and making contacts" [27]. | To assign a full-time coordinator(s) in the implementation of HPS |
| | Acting as a coordinator; being present | Local negotiations and being a link between school nurses and their decision makers was seen as an important part of the role… Being present in different situations was reported as a priority strategy for visualizing and profiling school health care in the municipalities [29]. | |
| | Interrupted collaboration; working part-time/ term-time only | "… you've [the school nurse] got six weeks [because you work only during term-time,] then where they [the schools/other supporting agencies] haven't got that support network or that contact… and I am thinking what am I going to walk into when I walk back in in *[sic]* September" [31]. | |
| | Getting support from peers | "Because we're all based in one place we're very lucky… whenever you come back to the office there'll be somebody there you know and if you've had a particular[ly] difficul chat with a young person there's usually somebody there that you can go back and offload [on]" [31]. | To acquire peer support |
| | Arranging education and training on topics of relationship building and maintenance, and conflict resolution | A good relationship among the school nurses, as well as continuing education… was seen as a priority strategy for strengthening the school nurses' profession… sometimes in conflict with the head teachers, the head school nurses regularly arranged priority meetings as well as education and training for school nurses in the municipality [29]. | To arrange education and training on topics of relationship building and maintenance and conflict resolution |

(such as the media and politicians), which could sometimes compensate for the lack of incentives [32]. Certificates awarded to the schools which "make the school achievements visible" also served this purpose [32].

While the health promoters perceived such recognition as crucial to their motivation in school health promotion, attitudes towards health or the culture of society also affect health promoters' motivation: "[health] gets pushed to the side… It's better that the child be fat than that the child get low marks. *Why?*

**Table 9.** Enabler 5 and supportive strategies through narrative synthesis.

| Synthesized theme | Examples of codes | Examples identified in original texts (author, year, page) | Possible supportive strategies |
|---|---|---|---|
| Enabler 5: continuing training and education in school health promotion | Unclear professional development pathway | "The head school nurses also described that there were no clear goals for their competence development. There were no formalized directives, study programmes or academic degrees for being a head school nurse" [29]. There was a general feeling that there were difficulties and limited opportunities to find suitable courses for developing their role as a head school nurse [29]. | To formulate professional developmental plan for school health promoters |
| | Lack of confidence related to perceived inadequate experiences and knowledge | "…well I [school nurse] said this but I'm not sure whether that was the right thing to say… it's just having that confidence that you are saying the right thing" [31]. "…I think we're worried about doing it wrong and we're worried about doing it badly" [31]. | To offer health promoters the opportunities of professional training and education in school health promotion |
| | Lack of confidence related to perceived inadequate experiences and knowledge (continued) | "You are really inexperienced when you start as a school health nurse, and it takes time before you've passed all the training courses. It would have been useful to have more skills related to the SHS included in the basic training" [30]. "I'd like to use the computer more to provide parents, colleagues and politicians with statistics on the well-being of our pupils. I don't know how to do that, but I'm supposed to be going on a training course" [30]. | To offer health promoters opportunities of professional training and education in school health promotion. |

Because society thinks [academic achievement] is more important, a lot of people anyway" [28, p. 1471, emphasis in original]. This culture might also be transmitted through the media: "Because then the media comes at you and says why aren't you teaching kids to read properly and we [teachers] get the blame" ([28], p. 1471).

Food suppliers' commitment contributes to the success of HPS. Keshavarz et al. [28] reported that "the banning of advertising and selling 'unhealthy food' in canteens led to the food suppliers' practice of providing more healthy options" ([28], p. 1471–1472). Therefore the school board management has to make policies to ensure that the food supplied and purchased is healthy for the children [28]. Gugglberger [32] found that the health promoters perceived that they obtained more support when consultation was given to their schools individually. Other support that the stakeholders could offer included health information and manuals, workshops and training in school health promotion, and symposia that facilitated exchange of knowledge and experiences [32].

## Enabler 3: Adopting a multidisciplinary, collaborative approach to implementing HPS

The health promoters believed that a multidisciplinary, collaborative approach brings "long-term and sustainable effects" in school health promotion [27,32]. It fosters the exchange of experiences and ideas in implementation of HPS [27,29,30,32]. Inchley et al. [27] reported that health promoters like to work in multidisciplinary teams within which experiences and resources can be shared. Some health promoters commented that different people in the team should have a "clear and distinct role" [27] or "a clear division of responsibilities" [30], so that they could focus on their professional areas, such as providing medical care by school nurses [29–31], managing catering services by catering managers [27], quality development for health promotion activities by activity managers [29], and administration and management by head school nurses, head teachers and principals [28,29]. Inchley et al. [27] also found that establishing a common understanding of underlying principles and values and negotiating mutually agreed goals and expectations are crucial in a multidisciplinary team.

Collaboration was not just restricted to adopting a whole-school approach within individual schools [27,32]. Gugglberger [32] reported that health promoters sought more cooperation and collaboration with other schools in different provinces and countries through various means such as regular meetings, information exchange, mutual sharing and learning, and discussion of problems and solutions. Inchley et al. [27] identified "three spheres" of collaboration: partnership working with external professionals, pupil participation and parental involvement. For example, catering staff were invited to share information about their school meal service at a "parents' evening", and a student council gathered student opinions and suggestions that informed changes and improvements in school facilities and policies [27].

## Enabler 4: Establishing professional networks and relationships

Professional networking and relationship building is an essential component in gaining support and consultation for the implementation of HPS [27,29–32]. Health promoters, particularly school nurses, indicated that they liked working with school doctors, paediatric specialists, skin specialists and ear specialists [30]. Some health promoters found it supportive to have a "coordinated school health nurse" [30] or external governmental agencies to help them in school health promotion and coordination, such as the "child and adolescent mental health service provision [CAMHS]" [31] and the "school health service [SHS]" [30]. In case of emergencies, the school nurses had to make appropriate referrals or seek professional advice from private practising specialists [30]. Sometimes the schools invited the specialists to gives presentations and lead discussions on students' problems [30].

Maintaining good relationships with colleagues within schools as well as with politicians and organizational leaders outside schools has been described as an essential element in the success of HPS [29,31]. A close working relationship also facilitated communication, information exchange, and sustaining continuous collaborative efforts between the schools and the community, especially when the health promoters responsible for the coordination worked only part-time or during term-time [31]. Further, a "trusting and good relationship" fosters peer supports in the workplace [31]. Inchley et al. noted that a coordinator in school health promotion is "the glue in keeping everything together and making contacts" ([27], p. 69).

## Enabler 5: Continuing training and education in school health promotion

According to the findings of studies included in this review, health promoters seek further training and education to overcome obstacles in implementing HPS projects [29–31]. The school nurses described their work as ranging from being lonely at work to having a well-functioning network and support system [30], such as the established professional networks and relationships mentioned in Enabler 4. Health promoters, particularly school nurses, reported a lack of confidence in school health promotion even though they had had training and possessed qualifications in health care [29]. For example, some health promoters asked themselves "how do I integrate this into everyday school life, how should I do this, how does it work?" ([32], p. 451), and a few school nurses expressed feelings of inadequacy in terms of their experience acting as a school health nurse" [30]. Some school nurses worried more about doing counselling or giving out inappropriate health advice to students than about the inaccuracy of their health knowledge [31]. This lack of confidence placed extra stress on health promoters with regard to delivering health promotions in schools [31].

Health promoters, especially school nurses, viewed continuing medical education and training in school health promotion as an important way to deliver quality health promotion in schools [29,30]. Some school nurses tried to gain more confidence by reading journals and research articles when they perceived a lack of theories and methods in their general health promotion work. However, health promoters might be discouraged from taking such expensive courses, thus financial support is important in this regard ([30], p.160).

## Discussions

This article reports a narrative review of qualitative evidence of the enablers in implementing HPS among health promoters. In this review, qualitative evidence from the included studies demonstrates that commitment from the school administration and management, parents' and students' participation, awards and recognition of successful efforts, and collaboration within schools and between schools and the community are important to the implementation of HSP. Communication and health promoters' competency are also major areas that were found by the studies in this review to determine the success of HPS. Note that due to the heterogeneity of the included studies, the five enablers were generated by synthesising the general concepts from the data presented in the included studies [22]. The themes might overlap each other and the implementation process of HPS is in a dynamic fashion, thus the codes and the data organised in Table 4–9 might also be interpreted differently by different readers.

The issue of the regional guidelines on development of HPS by the World Health Organization in 1996 has attracted more and more health promotion experts from both the education and health sectors to adopt the HPS framework in conducting school-based health intervention programmes and research [1]. During the literature review period in this systematic review, a number of review articles were noted, yet they are not included in the present narrative synthesis, for their data analysis was secondary in nature and they only included quantitative studies such as RCTs [1,2,15]. The aims of these reviews include evaluating the effectiveness of school-based promotion interventions [1,2], identifying methodologies and methodological gaps for evaluating HPS, establishing a conceptual framework for evaluating HPS in South Africa [15], and identifying the effects of student participation in school health promotion [9]. None of them aimed to explore the implementation process of HPS. The role of the school nurse and the concepts of HPS were investigated in a systematic review which included studies done in the 1990s [19] and a content analysis of school staff's views in Greece in 2008 [35]. All of these articles and reviews, although not included in the current narrative synthesis, are regarded as valuable in providing insightful contents for discussion.

## From policy and guideline establishment to the role delineation of health promoters

Schools possessed different health promotion policies and guidelines, but the interpretations varied among health promoters. Comments on these policies and guidelines ranged from stating that they gave the health promoters more autonomy in implementing HPS to complaining of vague and unclear interpretations that did not help very much in health promotion work and in turn affected the motivation of health promoters. The WHO HPS Framework [36] notes that the users of the guideline should implement it in a way that best fits the individual context and culture; however, as reported in this review, many societies tend to focus on academic achievement [28], which may result in enthusiastic health promoters compromising their motivation and intention in developing the school into a HPS. As evidence in the included studies, adaptation to HPS policies would require a re-prioritization of tasks [28,30]. The role of fulfilling class teaching by teachers often has to compete with sparing time for classroom health education; this supports the notion of incorporating health education and promotion into the school curriculum [1,2,15,33]. However, this strategy may not necessarily yield positive results, as some health promoters still think that health promotion is not their main role in schools [28,33]. Interestingly, although the collaborative approach of HPS has been largely emphasized in the included studies, it is seldom mentioned or elaborated how different health promoters see each others' roles or how they communicate, discuss or clarify among each other. None of the included articles address this possible gap in the perspective of school policy and management, nor could the existing literature provide correlative or comparative studies on this aspect due to the diversity of health promoters' roles, even among school nurses themselves [19]. For example, Morberg et al. reported that school nurses' autonomy and legitimacy for work, including school health promotion, actually depended on "trust and a good relationship between the head school nurse and the head teachers" ([29], p. 816), rather than being clearly delineated by existing policies or guidelines. Wainwright, Thomas & Jones [19] also argued that the transition from a teacher-led health promotion conscience to a nurse-led health promotion initiative still raises a lot of conflicts regarding role and professional boundaries. For example, it is not unusual for the existence of school nurses to be based not only on their functional role, but also on the fact that others think that they "bear full responsibility", and that still others even think that school nurses need not be present permanently in schools [33]. The purpose of the discussion at this point is not to judge whether the existence of certain healthcare professionals, such as school nurses and other specialists, is necessary or suitable in schools, but as a matter of fact that reflects the reality that mutual agreement on the role of different health promoters in implementing HPS has not yet been reached. The authors here argue that the existence of clear policies and guidelines for different health promoters which delineate clearly their roles and responsibilities would improve school nurses' role and autonomy in school health promotion.

## Coordination is the key to obtaining support and resources

In terms of committed support sought within schools, the top-down managerial approach and the bottom-up commitment approach have been identified from the included articles (Table 4–9) and discussed in the systematic reviews focusing on experimental studies only [1,2,9,15]. Principals and other senior staff who held the manager or supervisor role focused more on strategies for effective HPS implementation, which would draw resources from the community and other stakeholders [17–29,32], such as through marketing and obtaining awards and political recognition?. In contrast to junior teachers or school nurses, they were more focused on personal professional development, such as obtaining professional training and extending their career path [30,31]. The discussion here is not to compare different health promoters' position, their knowledge and professionalism or intelligence in any sense, but rather aims to emphasise the diversity and complexity of schools as organisations, in the same way that [28] proposed viewing HPS in light of the complex adaptive system. The authors here argue that in order for a school to obtain all the support required, as identified from the included studies, coordination is the key. While the WHO proposes the HPS as a whole-school approach, the United States Centers for Disease Control and Prevention [CDC] uses the term "Coordinated School Health" [37], which emphasizes the coordinated efforts within the schools and communities. In addition to the suggestion by the health promoters in the included studies to hire full-time school nurses, the CDC stresses hiring a full-time or part-time school health coordinator, who helps to "maintain active school health councils and facilitate health programming in the district and school and between the school and community", and to facilitate policy and cultural changes in the society [35]. The lack of such coordinated efforts was evidenced in the included studies, in which health promoters frequently lamented the lack of between-school communication, cross-provincial and international exchanges, social recognition and a favourable societal culture, but rarely assimilated the coordination role as their own task. This may be due partially to unsophisticated policies and guidelines, which restricted the potential of health promoters to attain the advanced coordination role, and partially to the current lack of financial support from schools and from the government [1,2,15,35]. However, in a more practical sense, the top-down approach would bring a more effective initiating force to introduce and support this coordination role, while the bottom-up commitment, including the participation of parents and students, is still critical for the sustaining the HPS [2,9]. The coordination role of health promoters, or the school health promotion coordinators, would thus serve as the medium to bridge the top-down and bottom-up efforts within schools, as well as a resource person who obtains support "horizontally" in the community.

### Limitations

Several limitations should be taken into account when assessing the contributions of the synthesized findings. Not all of the selected studies discussed and evaluated different types of support, even though financial or funding support is considered to be one of the most important factors for the successful implementation of HPS. One study [32] was conducted in a federalist political structure in which, as described by the author, the availability of resources and the financial and personnel autonomy of schools may be influenced under different conditions. Here the narrative synthesis articles have no political standing and therefore political inferences cannot be drawn.

Inchley et al.'s study [27] was drawn from a process evaluation of a 4-year project undertaken within the European Network of HPS in Scotland, although the schools were funded for a 2-year period only. There is no discussion of how the funding facilitated the implementation of HPS, or the effects on HPS after the funding ceased.

A further limitation concerned the range of the population. Included studies were restricted to the UK, Scotland, Sweden, Austria and Australia, and three of them included only school nurses (Table 1–3). This affects the transferability of the findings [38]. Not all of the studies described the details of the interview techniques used or showed the compositions of their participants, which also affected the 'thickness of data'. The data is 'thick' enough if the author includes detailed descriptions and contextual material from which judgements about the trustworthiness of a qualitative research can be made [36,37]. Therefore, the qualitative evidence presented in this article may be thin and the interpretations and transferability to other contexts may be limited.

Although the authors consider that the articles included here passed the quality appraisal of the CASP tool, their quality varied. Not all of the studies addressed in-depth reflexivity. In addition, the data analysis was not presented in a rigorous way in every study, limiting the interpretations that can be made. Due to the lack of data from these studies, a theory to describe the implementation strategies or process might not be possible at this stage.

## Conclusion

This narrative synthesis review provides qualitative evidence on the enablers and strategies contributing to the successful implementation of HPS. Approaches to implementing HPS may vary among countries and schools owing to the different contexts, thus school health policies that meet local health needs, contexts and cultures need to be formulated. This must involve mutual understanding and relationship building between the health and education sectors in order to promote health to children and adolescents. This article shows that the participation of and support from the school management, collaboration, relationship building and networking between schools and the community are all essential components of the successful implementation of HPS. As found and discussed in this review, health promoters seek a theoretical foundation in order to implement HPS. Further qualitative research is needed to provide a more in-depth understanding of the process of implementation of HPS. A grounded theory approach may be useful in order to develop a substantial theory to describe the process of the successful implementation of HPS.

## Author Contributions

Conceived and designed the experiments: TTMH VCLC AD RLTL. Analyzed the data: TTMH VCLC AD RLTL. Contributed reagents/materials/analysis tools: TTMH VCLC AD RLTL. Contributed to the writing of the manuscript: TTMH RLTL.

## References


1. Lister-Sharp D, Chapman S, Stewart-Brown S, Sowden A (1999) Health promoting schools and health promotion in schools: two systematic reviews. Health Technol Assess (Rockv) 3. Available: http://www.capmh.com/pubmed/10683593. Accessed 6 May 2013.
2. Stewart-Brown S (2006) What is the evidence on school health promotion in improving health or preventing disease and, speifically, what is the effectiveness of the health promoting schools approach? Copenhagen. Available: http://scholar.google.com/scholar?hl=en&btnG=Search&q=intitle:What+is+the+evidence+on+school+health+promotion+in+improving+health+or+preventing+disease+and+,+specifically+,+what+is+the+effectiveness+of+the+health+promoting+schools+approach+?#0. Accessed 6 May 2013.
3. Lee A, Cheng FFK, St Leger L (2005) Evaluating health-promoting schools in Hong Kong: development of a framework. Health Promot Int 20: 177–186. Available: http://www.ncbi.nlm.nih.gov/pubmed/15788527. Accessed 24 August 2013.
4. Leurs MTW, Schaalma HP, Jansen MWJ, Mur-Veeman IM, St Leger LH, et al. (2005) Development of a collaborative model to improve school health promotion in The Netherlands. Health Promot Int 20: 296–305. Available: http://www.ncbi.nlm.nih.gov/pubmed/15797902. Accessed 24 August 2013.
5. St Leger L (2006) Health Promotion and Health Education in Schools – Trends, Effectiveness and Possibilities. Victoria, Australia. Available: http://www.racv.com.au/wps/wcm/connect/fadf2a004da9bb7aa2c9fa54a1b45993/Health+Promotion+and+Health+Education+in+Schools.pdf?MOD=AJPERES&CACHEID=fadf2a004da9bb7aa2c9fa54a1b45993.
6. World Health Organization (2013) What is a health promoting school. Available: http://www.who.int/school_youth_health/gshi/hps/en/index.html.
7. Patton GC, Bond L, Carlin JB, Thomas L, Butler H, et al. (2006) Promoting social inclusion in schools: a group-randomized trial of effects on student health risk behavior and well-being. Am J Public Health 96: 1582–1587. Available: http://www.pubmedcentral.nih.gov/articlerender.fcgi?artid=1551970&tool=pmcentrez&rendertype=abstract. Accessed 8 October 2013.
8. Kolbe LJ (1986) Increasing the impact of school health promotion programs: Emerging research perspectives. Health Educ 17: 47–52. Available: http://www.ncbi.nlm.nih.gov/pubmed/3152360.
9. Griebler U, Rojatz D, Simovska V, Forster R (2014) Effects of student participation in school health promotion: a systematic review. Health Promot Int: 1–12. Available: http://www.ncbi.nlm.nih.gov/pubmed/24395957. Accessed 12 February 2014.
10. Marshall BJ, Sheehan MM, Northfield JR, Maher S, Carlisle R, et al. (2000) School-based health promotion across Australia. J Sch Health 70: 251–252.
11. St Leger L, Young I, Blanchard C (2012) Facilitating dialogue between the health and the education sectors to school health promotion and education. Scotland.
12. Sharma M, Romas JA (2008) Theoretical foundations of health education and health promotion. Burlington, MA: Jones & Bartlett Publishers. Available: http://doi.wiley.com/10.1111/j.1753-6405.2010.00489.x.
13. World Health Organization (1986) Ottawa Charter for Health Promotion.
14. Croghan E, Johnson C, Aveyard P (2004) School nurses: policies, working practices, roles and value perceptions. J Adv Nurs 47: 377–385. Available: http://www.ncbi.nlm.nih.gov/pubmed/15271156.
15. Mũkoma W, Flisher AJ (2004) Evaluations of health promoting schools: a review of nine studies. Health Promot Int 19: 357–368. Available: http://www.ncbi.nlm.nih.gov/pubmed/15306620. Accessed 12 April 2013.
16. Popay J, Roberts H, Sowden A, Petticrew M, Arai L, et al. (2006) Guidance on the conduct of narrative synthesis in systematic reviews: A product from the ESRC Methods Programme. Lancaster. Available: http://www.researchgate.

net/publication/233866356_Guidance_on_the_conduct_of_narrative_synthesis_in_systematic_reviews_A_product_from_the_ESRC_Methods_Programme.
17. Wells J, Barlow J, Stewart-Brown S (2003) A systematic review of universal approaches to mental health promotion in schools. Health Educ 103: 197–220. Available: http://www.emeraldinsight.com/10.1108/09654280310485546. Accessed 8 September 2013.
18. Education IU for HP and (2010) Promoting health in schools: From evidence to action.
19. Wainwright P, Thomas J, Jones M (2000) Health promotion and the role of the school nurse: a systematic review. J Adv Nurs 32: 1083–1091. Available: http://www.ncbi.nlm.nih.gov/pubmed/11114992.
20. Moher D, Liberati a, Tetzlaff J, Altman DG (2009) Preferred reporting items for systematic reviews and meta-analyses: the PRISMA statement. Bmj 339: b2535–b2535. Available: http://www.bmj.com/cgi/doi/10.1136/bmj.b2535. Accessed 1 March 2013.
21. Critical Appraisal Skills Programme (CASP) (2006) 10 questions to help you make sense of qualitative research. CASP Qual Checkl: 1–6. Available: http://media.wix.com/ugd/dded87_951541699e9edc71ce66c9bac4734c69.pdf.
22. Thomas J, Harden A (2008) Methods for the thematic synthesis of qualitative research in systematic reviews. BMC Med Res Methodol 8: 45. Available: http://www.pubmedcentral.nih.gov/articlerender.fcgi?artid=2478656&tool=pmcentrez&rendertype=abstract. Accessed 11 March 2013.
23. Sandelowski M, Barroso J (2007) Handbook for synthesizing qualitative research. New York: Springer Publishing Company.
24. Schools for Health in Europe (2007) Terms of reference SHE network. Available: http://www.schoolsforhealth.eu/upload/Terms_of_reference_SHE_network.pdf.
25. World Health Organization (1997) First conferences of the European Network of Health Promoting Schools: the Health Promoting School - an investment in education, health and democracy. Available: http://www.euro.who.int/__data/assets/pdf_file/0013/120307/E72971.pdf.
26. Gugglberger L (2011) Support for health promoting schools: a typology of supporting strategies in Austrian provinces. Available: http://www.ncbi.nlm.nih.gov/pubmed/21303788. Accessed 28 December 2012.
27. Inchley J, Muldoon J, Currie C (2006) Becoming a health promoting school: evaluating the process of effective implementation in Scotland. Available: http://www.ncbi.nlm.nih.gov/pubmed/17178755. Accessed 28 December 2012.
28. Keshavarz N, Nutbeam D, Rowling L, Khavarpour F (2010) Schools as social complex adaptive systems: a new way to understand the challenges of introducing the health promoting schools concept. Elsevier Ltd. Available: http://www.ncbi.nlm.nih.gov/pubmed/20207059. Accessed 19 November 2012.
29. Morberg S, Lagerström M, Dellve L (2009) The perceived perceptions of head school nurses in developing school nursing roles within schools. Available: http://www.ncbi.nlm.nih.gov/pubmed/19793238. Accessed 26 December 2012.
30. Reuterswärd M, Lagerström M (2010) The aspects school health nurses find important for successful health promotion. Available: http://www.ncbi.nlm.nih.gov/pubmed/19845886. Accessed 28 December 2012.
31. Pryjmachuk S, Graham T, Haddad M, Tylee A (2011) School nurses' perspectives on managing mental health problems in children and young people. Available: http://www.ncbi.nlm.nih.gov/pubmed/21883575. Accessed 6 March 2013.
32. Gugglberger L, Dür W (2011) Capacity building in and for health promoting schools: results from a qualitative study. Health Policy 101: 37–43. Available: http://www.ncbi.nlm.nih.gov/pubmed/20855125. Accessed 5 June 2013.
33. Whitehead D (2011) Before the cradle and beyond the grave: a lifespan/settings-based framework for health promotion. J Clin Nurs 20: 2183–2194. Available: http://www.ncbi.nlm.nih.gov/pubmed/21535458. Accessed 6 August 2014.
34. Layla A, Said H, Salama R (2013) Perceptions of school nurses and principals towards nurse role in providing school health services in Qatar. ... Egypt Public Heal ... 88: 19–25. Available: http://journals.lww.com/ephaj/Abstract/2013/04000/Perceptions_of_school_nurses_and_principals.5.aspx. Accessed 6 August 2014.
35. Alexandropoulou M (2013) The health promoting school and the school nurse: a content analysis of school staff's views. Br J Sch Nurs 8: 134–141.
36. World Health Organization (1996) WHO 1996 Regional guideline, development of health promoting schools a framework for action.
37. Centers for Disease Control and Prevention (2013) Coordinated school health. Available: http://www.cdc.gov/healthyyouth/cshp/.
38. Lincoln YS, Guba EG (1985) Naturalistic inquiry. London: SAGE. Available: http://linkinghub.elsevier.com/retrieve/pii/0147176785900628.

# 12

# Perception of Human Papillomavirus Infection, Cervical Cancer and HPV Vaccination in North Indian Population

**Showket Hussain[1], Vilas Nasare[1], Malasha Kumari[2], Shashi Sharma[3], Mohammad Aijaz Khan[4]*, Bhudev C. Das[5], Mausumi Bharadwaj[1]***

1 Division of Molecular Genetics & Biochemistry, Institute of Cytology & Preventive Oncology (ICMR), Noida, Uttar Pradesh, India, 2 Division of Clinical Oncology, Institute of Cytology & Preventive Oncology (ICMR), Noida, Uttar Pradesh, India, 3 Division of Biostatistics & Epidemiology, Institute of Cytology & Preventive Oncology (ICMR), Noida, Uttar Pradesh, India, 4 Division of Behaviour Oncology, Institute of Cytology & Preventive Oncology (ICMR), Noida, Uttar Pradesh, India, 5 Division of Molecular Oncology, Institute of Cytology & Preventive Oncology (ICMR), Noida, Uttar Pradesh, India

## Abstract

***Background:*** Human Papillomavirus (HPV) -associated cervical cancer is the second-most common cancer in women worldwide but it is the most frequent gynaecological cancer and cancer associated death in India women. The objective of this study was to assess knowledge about cervical cancer, HPV, HPV vaccine, HPV vaccine acceptance among school and undergraduates students and their parent's perception about acceptance of HPV vaccine in Northern part of India (Delhi and NCR regions).

***Materials and Methods:*** A qualitative questionnaire based survey among 2500 urban/rural students aged 12–22 years was conducted.

***Results:*** Overall, a low frequency (15%) of HPV and cervical cancer awareness was observed in students and their parents. However, the awareness was much higher in females belonging to urban setup compared to boys with a perception that HPV causes cervical cancer in women only. Additionally, only (13%) participants who were aware of cervical cancer and HPV) were willing to accept HPV vaccination. Apparently, parents of female students were two times more willing to accept HPV vaccination for their ward than male students ($p<0.001$; OR 95%CI = 2.09 (1.58–2.76).

***Conclusion:*** Cervical cancer and HPV awareness among school, undergraduate students and also to their parents was found to be very low in this part of India. The level of awareness and education appears to be insignificant determinants in rural compared to urban setup. Better health education will be needed to maximize public awareness for cervical cancer prevention.

**Editor:** Maria Lina Tornesello, Istituto Nazionale Tumori, Italy

**Funding:** The authors have no support or funding to report.

**Competing Interests:** The authors have declared that no competing interests exist.

* Email: bharadwajm@icmr.org.in (MB); madrkhan@gmail.com (MAK)

## Introduction

Cancer of the uterine cervix is the second-most common cancer in women worldwide but it is the most common health hazard in India [1]. 80% of sexually active women infected with persistent HPV infection leads invasive cervical cancer [1,2,3]. However, reduction of morbidity/mortality due to cervical cancer is early detection and treatment of cervical precancerous lesions. In developed countries, the mortality has reduced due to introduction of population-based cytological screening programme using Pap test [4]. In addition, screening for cervical infection of HPV has proved to be more effective and reliable [5].

Recently, two HPV vaccines quadrivalent "Gardasil" and bivalent "Cervarix" have been shown to be highly effective in preventing infection with high-risk type HPV16 and HPV18, the two most common oncogenic types. As these vaccines are highly effective before exposure to HPV, current guidelines prioritise adolescent girls as primary target group for HPV vaccination [6].

Though adolescents are the prime candidates for prophylactic HPV vaccination, several studies have shown that adolescents had very little knowledge about HPV vaccination [7,8,9]. The deficiency of such knowledge might adversely affect the vaccine acceptance. Therefore, there has been an exponential increase in the number of studies exploring acceptability of the vaccine since it became commercially available. Many studies have focused on parental willingness to vaccinate their children [1,10,11,12,13,14]. But only few studies have evaluated the knowledge of HPV vaccine, attitudes and intentions of young women [15,16,17,18]. Recent reviews [19,20,21,22] showed that acceptance of the vaccine is high among those who are aware of the relationship between HPV and cervical cancer.

The deficiency of knowledge of causal relationship between HPV and cervical cancer might adversely affect the vaccine acceptance in India. Several studies have been undertaken to evaluate women's awareness and knowledge level about cervical cancer and HPV vaccine [23,24,25]. A report from rural India

**Table 1.** Demographic characteristics of the population studied.

| Characteristics | No. of Participants (N = 2500) | Percent Distribution (%) |
|---|---|---|
| **Age** | | |
| 12–15 | 320 | 12.8 |
| 16–18 | 713 | 28.52 |
| 19–22 | 1467 | 58.68 |
| **Sex** | | |
| Female | 1570 | 62.8 |
| Male | 930 | 37.2 |
| **Education** | | |
| Standard 6–8 | 286 | 11.44 |
| Standard 9–11 | 813 | 32.52 |
| Standard 12-undergraduate | 1401 | 56.04 |
| **Religion** | | |
| Muslim | 786 | 31.44 |
| Hindu | 1714 | 68.56 |

among nursing staff showed that 74% know that pap smear is used for detection of cervical cancer but only 59% know that pap smear can detect both cancerous as well as precancerous lesions of cervix. Surprisingly, only 18% know about HPV vaccine [25].

Preliminary study among 8–17 years old adolescents and their parents in India, suggested that majority of them are unaware of cervical cancer, HPV and HPV vaccines [26]. In view of this, we conducted a study among students from high-school up to undergraduate students to evaluate their knowledge about knowledge of cervical cancer, HPV awareness, willingness of HPV vaccine acceptance among adolescents and their parents and to identify predictors of girls receiving the HPV vaccine.

## Materials and Methods

A pre-designed questionnaire-based survey was conducted and a total of 2600 participants aged between 12–22 years were enumerated from June 2009–June 2011 that included both urban and rural school population of Noida and Delhi. Out of 2600 participants, only 2500 participants completed the questionnaire. The study was approved by Ethics Committee of Institute of Cytology & Preventive Oncology (ICPO/IEC/2008-09/05). Written consent was taken from all participants and guardians in case of minors.

First part of the questionnaire was to collect information on age, sex, study stream, level of study, place of permanent residence, family income, family size and religion etc. were noted. The remaining part a self-administered questionnaire was used for this study, which were to be filled in individually by the participants under the strict vigilance of the teachers/researchers/mentors which serves as invigilators to monitor the influence on answers by the students. The questionnaire contained questions regarding knowledge of cervical cancer, HPV and awareness about HPV vaccine. In addition, there is question on parent's opinion about HPV vaccine acceptance. The questions were developed based on previous established facts for cervical cancer [27,28,29,30]. The most of the questions "yes", "no", or appropriate multiple choices were given as answers. The data from questionnaire were processed anonymously. Furthermore, the data was again validated by revisiting the same school after one, three and six months of the 1st visit to access the knowledge and awareness among participants. Data were analysed using SPSS software version 14.0 to assess the association between demographic factors and HPV awareness and cervical cancer.

## Results

A total of 2600 students participated in the study. Sixty eight (68) participants did not complete the personal information details and thirty two (32) were having incomplete questionnaires. Therefore, a total of 2500 participants could complete the questionnaire, out of which 930 (37.2%) were male and 1570 (62.8%) were female. Most of them 56% were from rural set up where as 44% were of urban region. Most of students 58.7% were in the age group of 19–22 years, 28.5% belonged to16–18 years, while 12.8% were of age group 12–15 years. The participation rate of female students was higher (62.8%) as compared to male students (37.2%). Two hundred eighty six (11.44%) students were in the education group of 6–8th standard, eight hundred thirteen (32.52%) students were of 10–11th standard whereas fourteen hundred and one (56.04%) students were of 12th standard as well as of undergraduate level respectively. Further stratification of data with respect to religion revealed a higher participation rate of Hindu students (68.56%) which was evident as majority of Hindu population is dominant in these areas whereas 31.44% were of Muslim students. Detailed demographic characteristics of the participants are presented in Table 1.

Table 2, 3 and 4 describes the awareness of the participants.

### Knowledge about cervical cancer

In order to examine the knowledge/awareness about cervical cancer, HPV and HPV vaccines, a short type questions in local as well as in English language were asked to the students and their parents (Table 2). In general, three hundred seventy five (15%) participants were only well aware of cervical cancer. Of these, two hundred fifty seven (69%) female students were aware of cervical cancer whereas 118 (31%) male students knew about cervical cancer. A significant correlation of cervical cancer awareness was

**Table 2.** Awareness about cervical cancer, HPV and HPV vaccine.

| Parameters | Awareness among participants | |
|---|---|---|
| | Frequency | Percentage |
| Knowledge about cervical cancer (n = 2500) | 375 | 15 |
| Knowledge about HPV infection causes genital cancer (n = 375) | 275* | 73.3 |
| HPV vaccine awareness (n = 275) | 225 | 81.8 |
| HPV vaccine willingness (n = 275) | 175** | 63.6 |
| Parents opinion about HPV vaccine (n = 2500) | 325*** | 13 |

*Number indicate participants who had knowledge about cervical cancer and know the causative agent.
**Number indicate participants who had both knowledge and know the causative agent.
***General opinion among all participants.

observed with respect to female students ($p<0.05$) and this could be attributed due to more female participation. Thus, cervical cancer knowledge was apparently more in female participants when compared to male participants ($p<0.05$, OR = 1.35, 95%CI = 1.06–1.72) (Table 3). Furthermore, data demonstrate that 235 students (63%) belonged to rural area whereas 140 (37%) were of urban and had a knowledge about cervical cancer. On the other hand, a significant difference was also observed when the comparison was made between rural and urban residence of students. Certainly, a more knowledge about cervical cancer was observed in participants who belonged to urban setup, ($p<0.001$, OR = 1.38; 95%CI = 1.10–1.75) (Table 4).

## Knowledge of HPV causes genital cancer

Of the total participants (375) who had knowledge about cervical cancer, two hundred seventy five (73%) participants were having knowledge that cervical cancer is caused due to HPV infection (Table 2). A significant difference was observed between male: female and rural vs urban participants, as one hundred seventy two (63%) females and one hundred three (37%) males were aware that HPV infection causes genital cancer (Table 3).

## HPV vaccine awareness

Furthermore, the students were asked to know whether or not they are aware that HPV vaccines are commercially available, two hundred twenty five participants were aware of availability of vaccines. Among them, one hundred sixty two (72%) were female students and sixty three (28%) were male students. Therefore, the correlation of gender of the students with HPV vaccine awareness was observed and found to be statistically significant ($p = 0.004$; OR = 1.57, 95%CI = 1.14–2.14). Interestingly, vaccine availability awareness was also attributed to urban population 65% (143/225) (Table 4).

## HPV vaccine willingness

Students were educated about the risk factors associated with cervical cancer and how it could be prevented through vaccination and other practices, the willingness of HPV vaccination was found to be 70% in females and 64% in urban populations (Table 3 and Table 4).

## Parent's opinion about HPV vaccine

Last but not the least, parents opinion was also taken into consideration with respect to vaccine implementation program in North-Indian population. 13% of the parents agreed to vaccinate their wards (Table 2).

## Validation of questionnaire

After completion of questionnaire by participants, a brief power point presentation was addressed among all subjects which included introduction to cervical cancer, incidence rate both in India and world wide, diagnostic modalities: Pap-test, liquid based cytology (LBC), visual inspection (VIA, VILI), colposcopy etc. and HPV DNA test by hybrid capture 2 (HC2), reverse line blot, real-time PCR etc., prevention and management. In order to evaluate the impact of awareness made available to participants, three times visits ($1^{st}$ month, $3^{rd}$ month and $6^{th}$ month) was made to the same school. A semi-structured qualitative interview was conducted to collect the information regarding awareness, knowledge, disease exposome and vaccination programme etc. All the answers were recorded and reviewed. A good awareness response was observed among participants regarding the knowledge and awareness of

**Table 3.** Comparison of awareness among Females and Males.

| Parameters | Sex | | P-value | Odd ratio (95%CI) |
|---|---|---|---|---|
| | Female | Male | | |
| **Knowledge about cervical cancer (n = 375)** | 257(68.5%) | 118(31.5%) | 0.13 | 1.35 (1.06–1.72) |
| **Knowledge about HPV infection causes genital cancer (n = 275)** | 172(62.5%) | 103(37.4%) | 0.93 | 0.99 (0.76–1.29) |
| **HPV vaccine awareness (n = 225)** | 162(72%) | 63(28%) | **0.004** | 1.57 (1.14–2.14) |
| **HPV vaccine willingness (n = 175)** | 123(70.2%) | 52(29.7%) | **<0.001** | 5.2 (3.45–9.01) |
| **Parents opinion about HPV vaccine (n = 325)** | 248(15.79%) | 77(8.27%) | **<0.001** | 2.09 (1.58–2.76) |

**Table 4.** Awareness about cervical cancer and HPV according to living area.

| Factors | Knowledge | Living area | | P-value | Odd ratio; (95%CI) |
|---|---|---|---|---|---|
| | | Urban | Rural | | |
| **Knowledge about cervical cancer (n = 375)** | Yes | 235 (62.6) | 140 (37.3) | **<0.001** | 2.82 (2.07–3.83) |
| **Knowledge about HPV infection causes genital cancer (n = 275)** | Yes | 172 (62.5%) | 103 (37.45%) | 0.02 | 1.36 (1.04–1.77) |
| **HPV vaccine awareness (n = 225)** | Yes | 143 (63.5%) | 82 (36.45%) | 0.02 | 1.41 (1.05–1.89) |
| **HPV vaccine willingness (n = 175)** | Yes | 113 (64.5%) | 62 (35.4%) | 0.02 | 1.47 (1.05–2.05) |
| **Parents opinion about HPV vaccine (n = 325)** | Yes | 213 (65.53%) | 112 (34.46%) | **<0.001** | 1.58 (1.23–2.04) |

cervical cancer and HPV. However, a negative response was documented with respect to implementation of vaccination programme in India due to adverse effects of vaccine related deaths recently. Consequently, a negative response which includes anxiety, physco-social distress and high cost of current vaccines was observed. In order to reduce the burden of cervical cancer and perhaps other disease prevalent in India, awareness through print and electronic – mass media is warranted.

## Discussion

As per our knowledge the present study is the first report to evaluate the knowledge of cervical cancer, HPV and HPV vaccine among the high-school and under graduate students in NCR (Noida) and Delhi region of India. It provides the useful information which may help in designing HPV vaccine programs and public health policy making in India. The school/college based studies of HPV awareness are very few and we observed an interesting correlation between increasing age and HPV awareness. Our result is in consistent with the other studies in India that showed low level of cervical cancer and HPV knowledge (15%) in graduate, postgraduate and even in medical students [24,31]. But in contrast, another study from India showed that majority of the participants were well aware (89.6%) of several risk factors of cervical cancer development and its causal relation with HPV because of the study was conducted among medical students [32].

A study from Korea showed a mere 9.5% of female high school and university students had ever heard of HPV [33] But another study from Mexico among college students, aged 17–25 years, showed that most of the students have heard of HPV, although they had limited knowledge about the causal relation with virus and the preventive strategies [34]. Similarly, another study among college students aged 18–35 years in Ghana noted very low awareness (7.9%) regarding the link between HPV and cervical cancer [35]. Even a study from US showed that 21.5% of the college women have never heard of HPV [36]. Racial differences in HPV knowledge was also reported among US rural ethnic (29% in Blacks and 42% in Whites) populations [37]. Another study reported that 53.3% of the undergraduate female students had heard about cervical cancer and 37.8% knew about HPV in Durban, South Africa [38]. Similarly, another study from Taiwan among 953 undergraduate women aged 17–36 years in five universities in southern Taiwan reported that 70% of undergraduate women had limited knowledge of cervical cancer and 49% were having HPV awareness [39]. Therefore, it was reported that general public has low level of knowledge on HPV infection [20]. Similar to this study, another report from developing countries (India, Peru, Uganda, and Vietnam) showed low level of knowledge of HPV among children, parents, teachers, community leaders, and even health service providers of these four countries [40]. But in contrast, a study among the female educated youths in India, Nepal and Srilanka concluded that the awareness of cervical cancer was 66% in India, 58.8% in Nepal and 57.7% in Srilanka respectively [41]. Another study from Turkey among nursing students (age16–27 yrs) in tertiary hospital reported that they have theoretical knowledge but not aware that routine gynaecological examination and pap smears can be taken for prevention of cervical cancer [42]. There is a separate study in Polish population among female students (age 18–26 yrs) showed that general knowledge about cervical cancer and their causative agent of HPV is very high but they have poor knowledge about HPV vaccine and cytological screening [43]. But in contrast, a study from Greece among female University and technological institute students (age 18–26 years) reported that 59.1% students are aware of HPV vaccine and this high level of knowledge is positively associated with vaccine uptake [44].

In the present study, the male students were found to be less knowledgeable about HPV than the female students. This indicates that the female students were much aware about the cervical cancer. Similar to our findings, a study among Australian women and men between the ages 18 and 70 years showed that 62.8% of women and only 38.3% of men had heard of HPV [45]. In contrast, the studies from developing countries demonstrated that participants, aged 15–45 years, from both rural and urban settings have a low level of awareness about HPV [46]. Only one study from India among medical students showed that majority (89.6%) of the participates were aware of preventable nature of cervical cancer [32]. It was noticed from the other studies that gender also appears to have influenced knowledge and awareness, especially for HPV to some extent [47,48]. Significant gender differences were observed, with females having better awareness and knowledge than males. Although the data are limited as not all studies reported results separately for males and females, these findings, could be reflective of the way awareness campaigns, for example on HPV, have been targeted more at females than at males.

The results of the present study also showed that Muslim students have very less knowledge as compared to Hindu students. It is important to note that presence of HPV and cervical cancer is relatively much lower in Muslim population. In this regards, the regional differences may be due to cultural, religious, social, ethnic variation [1]. Our results reflected that the HPV awareness is influenced by age, education, gender and community also.

The present study is also able to determine the parent's opinion about HPV and HPV related information. Our previous study [26] demonstrated that parental literacy has a tremendous influence on the knowledge of cervical cancer (17%) and HPV infection (8%) for their school- aged children in India. In this study we found that knowledge about HPV infection causes genital cancer in male has little more knowledge than the female and in contrast the knowledge about cervical cancer is higher in females than in males. In another study from India reported that 41% participants were aware of a link between sexual activity and cervical cancer [24]. Similarly, a Korean survey [49] showed that 31.5% women aged more than 20 years were aware that sexually transmitted infections (STIs) can cause cervical cancer. But in contrast, few studies from Asian countries also reported of low knowledge levels of public on etiologic involvement of STIs and HPV in cervical cancer development [50,51].

Study demonstrated that the area wise, urban dwellers had higher knowledge about "HPV infection causes genital cancer" than rural belt and similarly we found that knowledge about "cervical cancer" is higher in urban than rural. This study also showed that more attention is needed to educate the rural populations. In this regard, Li et al reported that (51.1%) urban women knew that HPV is related to cervical cancer in compare to their rural counterpart (41.6%). Even fewer (8.1%) knew that it is associated with genital warts with the similar rate of both geographies [52]. Poor knowledge and awareness of cervical cancer among women and other characteristics has been reported from many different geographic regions [35,53,54,55]. This low level knowledge is consistent with the findings from another study of Chinese women in Hong Kong, which reported 10% of women were aware of HPV but had limited specific knowledge of HPV [51]. In some other developed countries with well integrated cervical cancer screening program with the Pap test, such as UK and US, the depth of knowledge about HPV were also reported to be very low [56,57,58]. In contrast, a relatively high rate of HPV awareness (51.2%) was reported from a study from Australia, which may be due to the increased media coverage, particularly in relation to the development of an HPV vaccination program [59]. As lack of knowledge is regarded as one of the major barriers that pose challenges to widespread implementation of HPV vaccine in developing countries [60], increased knowledge of education and health care providers; social workers may help to increase the general knowledge of HPV and HPV related diseases in India.

Our data represents that overall HPV vaccine awareness is very low both in female and male as well as dwellers of rural and urban origin. But in contrast, few studies reported that high vaccine acceptance among parents and adolescents in the general population [11,57,61,62,63,64] found that 84% of participants would accept a free HPV vaccine, whereas 47% were unconcerned about future personal HPV infection risk. Males were less likely to accept a free HPV vaccine and to be concerned about future personal HPV infection risk. Among young women the acceptability of the vaccines is greater if they know that the latter give protection against genital warts [65]. But in most populations, knowledge of HPV and related vaccines is low but vaccine acceptance is high.

In our study majority of participants was unwilling to be vaccinated due to lack of knowledge of HPV vaccine and its safety which were the major reasons for them. This is consistent with studies from other areas and countries [14,51,66]. Our previous report [26] showed that some parents had diverse opinions that HPV vaccines would make sex safe, leading to freedom for promiscuity and risky sexual behaviour, which is not very common in this region of the globe due to sociocultural factors. They also thought that this would cause social stigmas and tarnish their family's prestige, which has lead to widespread. Therefore, it is extremely important to raise general awareness about HPV, de-stigmatization of HPV infection and subsequently to gain acceptance for a mass vaccination program for pre-adolescent and adolescent girls in India.

In the present study parents decision between mother (15.8%) and father (8.3%) were very low about HPV vaccine as they are decision maker as vaccination takes place within the family unit, generally by one or both parents. We also observed that father's roles in decision making are also important for finances or critical health events. Although several other studies have examined the preferences for the HPV vaccine among parents [19,60,66,67,68,69] and among girls or young women [8,47,70], but none have compared parental preferences with adolescent preferences.

The strength of our study lies in the selection of study population of both rural and urban set up. But still there is limitation of our study. Findings of the present study could not be generalised to the large Indian population. Hence, an awareness regarding cervical cancer, its prevention and management is warranted.

In conclusion, in order to reduce the burden of cervical cancer and implementation of vaccination program, awareness is required which can be achieved by print and electronic media by raising slogans, conducing free camps in rural sectors for cancer screening and most importantly to sensitize Indian population for vaccine acceptance. Thus, there is a need with immediate effect to educate and aware the young population through print and/ electronic media, NGOs, Hollywood, Bollywood stars and famous sports personalities about ill- myths associated with cervical cancer vaccination program in India.

## Acknowledgments

The authors would like to thank all schools students, teachers and their parents for their support and cooperation. Also anonymous reviewers of this manuscript are greatly acknowledged for their critical comments and suggestions.

## Author Contributions

Conceived and designed the experiments: MB. Contributed reagents/ materials/analysis tools: SH VN. Wrote the paper: SH MAK MB. Supervision of the study: MB. Collection of data: VN MK. Compilation of data: VN. Statistical analysis: SS SH. Interpretation of data: SH. Critical revision of the manuscript: BCD.

## References

1. Das BC, Hussain S, Nasare V, Bharadwaj M (2008) Prospects and prejudices of human papillomavirus vaccines in India. Vaccine 26: 2669–2679.
2. Kohaar I, Thakur N, Salhan S, Batra S, Singh V, et al. (2007) TNFalpha-308G/A polymorphism as a risk factor for HPV associated cervical cancer in Indian population. Cell Oncol 29: 249–256.
3. Kohaar I, Hussain S, Thakur N, Tiwari P, Nasare V, et al. (2009) Association between human leukocyte antigen class II alleles and human papillomavirus-mediated cervical cancer in Indian women. Hum Immunol 70: 222–229.
4. Wheeler CM (2007) Advances in primary and secondary interventions for cervical cancer: human papillomavirus prophylactic vaccines and testing. Nat Clin Pract Oncol 4: 224–235.

5. Sehgal A, Singh V (2009) Human papillomavirus infection (HPV) & screening strategies for cervical cancer. Indian J Med Res 130: 234–240.
6. Kim JJ, Ortendahl J, Goldie SJ (2009) Cost-effectiveness of human papillomavirus vaccination and cervical cancer screening in women older than 30 years in the United States. Ann Intern Med 151: 538–545.
7. Cates JR, Ortiz R, Shafer A, Romocki LS, Coyne-Beasley T (2012) Designing messages to motivate parents to get their preteenage sons vaccinated against human papillomavirus. Perspect Sex Reprod Health 44: 39–47.
8. Caskey R, Lindau ST, Alexander GC (2009) Knowledge and early adoption of the HPV vaccine among girls and young women: results of a national survey. J Adolesc Health 45: 453–462.
9. Hilton S, Smith E (2011) "I thought cancer was one of those random things. I didn't know cancer could be caught...": adolescent girls' understandings and experiences of the HPV programme in the UK. Vaccine 29: 4409–4415.
10. Bair RM, Mays RM, Sturm LA, Zimet GD (2008) Acceptability of the human papillomavirus vaccine among Latina mothers. J Pediatr Adolesc Gynecol 21: 329–334.
11. Lenselink CH, Gerrits MM, Melchers WJ, Massuger LF, van Hamont D, et al. (2008) Parental acceptance of Human Papillomavirus vaccines. Eur J Obstet Gynecol Reprod Biol 137: 103–107.
12. Ogilvie GS, Remple VP, Marra F, McNeil SA, Naus M, et al. (2007) Parental intention to have daughters receive the human papillomavirus vaccine. Cmaj 177: 1506–1512.
13. Sperber NR, Brewer NT, Smith JS (2008) Influence of parent characteristics and disease outcome framing on HPV vaccine acceptability among rural, Southern women. Cancer Causes Control 19: 115–118.
14. Woodhall SC, Lehtinen M, Verho T, Huhtala H, Hokkanen M, et al. (2007) Anticipated acceptance of HPV vaccination at the baseline of implementation: a survey of parental and adolescent knowledge and attitudes in Finland. J Adolesc Health 40: 466–469.
15. Crosby R, Schoenberg N, Hopenhayn C, Moore G, Melhan W (2007) Correlates of intent to be vaccinated against human papillomavirus: an exploratory study of college-aged women. Sex Health 4: 71–73.
16. D'Urso J, Thompson-Robinson M, Chandler S (2007) HPV knowledge and behaviors of black college students at a historically black university. J Am Coll Health 56: 159–163.
17. Gerend MA, Lee SC, Shepherd JE (2007) Predictors of human papillomavirus vaccination acceptability among underserved women. Sex Transm Dis 34: 468–471.
18. Gerend MA, Magloire ZF (2008) Awareness, knowledge, and beliefs about human papillomavirus in a racially diverse sample of young adults. J Adolesc Health 42: 237–242.
19. Brewer NT, Fazekas KI (2007) Predictors of HPV vaccine acceptability: a theory-informed, systematic review. Prev Med 45: 107–114.
20. Klug SJ, Hukelmann M, Blettner M (2008) Knowledge about infection with human papillomavirus: a systematic review. Prev Med 46: 87–98.
21. Zimet GD, Liddon N, Rosenthal SL, Lazcano-Ponce E, Allen B (2006) Chapter 24: Psychosocial aspects of vaccine acceptability. Vaccine 24 Suppl 3: S3/201-209.
22. Bharadwaj M, Hussain S, Nasare V, Das BC (2009) HPV & HPV vaccination: issues in developing countries. Indian J Med Res 130: 327–333.
23. Sankaranarayanan R, Nene BM, Shastri SS, Jayant K, Muwonge R, et al. (2009) HPV screening for cervical cancer in rural India. N Engl J Med 360: 1385–1394.
24. Saha A, Chaudhury AN, Bhowmik P, Chatterjee R (2010) Awareness of cervical cancer among female students of premier colleges in Kolkata, India. Asian Pac J Cancer Prev 11: 1085–1090.
25. Singh E, Seth S, Rani V, Srivastava DK (2012) Awareness of cervical cancer screening among nursing staff in a tertiary institution of rural India. J Gynecol Oncol 23: 141–146.
26. Hussain S, Bharadwaj M, Nasare V, Kumari M, Sharma S, et al. (2012) Human papillomavirus infection among young adolescents in India: impact of vaccination. J Med Virol 84: 298–305.
27. Brinton LA (1992) Epidemiology of cervical cancer–overview. IARC Sci Publ: 3–23.
28. Parazzini F, La Vecchia C, Negri E, Cecchetti G, Fedele L (1989) Reproductive factors and the risk of invasive and intraepithelial cervical neoplasia. Br J Cancer 59: 805–809.
29. Holly EA (1996) Cervical intraepithelial neoplasia, cervical cancer, and HPV. Annu Rev Public Health 17: 69–84.
30. Brinton LA, Reeves WC, Brenes MM, Herrero R, de Britton RC, et al. (1989) Parity as a risk factor for cervical cancer. Am J Epidemiol 130: 486–496.
31. Mehta S, Rajaram S, Goel G, Goel N (2013) Awareness about Human Papilloma Virus and its Vaccine Among Medical Students. Indian J Community Med 38: 92–94.
32. Pandey D, Vanya V, Bhagat S, Vs B, Shetty J (2012) Awareness and attitude towards human papillomavirus (HPV) vaccine among medical students in a premier medical school in India. PLoS One 7: e40619.
33. Han YJL, Kang SR, Kim EJ, Kim MK, Kim NH, et al. (2007) Knowledge regarding cervical cancer, human Papillomavirus and future acceptance of vaccination among girls in their late teens in Korea. Korean J Obstet Gynecol 50: 1090–1099.
34. Vogtmann E, Harlow SD, Valdez AC, Valdez JC, Ponce EL (2011) HPV knowledge in Mexican college students: implications for intervention programmes. Health Soc Care Community 19: 148–157.
35. Abotchie PN, Shokar NK (2009) Cervical cancer screening among college students in ghana: knowledge and health beliefs. Int J Gynecol Cancer 19: 412–416.
36. Lopez RM, McMahan S (2007) College women's perception and knowledge of human papillomavirus (HPV) and cervical cancer. Californian Journal of Health Promotion 5: 12–25.
37. Cates JR, Brewer NT, Fazekas KI, Mitchell CE, Smith JS (2009) Racial differences in HPV knowledge, HPV vaccine acceptability, and related beliefs among rural, southern women. J Rural Health 25: 93–97.
38. Hoque ME (2013) Awareness of cervical cancer, Papanicolau's smear and its utilization among female, final year undergraduates in Durban, South Africa. J Cancer Res Ther 9: 25–28.
39. Hsu YY, Cheng YM, Hsu KF, Fetzer SJ, Chou CY (2011) Knowledge and beliefs about cervical cancer and human papillomavirus among Taiwanese undergraduate women. Oncol Nurs Forum 38: E297–304.
40. Bingham A, Drake JK, LaMontagne DS (2009) Sociocultural issues in the introduction of human papillomavirus vaccine in low-resource settings. Arch Pediatr Adolesc Med 163: 455–461.
41. Joy T, Sathian B, Bhattarai C, Chacko J (2011) Awareness of cervix cancer risk factors in educated youth: a cross-sectional, questionnaire based survey in India, Nepal, and Sri Lanka. Asian Pac J Cancer Prev 12: 1707–1712.
42. Uzunlar O, Ozyer S, Baser E, Togrul C, Karaca M, et al. (2013) A survey on human papillomavirus awareness and acceptance of vaccination among nursing students in a tertiary hospital in Ankara, Turkey. Vaccine 31: 2191–2195.
43. Kamzol W, Jaglarz K, Tomaszewski KA, Puskulluoglu M, Krzemieniecki K (2013) Assessment of knowledge about cervical cancer and its prevention among female students aged 17–26 years. Eur J Obstet Gynecol Reprod Biol 166: 196–203.
44. Donadiki EM, Jimenez-Garcia R, Hernandez-Barrera V, Carrasco-Garrido P, Lopez-de Andres A, et al. (2012) Knowledge of the HPV vaccine and its association with vaccine uptake among female higher-education students in Greece. Hum Vaccin Immunother 9.
45. Pitts MK, Heywood W, Ryall R, Smith AM, Shelley JM, et al. (2010) Knowledge of human papillomavirus (HPV) and the HPV vaccine in a national sample of Australian men and women. Sex Health 7: 299–303.
46. Nnodu O, Erinosho L, Jamda M, Olaniyi O, Adelaiye R, et al. (2010) Knowledge and attitudes towards cervical cancer and human papillomavirus: a Nigerian pilot study. Afr J Reprod Health 14: 95–108.
47. Gottvall M, Larsson M, Hoglund AT, Tyden T (2009) High HPV vaccine acceptance despite low awareness among Swedish upper secondary school students. Eur J Contracept Reprod Health Care 14: 399–405.
48. Pelucchi C, Esposito S, Galeone C, Semino M, Sabatini C, et al. (2010) Knowledge of human papillomavirus infection and its prevention among adolescents and parents in the greater Milan area, Northern Italy. BMC Public Health 10: 378.
49. Oh JK, Lim MK, Yun EH, Lee EH, Shin HR (2010) Awareness of and attitude towards human papillomavirus infection and vaccination for cervical cancer prevention among adult males and females in Korea: a nationwide interview survey. Vaccine 28: 1854–1860.
50. Dinh TA, Rosenthal SL, Doan ED, Trang T, Pham VH, et al. (2007) Attitudes of mothers in Da Nang, Vietnam toward a human papillomavirus vaccine. J Adolesc Health 40: 559–563.
51. Lee PW, Kwan TT, Tam KF, Chan KK, Young PM, et al. (2007) Beliefs about cervical cancer and human papillomavirus (HPV) and acceptability of HPV vaccination among Chinese women in Hong Kong. Prev Med 45: 130–134.
52. Li J, Li LK, Ma JF, Wei LH, Niyazi M, et al. (2009) Knowledge and attitudes about human papillomavirus (HPV) and HPV vaccines among women living in metropolitan and rural regions of China. Vaccine 27: 1210–1215.
53. Lambert EC (2001) College students' knowledge of human papillomavirus and effectiveness of a brief educational intervention. J Am Board Fam Pract 14: 178–183.
54. Ralston JD, Taylor VM, Yasui Y, Kuniyuki A, Jackson JC, et al. (2003) Knowledge of cervical cancer risk factors among Chinese immigrants in Seattle. J Community Health 28: 41–57.
55. Wong LP, Wong YL, Low WY, Khoo EM, Shuib R (2009) Knowledge and awareness of cervical cancer and screening among Malaysian women who have never had a Pap smear: a qualitative study. Singapore Med J 50: 49–53.
56. Dell DL, Chen H, Ahmad F, Stewart DE (2000) Knowledge about human papillomavirus among adolescents. Obstet Gynecol 96: 653–656.
57. Marlow LA, Waller J, Wardle J (2007) Parental attitudes to pre-pubertal HPV vaccination. Vaccine 25: 1945–1952.
58. Tiro JA, Saraiya M, Jain N, Liddon N, Cokkinides V, et al. (2008) Human papillomavirus and cervical cancer behavioral surveillance in the US. Cancer 113: 3013–3030.
59. Pitts MK, Dyson SJ, Rosenthal DA, Garland SM (2007) Knowledge and awareness of human papillomavirus (HPV): attitudes towards HPV vaccination among a representative sample of women in Victoria, Australia. Sex Health 4: 177–180.
60. Dempsey AF, Zimet GD, Davis RL, Koutsky L (2006) Factors that are associated with parental acceptance of human papillomavirus vaccines: a

randomized intervention study of written information about HPV. Pediatrics 117: 1486–1493.
61. Di Giuseppe G, Abbate R, Liguori G, Albano L, Angelillo IF (2008) Human papillomavirus and vaccination: knowledge, attitudes, and behavioural intention in adolescents and young women in Italy. Br J Cancer 99: 225–229.
62. Kahn JA, Rosenthal SL, Jin Y, Huang B, Namakydoust A, et al. (2008) Rates of human papillomavirus vaccination, attitudes about vaccination, and human papillomavirus prevalence in young women. Obstet Gynecol 111: 1103–1110.
63. Walsh CD, Gera A, Shah M, Sharma A, Powell JE, et al. (2008) Public knowledge and attitudes towards Human Papilloma Virus (HPV) vaccination. BMC Public Health 8: 368.
64. Chelimo C, Wouldes TA, Cameron LD (2010) Human papillomavirus (HPV) vaccine acceptance and perceived effectiveness, and HPV infection concern among young New Zealand university students. Sex Health 7: 394–396.
65. Hoover DR, Carfioli B, Moench EA (2000) Attitudes of adolescent/young adult women toward human papillomavirus vaccination and clinical trials. Health Care Women Int 21: 375–391.
66. Brabin L, Roberts SA, Farzaneh F, Kitchener HC (2006) Future acceptance of adolescent human papillomavirus vaccination: a survey of parental attitudes. Vaccine 24: 3087–3094.
67. Constantine NA, Jerman P (2007) Acceptance of human papillomavirus vaccination among Californian parents of daughters: a representative statewide analysis. J Adolesc Health 40: 108–115.
68. Fazekas KI, Brewer NT, Smith JS (2008) HPV vaccine acceptability in a rural Southern area. J Womens Health (Larchmt) 17: 539–548.
69. Morison LA, Cozzolino PJ, Orbell S (2010) Temporal perspective and parental intention to accept the human papillomavirus vaccination for their daughter. Br J Health Psychol 15: 151–165.
70. Conroy K, Rosenthal SL, Zimet GD, Jin Y, Bernstein DI, et al. (2009) Human papillomavirus vaccine uptake, predictors of vaccination, and self-reported barriers to vaccination. J Womens Health (Larchmt) 18: 1679–1686.

# 13

# A Pilot RCT of Psychodynamic Group Art Therapy for Patients in Acute Psychotic Episodes: Feasibility, Impact on Symptoms and Mentalising Capacity

**Christiane Montag[1]*, Laura Haase[1], Dorothea Seidel[1,2], Martin Bayerl[1], Jürgen Gallinat[1], Uwe Herrmann[2], Karin Dannecker[2]**

**1** Charité University Medicine Berlin (Charité Universitätsmedizin Berlin), Department of Psychiatry and Psychotherapy, Campus Mitte, Berlin, Germany, **2** Weissensee School of Art (Kunsthochschule Berlin-Weißensee), Art Therapy Department, Berlin, Germany

## Abstract

This pilot study aimed to evaluate the feasibility of an assessor-blind, randomised controlled trial of psychodynamic art therapy for the treatment of patients with schizophrenia, and to generate preliminary data on the efficacy of this intervention during acute psychotic episodes. Fifty-eight inpatients with DSM-diagnoses of schizophrenia were randomised to either 12 twice-weekly sessions of psychodynamic group art therapy plus treatment as usual or to standard treatment alone. Primary outcome criteria were positive and negative psychotic and depressive symptoms as well as global assessment of functioning. Secondary outcomes were mentalising function, estimated with the Reading the mind in the eyes test and the Levels of emotional awareness scale, self-efficacy, locus of control, quality of life and satisfaction with care. Assessments were made at baseline, at post-treatment and at 12 weeks' follow-up. At 12 weeks, 55% of patients randomised to art therapy, and 66% of patients receiving treatment as usual were examined. In the per-protocol sample, art therapy was associated with a significantly greater mean reduction of positive symptoms and improved psychosocial functioning at post-treatment and follow-up, and with a greater mean reduction of negative symptoms at follow-up compared to standard treatment. The significant reduction of positive symptoms at post-treatment was maintained in an attempted intention-to-treat analysis. There were no group differences regarding depressive symptoms. Of secondary outcome parameters, patients in the art therapy group showed a significant improvement in levels of emotional awareness, and particularly in their ability to reflect about others' emotional mental states. This is one of the first randomised controlled trials on psychodynamic group art therapy for patients with acute psychotic episodes receiving hospital treatment. Results prove the feasibility of trials on art therapy during acute psychotic episodes and justify further research to substantiate preliminary positive results regarding symptom reduction and the recovery of mentalising function.

***Trial Registration:*** ClinicalTrials.gov NCT01622166

**Editor:** Yiru Fang, Shanghai Mental Health Center, Shanghai Jiao Tong University School of Medicine, China

**Funding:** The study was financially supported by the Weissensee School of Art. The funders had no role in study design, data collection and analysis, decision to publish, or preparation of the manuscript.

**Competing Interests:** The authors have declared that no competing interests exist.

* Email: christiane.montag@charite.de

## Introduction

Art therapy (AT) has a long tradition for the understanding and the treatment of patients with severe mental disorders [1–4], and group art therapy has become a common adjunctive intervention in hospital settings [5]. After early attempts to use the artifacts of psychiatric patients as a diagnostic medium and to gain access to their unconscious inner life, contemporary art therapy is valued as a non-verbal, ressource-oriented "form of therapy in which the making of visual images… in the presence of a qualified art therapist contributes towards externalisation of thoughts and feelings which may otherwise remain unexpressed" [6]. The development of art therapy was inextricably linked to the treatment of psychotic patients, which on the one hand can be seen as a consequence of the long-standing interest in their creative expressions [7], but on the other must be related to the unique properties of art therapy itself, rendering it perhaps more suitable for acutely psychotic persons than other forms of exploratory psychotherapy [8]. The creative space offers the opportunity to express and communicate even unusual experiences in a validating and non-judgmental environment. The tripartite relationship between the patient/creator, the therapist and the artifact allows a finely nuanced regulation of interpersonal contact and intensity [9]. Art therapy has been considered particularly helpful to patients who are unable to express their inner life verbally - may it be because of its 'abnormal' or 'unspeakable' contents [9], formal thought disorder, alexithymia [10], or fear of being overwhelmed by emotion [3]. Moreover, creating artworks may affirm the vulnerable sense of self and ownership in psychoses [8,11], foster benign self-awareness [12,13] and strengthen self-efficacy in the process of recovery [14]. Art therapy in psychotic people can help to restore orientation and structure within internal and external experiences, and the artistic 'externalisation' of inner states or experiences can become subject to cautious distancing and reality-testing [4]. In contrast to normal symbol-formation, images in acute schizophrenia may not always have an 'as-if' quality. This may correspond to the large body of evidence reporting a reduced mentalising capacity, or deficits in theory of mind, empathy and the understanding of metaphor in this disorder [15–19]. Previous findings suggest that mentalising deficits are detectable in all stages and the entire spectrum of psychotic disorders, but underlie substantial alterations during acute phases of illness [20]. Art therapy might, like any other psychotherapy, but even more so through the reflection of images and artifacts, help to recover mentalising function in psychosis by promoting the formation of mental representations of thoughts and feelings and to develop a "language for mental content which supports mentalisation" [13]. To jointly reflect about and to share the experience of art can invite to adopt the perspective of others [4].

Under the umbrella of creative therapies and based on a meta-analysis compassing art, music, drama and dance movement therapies, art therapy was integrated in international treatment recommendations for schizophrenia like the British NICE guidelines [21]. The recently issued guideline on psychosocial therapies in severe mental disorders of the German Society for Psychiatry, Psychotherapy and Neurology endorsed art therapy with a recommendation grade B [22]. However, compared to the wealth of clinical experience, naturalistic reports and subjective accounts of the healing properties of artmaking, the body of scientific evidence from controlled research is still small [23,24]. Ruddy and Milnes' systematic review identified 61 studies, but reported only two randomised controlled trials (RCT; total n = 137) comparing art therapy plus treatment as usual (TAU) with standard care alone in outpatients with schizophrenia or schizophrenia-like illness [8], which tentatively indicated positive effects of art therapy on self-esteem [12] and negative symptoms [25], but did not show any impact on psychosocial functioning or quality of life. Only one study was conducted in inpatients and reported positive effects of group art therapy compared to treatment as usual on social functioning [26]. In contrast, the largest and most recently published three-arm RCT of art therapy (MATISSE trial, [27]) in 417 patients with schizophrenia randomised to art therapy or an activity control intervention plus TAU or TAU alone, could not prove any additional benefit regarding global assessment of functioning or positive and negative symptoms scores at 12 and 24 months. However, this study included stabilised outpatients and reported substantial problems of attendance - median level of attendance was 11 sessions in the AT group over a 1-year period - as well as very low group sizes that might have limited the interaction between participants. Short term outcome data were not recorded, so that benefits during or shortly after the intervention could not be registered. As a conclusion, the authors recommended to study the impact of AT delivered in inpatient settings [27]. Therefore, the main purpose of the presented pilot study was to investigate the feasibility of an efficacy trial of art therapy for inpatients with schizophrenia during acute psychotic episodes and to generate preliminary data on the effects of art therapy on psychotic symptoms and global functioning. On an exploratory basis, we aimed to elucidate the influence of art therapy on measures of mentalising like cognitive empathy and levels of emotional awareness, as well as on self-efficacy, quality of life and satisfaction with care. For this reason a single-blind, parallel-group RCT was conducted, comparing a 6 week-course of 90 minutes of art therapy twice weekly in addition to TAU with standard treatment alone in patients with schizophrenia during acute episodes that required hospitalisation.

## Methods

### 2.1. Ethics and Registration

The study was approved by the local ethics committee (Charité Universitätsmedizin Berlin, EA1/104/11, positive vote: May 12, 2011) and conducted according to the principles expressed in the Declaration of Helsinki; all subjects gave written informed consent. Capacity to consent was assessed according to the principles defined by Helmchen and Lauter [28]. No patients who were unable to consent were included. In addition, legal representatives of patients, if present, were informed about study participation. The trial was registered at www.ClinicalTrials.gov (identifier: NCT01622166). Due to technical reasons, the study was registrated after enrolment started. The authors confirm that all ongoing and related trials for this intervention are registered. The protocol for this trial and supporting CONSORT checklist are available as supporting information; see **Protocol S1** and **Checklist S1**. The study started later and recruitment took substantially longer than expected at the time when the protocol was prepared.

### 2.2. Participants

Between 8/2011 and 9/2012, 122 inpatients of the Charité Universitätsmedizin Berlin (Psychiatric University Hospital at St. Hedwig Krankenhaus), aged between 18 and 64 years and diagnosed with schizophrenia according to DSM-IV, were screened and recruited by the treating psychiatrists with structured interviews (Structured Clinical Interview I and II (questions 103–117 for antisocial personality disorder) for DSM-IV, [29]) in order to exclude axis-I disorders other than schizophrenia and antisocial personality disorder. Other exclusion criteria were insufficient German language competence, any other psychiatric disorder apart from schizophrenia, relevant use of alcohol or illegal substances, organic brain disease or severe somatic disease impairing cerebral function, inability to give informed consent, acute suicidal intention, aggression and hospitalisation according to Berlin Mental Health Law (PsychKG). Patients were also excluded, when treatment in a group setting was impeded by 1) severe psychomotor agitation or impulsivity, 2) marked hostility and aggression, 3) severe paranoid ideation related to the setting or group members. Diagnoses according to DSM-IV-TR comprised paranoid (n = 45), disorganised (n = 4) and undifferentiated schizophrenia (n = 5), and first episodes of schizophreniform disorder (n = 4). Distribution of diagnoses did not differ between groups - neither in randomised patients nor in completers. Patients who were professionally involved in the making or the reception of art, or had attended art therapy as an outpatient before admission, were not included. Moreover, patients were asked to rate both their active and passive interest in art on a 4-point Likert scale (not at all - occasionally - regularly - passionate). There were no differences between groups, neither at randomisation nor in the per-protocol sample, and none between completers and dropouts.

### 2.3. Randomisation, concealment and masking

Fifty-eight patients were randomised using a randomisation list provided by the Charité central pharmacy. The allocation sequence was concealed until assignment by telephone. Participants and clinical staff involved in the administration and supervision of art therapy (D.S., L.H., K.D., U.H.) were aware of allocation status. Clinical ratings and scoring of Levels of emotional awareness scale (LEAS) transscripts were performed by psychiatrists (M.B., C.M.) not involved in the direct treatment of patients and blind to randomisation. Patients were instructed not to inform the assessors of their allocation status. Neuropsychological tests and questionnaires were administered by a researcher aware of therapy assignment (L.H.).

## 2.4. Interventions

Art therapy was administered in 12 sessions of 90 minutes for 6 weeks. Groups included between 3 and 6 patients. The setting was a room designed as an art studio in the clinic. It contained working tables, a variety of art materials such as water colour and poster paint, pencils, color pencils, markers, crayons, pastels, different size paper and brushes, drawing boards, clay, tools, an easel and storage facilities. The approach was non-directive – patients could choose to create whatever they wanted and use any available material they liked. They were encouraged to find their own image at their own pace. Interventions by the art therapist aimed at supporting the art process and helping to understand the image. The last 30 minutes of a session were reserved for a shared viewing and reflecting on the images. Each patient was asked if he/she wanted to present his/her image and to talk about it. Other patients were invited to comment and share their observations and ideas. If a patient did not want to share his image, this wish was respected. The patient's autonomous decision-making about the handling of his or her art work was crucial. For a thorough description of therapeutic attitude, specific interventions and their rationale we refer to Dannecker (2010 [4]), serving as a therapeutic guideline for the art therapist.

One art therapist (D.S.) conducted the AT intervention and was accompanied by a co-worker who video-taped the sessions. All AT sessions were video-taped to assure treatment fidelity that was also confirmed during regular, joint video-based supervisions (K.D., U.H.), and to allow for qualitative analyses, which will be reported elsewhere. Patients assigned to the control group received TAU without an offer of art therapy. All patients were demanded to refrain from taking part in any other visual artistic activity apart from the sessions provided in the hospital during the trial phase. Patients who were discharged or transferred to a day clinic within the 12-session course were actively encouraged to attend all sessions. All patients received a designed reminder card of the session dates and were also motivated by personal contact and phone calls to participate.

Patients receiving TAU were also actively reminded of the follow-up examinations. In addition to supportive contact and pharmacotherapy, TAU covered a broad spectrum of verbal targeted psychotherapies for patients with psychoses like cognitive-behavioural therapy and modified psychodynamic interventions in individual and group settings, as well as occupational therapy, music therapy, cognitive and social skills training, excursions, relaxation and sports.

## 2.5. Outcome measures

Primary outcome measures were psychotic and depressive symptoms, measured by semi-structured interviews, which comprised composite scores of the Scale for the assessment of negative symptoms (SANS, [30]) and the Scale for the assessment of positive symptoms (SAPS, [31]), the Calgary depression scale for schizophrenia (CDSS, [32]), as well as psychosocial outcome, measured by the Global assessment of functioning scale of the DSM-IV-TR (GAF, [33]).

Secondary outcome measures were parameters of mentalising function, self-efficacy/locus of control, quality of life and satisfaction with care.

Mentalising was covered by the constructs of 1) cognitive empathy, determined with the Reading the mind in the eyes test (RME, [34]; German translation [35]) that requires the inference of complex affective mental states from photographs depicting the eye regions of 36 persons, and 2) the Levels of emotional awareness scale (LEAS, [36]; German version [37]), assessing the ability to imagine, to recognize and to express one's own and others' emotions when presented with 10 emotionally evocative written scenarios. Two parallel versions were used for testing at baseline and post-treatment visits in a balanced manner. The development of the LEAS was based on Piaget's model of emotional-cognitive development, which comprises 5 hierarchically ascending levels [38]. The increasing complexity and elaboration of emotional awareness of both own and others' emotional mental states is reflected by higher scores of the LEAS-self and LEAS-other scales, respectively, that were determined from transscripts of participants' answers using a detailed scoring manual and glossary. The 2 versions of the LEAS have shown a sufficient internal, inter-rater and test-retest reliability [37] and were also shown to capture changes in emotional awareness in the course of psychotherapeutic treatment [39]. LEAS-other scores correlated with tests of higher-order mentalising in patients with somatoform disorder [40]. From a first study in schizophrenic patients, Baslet et al. reported lower levels of emotional awareness of others in patients compared to healthy controls [41].

Self-efficacy and locus of control were evaluated by the Questionnaire for competence and control (Fragebogen zu Kompetenz- und Kontrollüberzeugungen, FKK, [42]), a translation and extension of Levenson's IPC scales [43]. The FKK consists of 4 8-item scales, named self-concept of own ability, internality, social externality and fatalistic externality. Two secondary scales were calculated by adding two primary subscales and used for analysis: The self-concept of own ability and internality scales estimate global self-efficacy, and a sum score of the 2 externality scales reflects overall externality. Internality was found related to successful recovery in schizophrenia [14].

Quality of life during the past 4 weeks was evaluated using the core module of the Modular system for quality of life (MSQoL, [44]).

General satisfaction with hospital care was self-rated on an 8-item questionnaire (Fragebogen zur Patientenzufriedenheit, ZUF-8 [45]).

Potential confounders like verbal intelligence and verbal working memory and learning were estimated by a multiple choice vocabulary test (Mehrfachwahl-Wortschatztest, MWT-B, [46]) and the Auditory Verbal Learning Test (AVLT, [47]).

## 2.6. Procedure

Patients randomised to art therapy then were offered a trial AT session in which they were introduced to the setting and the circumstances of video-taping the sessions. Post-intervention, after approximately 6 weeks, a second examination was performed, including psychopathology, GAF, social-cognitive and emotional measures, locus of control and quality of life. Psychopathology, GAF, self-efficacy and quality of life measures were re-evaluated at a 12 weeks follow-up in both samples.

The progress through the phases of the trial of the two groups, as well as numbers and reasons for dropout are depicted in the CONSORT 2010 flow diagram (http://www.consort-statement.org/consort-statement/flow-diagram0/; **Figure 1**).

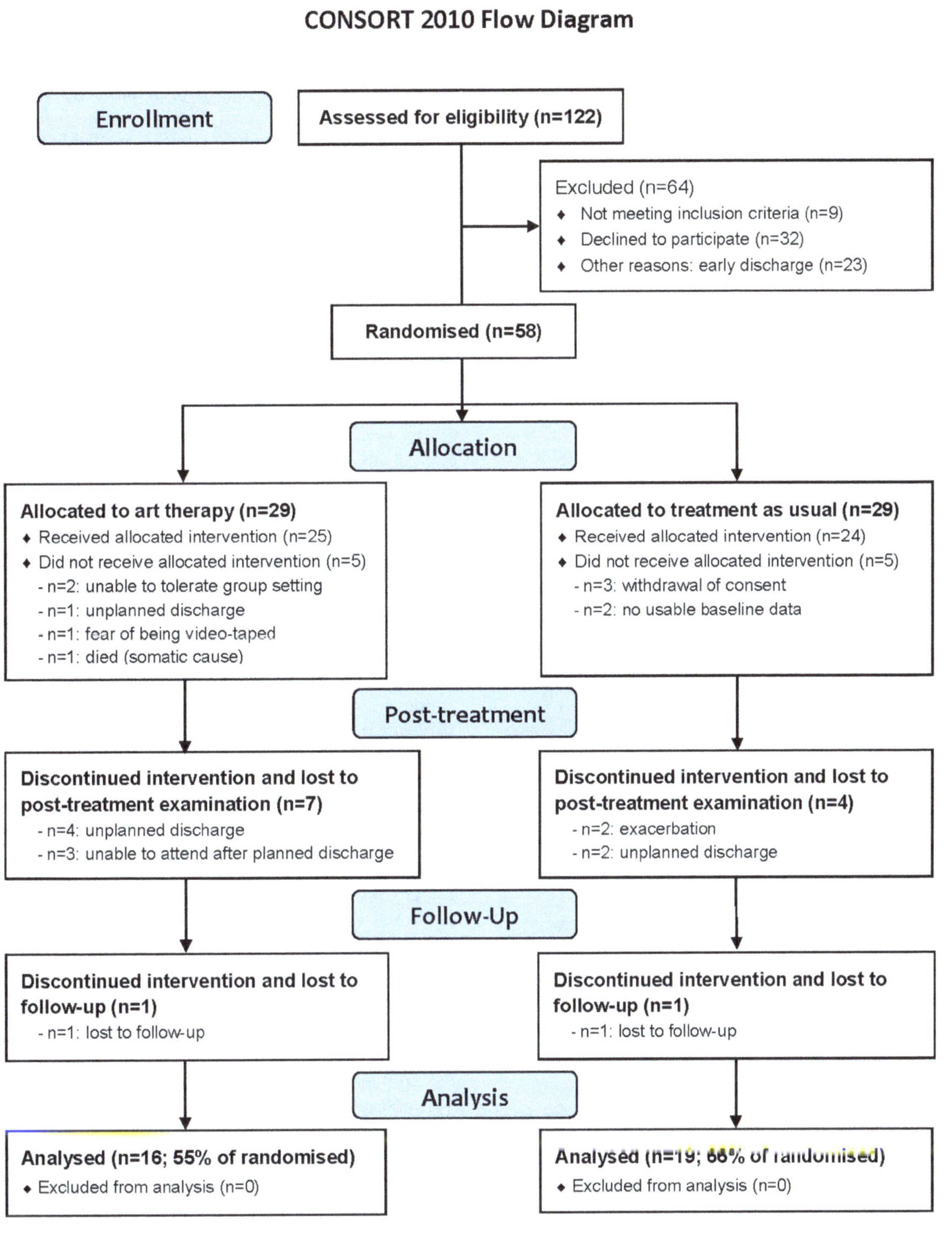


**Figure 1. CONSORT 2010 flow diagram.**

## 2.7. Statistical analyses

In this pilot study, no sample size calculation was performed. Statistical calculations were carried out as indicated in the results section using SPSS for Windows 20.0. All tests were performed with a 2-sided $p<0.05$. Data were tested for normality using the Kolmogorov-Smirnov-Test. The main analyses were performed on completer's data (per-protocol sample). T- and Chi$^2$-tests were used to determine group differences of demographic and illness parameters. To account for possible regression to the mean and differences in baseline ratings, the primary outcome parameters SANS, SAPS, CDSS and GAF were compared between groups by ANCOVAs of both post-treatment and follow-up scores of SANS, SAPS, CDSS or GAF as dependent variables, intervention and gender as factors as well as the respective baseline scores and verbal IQ as covariates. Homoscedasticity was confirmed by Levene tests ($p<0.05$). Partial $\eta^2$ values, reflecting the proportion of the total variance attributable to the intervention factor of the variance remaining after excluding variance explained by other predictors, are given as a rough estimate of effect size, with partial $\eta^2>0.14$ representing small, $\eta^2>0.36$ medium, and $\eta^2>0.51$ large effects [48], p56. Secondary outcome parameters were analysed in the same manner. As social-cognitive function partly depends on neurocognition, $AVLT^{(1-5)}$ scores were introduced as additional covariates for the group comparisons of social-cognitive measures. Group differences of overall satisfaction at post-treatment were determined by ANCOVA with the factors treatment group and gender, and the covariate verbal IQ. Multiple imputation was used to estimate missing post-treatment and follow-up scores to allow for an additional intention-to-treat analysis of primary outcome measures. Group differences were determined by mixed-model ANCOVA with intervention and baseline scores of the dependent variable as covariates. F-tests of 50 imputed data sets were pooled according to [49] using SPSS syntax by [50].

## Results

### 3.1. Sample characteristics and attendance

In total, 58 patients completed the baseline examination; 29 patients received art therapy and TAU; 29 patients were assigned to TAU. Twelve patients (1 female) left the AT group after an average of 2.2±1.8 sessions for reasons stated in **Figure 1**, five of which did not complete the introductory session. In 3 patients, the AT or trial setting was related to dropout (fear of video-taping, inability to tolerate group setting) - in all other cases reasons for dropout were unrelated to the setting. Nine patients (0 female) dropped out of the control group, 3 of which withdrew consent after being randomised to the control group. Two patients had no usable baseline data. Dropouts did not differ from completers in symptom severity at baseline, educational years or duration of illness. Only 3 patients completed less than 12 AT sessions, but 8, 8, and 9 sessions respectively. Two individuals were lost to 12-weeks follow-up. One patient died from a somatic cause unrelated to AT. No other serious adverse events were recorded.

Baseline demographic, illness characteristics and neuropsychological data are given in **Table 1**. When analysing completers only, patients in the AT + TAU group differed significantly from controls with regard to gender and verbal IQ at baseline. In the intention-to-treat sample, baseline SANS values in the AT group were significantly higher than in controls ($T_{[51]} = -2.940$, $p<0.01$; **Table 2**).

### 3.2. Primary outcome measures

ANCOVAs with post-treatment and follow-up scores of SAPS, SANS, CDSS and GAF as dependent variables were performed, controlling for gender, verbal IQ and the baseline score of the respective dependent variable (**Table 2**). In the per-protocol sample, patients who had received AT had a significantly greater mean reduction of positive and negative symptoms at 12-week follow-up than patients treated as usual. Greater reductions of SAPS scores in the AT group already appeared at post-treatment and were maintained in the intention-to-treat analysis. The significance of the group difference in negative symptoms at 12 weeks was reduced to a trend. In the per-protocol sample, global assessment of functioning was significantly higher in the AT group at both visits, but not in the intention-to-treat sample. There were no group differences regarding depressive symptoms (**Table 2**), and were no significant interactions between intervention group and gender.

### 3.3. Secondary outcome measures

LEAS scores differed significantly between groups at post-treatment, favoring AT (LEAS-self: $T_{[34]} = -2.186$, $p<0.05$; LEAS-other: $T_{[34]} = -2.596$, $p<0.05$); however, after control for verbal IQ, $AVLT^{(1-5)}$ and baseline values significance was maintained for LEAS-other scores only (**Table 3**). No group differences were detected for cognitive empathy at the Reading the mind in the eyes test. Patients receiving TAU showed significantly higher scores for generalised self-efficacy at post-treatment ($T_{[35]} = 2.585$, $p<0.05$) and at follow-up ($T_{[33]} = 2.455$, $p<0.05$), but this was not maintained at ANCOVA. There were no significant group differences in FKK generalised externality, quality of life and overall satisfaction with hospital care (**Table 3**).

## Discussion

This pilot project aimed to investigate the feasibility of an efficacy study of art therapy in addition to TAU compared to stardard treatment alone in an assessor-blind, randomised controlled design in acutely psychotic, hospitalised patients diagnosed with schizophrenia.

### 4.1. Feasibility

Study design had to consider both the necessity of a relatively brief intervention period due to the shortness of an average hospital stay and the high initial symptom load of patients. Inability to consent and the cognitive demands of the baseline examination limited recruitment. Substantial numbers of screened patients were either discharged early or declined to participate for various reasons. Despite of this, recruitment and randomisation of participants was practicable. Future inclusion of an attractive, active control group might even facilitate recruiting, as patients were looking forward to the intervention. The non-pharmacological focus of the study was well-accepted, and helped to develop trust. Dropout occurred mainly in case of unplanned discharge from hospital or when patients were unable to attend the group as outpatients because of alternative occupations. Attendance of the AT group was good as soon as participants were engaged in the group and as long as they stayed in the hospital. At post-treatment, 59% of patients randomised to art therapy and 69% receiving TAU were examined, and 55% of patients treated with AT versus 66% of participants in the control group completed the follow-up examination at 12 weeks. Compared to the trials conducted in chronic outpatients, attrition rates of our acute patients tended to be higher. Green et al. reported 40% attrition at 20 weeks and 65% at 9-months follow-up [12], in the study of Richardson et al., 19% of patients had left at 12 weeks and 60% at 6-months follow-up [25]. Only 31% of the AT patients of Crawford et al. had attended 10 or more groups at 12 months [27]. Attrition rates can be considered as satisfactory, if the exacerbated state of the participants and the ubiquitous wish to leave the hospital as early as possible is kept in mind. (Unfortunately, the only other study of AT in inpatients was published in Chinese, and detailed data are not available [26]). Although statistically non-significant, a higher number of patients receiving AT than controls left the study early. Similar attrition rates across groups were found by Crawford et al. [27] and Richardson et al. [25], while Green et al. [12] reported higher attrition in the control group. Compared to these studies of stabilised outpatients, the greater demands of the AT sessions theoretically might have caused dropout of acutely psychotic patients, while patients in the control group had the chance to avoid intense therapeutic interactions if they wished to. However, only 3 out of 29 patients randomised to AT left early for study-related reasons. Otherwise the setting was well tolerated, and apart

**Table 1.** Baseline demographic and neuropsychological parameters, and illness characteristics in patients receiving art therapy or treatment as usual.

| | Per-protocol sample | | | Intention-to-treat sample | | |
|---|---|---|---|---|---|---|
| | AT (n=16) | TAU (n=19) | Statistics | AT (n=29) | TAU (n=24) | Statistics |
| Gender (m/f) | 7/9 | 15/4 | **4.609**[1]* | 19/10 | 19/5 | 1.206[1] |
| age (yrs) | 38.8±11.9 | 39.6±10.6 | 0.231 | 37.4±11.2 | 38.8±10.4 | 0.473 |
| education (yrs) | 15.3±4.6 | 13.2±4.1 | −1.438 | 14.2±4.6 | 13.7±4.0 | −0.460 |
| verbal IQ | 116.6±14.5 | 105.5±13.5 | **−2.339*** | 107.2±17.7 | 108.6±14.5 | 0.314 |
| AVLT $^{(1-5)}$ | 8.0±3.2 | 6.3±2.7 | −1.655 | 7.4±3.0 | 6.6±2.9 | −0.934 |
| AVLT $^{(int)}$ | 3.3±2.7 | 3.6±2.6 | 0.428 | 3.0±2.4 | 3.6±2.4 | 0.940 |
| duration of illness (yrs) | 12.1±12.1 | 15.2±9.3 | 0.839 | 11.3±10.8 | 13.9±9.2 | 0.932 |
| age of onset (yrs) | 26.6±9.2 | 24.5±8.7 | −0.713 | 25.6±7.6 | 24.4±8.8 | −0.497 |
| CPZ equiv. [mg] | 352.5±264.1 | 522.0±298.4 | 1.763 | 451.0±362.7 | 501.8±326.2 | 0.531 |

T-test for independent samples;
[1]: $\chi^2$-test;
*: p<005 (AT: art therapy; TAU: treatment as usual; AVLT: Auditory verbal learning test; CPZ equiv.: antipsychotic dose converted to chlorpromazine equivalents).

from one patient who died from a somatic cause that was unlikely to be related to AT, no adverse events were noticed in the AT group.

## 4.2. Primary outcome measures

As most patients were lost to follow-up after dropout, the main analysis of primary outcome parameters had to refer to the per-protocol sample. Results of this tentative analysis suggest a greater mean reduction of positive symptoms in patients receiving AT at post-treatment and at 12-week follow-up, even if baseline scores were controlled. Negative symptoms were lower in the AT group at follow-up. Results were partly maintained in the intention-to-treat analysis. There were significantly higher GAF mean scores in the AT group at post-treatment and follow-up, but no significant group differences as for depression ratings. Although in contrast to the methodologically rigorous MATISSE trial [27] that did not report any benefit of weekly AT at 12 and 24 months, our preliminary results point in a similar direction as findings of Richardson et al., who reported a reduction in SANS scores and better social functioning in 43 patients randomised to AT after 12 sessions and at 6 months follow-up compared to TAU (n=47), and of Meng et al., who found an increase in overall mental health and social functioning associated with twice-weekly group art therapy over 15 weeks vs. TAU [25,26]. Corroborating evidence from other creative therapies [51–53], our results support the notion that the arts therapies might be helpful in reducing negative symptoms in psychosis. Moreover, in the follow-up period SANS scores in the AT group further improved, while they deteriorated again in the control group. It therefore might be speculated that the experience of AT during acute psychotic episodes might possibly prevent an increase of negative symptoms after remission of acute psychosis.

The decrease of positive symptoms in the AT compared to the TAU group at post-treatment and follow-up should inspire further investigation: Our results contradict the notion that psychodynamic therapies may lead to high emotional intensities and deleterious aftermaths in psychotic patients [5,54]. Our findings may correspond to subjective accounts of patients, who experienced stress reduction during AT sessions, and to the view that the AT setting and the artwork may "contain rather than stimulate anxiety" in psychotic patients [3,5,55].

## 4.3. Secondary outcome measures

Art therapy might counteract core negative symptoms like anhedonia, lack of motivation and affective blunting, but might also exert protective effects on self-esteem, self-efficacy and a creative sense of agency in the course of recovery. Beside a number of case reports and uncontrolled research [56–58], also Green et al. reported significant improvement of patients receiving AT in their attitudes towards themselves, which was correlated with self-esteem, and their ability to get along with others [12]. Meng et al reported higher values on the Tennessee Self Concept Survey, indicating that patients who received AT viewed themselves as more competent and valuable [26]. However, though externality scores nominally decreased in our AT group until follow-up, but did not so in controls, no significant influence of AT on externality or self-efficacy was determined in this study. Moreover, groups did not differ with regard to depressive psychopathology. Beside insufficient statistical power to detect minor effects in small-sized samples, findings might also indicate that the beneficial effects of AT in acute, compared to remitted psychoses might be associated with other mechanisms than an action on locus of control and depression.

Another exploratory focus of this study was directed to possible changes of mentalising abilities in the course of AT. Mentalising deficits, e. g. difficulties to recognize, to infer and to reflect about one's own and other's mental states have consistently been reported in schizophrenia [15], are related to symptom expression [19] and crucially linked to psychosocial outcome [59,60]. While neuroscientific research tended to investigate the social-cognitive aspects of mentalising like theory of mind and social perception, psychotherapeutic approaches concentrate on mentalisation of affective experiences, its developmental origins and interplay with affect regulation [61], and have extended to the field of psychoses [62,63]. While no group differences were detected for cognitive empathy [34] in our study, patients in the AT group showed higher levels of emotional awareness scores, in particular regarding others' emotions, at the end of the intervention period compared to patients treated as usual. This is interesting, as theoretical

**Table 2.** Means, standard deviations, and group comparisons between art therapy and treatment as usual for psychopathological symptoms (SAPS, SANS, CDSS) and global assessment of functioning (GAF) in per-protocol and intention-to-treat samples at post-treatment and follow-up visits.

| | baseline (0 wks) | | post-treatment (6 wks) | | follow-up (12 wks) | | post-treatment (6 wks) | $\eta^2_p$ | follow-up (12 wks) | $\eta^2_p$ |
|---|---|---|---|---|---|---|---|---|---|---|
| | AT | TAU | AT | TAU | AT | TAU | AT vs.TAU | | AT vs.TAU | |
| **per-protocol** | [1] | [1] | [2] | [2] | [1] | [1] | [2] | | [1] | |
| SAPS | 60.0±26.2 | 55.3±26.7 | 19.1±19.8 | 37.1±23.1 | 13.3±16.4 | 35.0±30.9 | **$F_{[1;\,32]}=11.698^{**}$** (underlined) | **0.268** | **$F_{[1;\,30]}=6.960^{*}$** | **0.188** |
| SANS | 48.9±20.6 | 38.1±19.2 | 24.1±15.6 | 27.9±16.2 | 15.9±13.8 | 30.8±18.1 | $F_{[1;\,32]}=1.441$ | 0.043 | **$F_{[1;\,30]}=7.820^{**}$** (underlined) | **0.207** |
| CDSS | 7.9±5.4 | 7.4±4.7 | 5.6±4.2 | 5.9±4.5 | 4.7±4.7 | 5.1±3.9 | $F_{[1;\,32]}=1.425$ | 0.043 | $F_{[1;\,30]}=0.372$ | 0.012 |
| GAF | 38.2±13.3 | 37.8±12.1 | 59.6±16.8 | 47.3±14.1 | 62.0±15.2 | 51.3±13.9 | **$F_{[1;\,32]}=5.218^{*}$** | **0.140** | **$F_{[1;\,30]}=5.005^{*}$** | **0.143** |
| **intention-to-treat** | [3] | [3] | [3] | [3] | [3] | [3] | [3] | | [3] | |
| SAPS | 65.0±26.8 | 55.3±24.9 | 27.2±23.5 | 36.7±22.2 | 23.2±24.5 | 34.1±28.6 | **$F_{[1;\,37.750]}=4{,}462^{*}$** | - | $F_{[1;\,37.349]}=2.858$ | - |
| SANS | 53.9±22.0 | 37.3±17.4 | 27.6±16.8 | 27.1±15.5 | 24.6±19.1 | 29.3±17.4 | $F_{[1;\,39.205]}=0.768$ | - | *$F_{[1;\,34.770]}=3.291^{\dagger}$* | - |
| CDSS | 7.4±5.5 | 6.7±4.5 | 6.4±4.5 | 5.9±3.9 | 5.3±4.5 | 5.3±3.9 | $F_{[1;\,33.011]}=0.024$ | - | $F_{[1;\,30.793]}=0.031$ | - |
| GAF | 37.0±12.8 | 38.4±11.0 | 52.4±17.2 | 48.0±14.0 | 55.8±17.8 | 51.2±14.4 | $F_{[1;\,38.297]}=1.114$ | - | $F_{[1;\,35.663]}=1.036$ | - |

[1]: $n_{AT}=16/n_{TAU}=19$;
[2]: $n_{AT}=16/n_{TAU}=20$;
[3]: $n_{AT}=24/n_{TAU}=29$.
Per-protocol sample: ANCOVA factors: intervention, gender; covariates: verbal IQ, baseline value of dependent variable; $F_{[df]}$; *: $p<0.05$; **: $p<0.01$; $\eta^2_p$; corrected p-value (Bonferroni) $p<0.0125$ (significant results underlined). Intention-to treat sample: descriptive statistics and ANCOVA on multiply imputed data (m = 50): covariates: intervention, baseline value of dependent variable; pooled $F_{[df]}$; *: $p<0.05$; †: $p=0.078$ (AT: art therapy; TAU: treatment as usual; SANS: Scale for the assessment of negative symptoms; SAPS: Scale for the assessment of positive symptoms; CDSS: Calgary depression scale for schizophrenia; GAF: Global assessment of functioning).

**Table 3.** Means, standard deviations, group differences ($F_{[df]}$) and effect sizes ($\eta^2_{p}$) between art therapy and treatment as usual for social cognition (LEAS, RME), self-efficacy/locus of control (FKK), quality of life (MSQoL) and satisfaction with care (ZUF-8) scores in the per-protocol sample.

| | baseline (0 weeks) | | post-treatment (6 weeks) | | follow-up 12 weeks) | | post-treatment (6 weeks) | follow-up (12 weeks) |
|---|---|---|---|---|---|---|---|---|
| | AT | TAU | AT | TAU | AT | TAU | AT vs. TAU | AT vs. TAU |
| per protocol | [1] | [1] | [1] | [1] | [2] | [2] | [1] | [2] |
| LEAS-self [3] | 23.6±6.5 | 22.2±8.0 | 29.3±5.4 | 24.8±6.5 | | - | $F_{[1;29]}=2{,}129$ | - |
| LEAS-other[3] | 18.9±6.8 | 19.4±9.2 | 26.9±6.5 | 20.6±7.9 | | - | **$F_{[1;29]}=5.632$*** | - |
| RME[3] | 20.5±5.5 | 20.6±5.9 | 22.3±4.3 | 20.7±5.5 | | - | $F_{[1;30]}=0.653$ | - |
| FKK SKI[3] | 60.5±15.1 | 68.3±12.9 | 56.4±9.3 | 64.6±10.0 | 58.9±10.7 | 67.93±10.3 | $F_{[1;30]}=1.646$ | $F_{[1;28]}=0.561$ |
| FKK PC[3] | 62.4±18.2 | 60.7±13.5 | 55.6±13.0 | 54.4±16.5 | 52.4±10.8 | 57.5±13.2 | $F_{[1;30]}=0.782$ | $F_{[1;28]}=3.989$ |
| MSQoL[4] | 183.9±40.8 | 194.7±46.8 | 202.6±42.2 | 218,3±33.3 | 224.1±36.4 | 214.3±34.7 | $F_{[1;31]}=0.098$ | $F_{[1;29]}=3.251$ |
| ZUF-8[4] | | - | 16.7±4.5 | 14.1±4.4 | | - | $F_{[1;31]}=1.522$ | - |

[1]: $n_{AT}=16/n_{TAU}=20$;
[2]: $n_{AT}=16/n_{TAU}=19$;
[3]: ANCOVA factors: intervention, gender; covariates: verbal IQ, AVLT$^{(1-5)}$, baseline value of dependent variable.
[4]: ANCOVA factors: intervention, gender; covariates: verbal IQ, baseline value of dependent variable; (post hoc) $F_{[df]}$; *: $p<0.05$; corrected p-value (Bonferroni) $p<0.007$.
(LEAS: Levels of Emotional Awareness Scale; RME: Reading the Mind in the Eyes Test; FKK SKI: sum score self-efficacy; FKK PC: sum score externality; MSQoL: Modular system for quality of life; ZUF-8: satisfaction with care).

considerations suggest that AT may mediate between concrete and symbolic ways of thinking [64]. Although mental state reflection is an active ingredient of any form of psychotherapy and already targeted in a variety of therapies for schizophrenia [65–67], AT may bear additional benefits. Psychotic patients may externalise their inner states in a concrete physical way - the artwork than allows to reflect upon, to clarify and to re-internalize meaning of internal states, and to develop a mentalising stance; the intentional use of symbolic representations is encouraged. Self-exploration and insight are facilitated together with a strengthening of a creative sense of self [56], thus preventing self-stigma. Moreover, art-sharing and communication with the art therapist and group members may help to appreciate the perspective of others [4], to find a language for mental content and thus to facilitate explicit mentalising [13,68]. This process may find its reflection in the levels of emotional awareness concept inspired by Piaget [69]. AT has been integrated in mentalisation-based treatment programmes for patients with Borderline personality disorder [70], in juvenile offenders [71] and was found to promote parental mentalisation [72]. Moreover, Kidd and Castano [73] showed that in healthy adults also the non-therapeutic engagement with works of art like literary fiction may positively influence theory of mind. The finding of more mature levels of emotional awareness after 6 weeks of AT might be associated with a recovery of the ability to reason about own and other's emotional mental states in psychotic patients. In contrast, no changes were detected for cognitive empathy. This might be explained by the fact that AT more intensely trains emotional awareness by introspection and imagination, compared to the ability to recognize emotions from facial expressions. However, our result is a preliminary indication from a first quantitative research attempt on the effects of AT on mentalising that requires further substantiation.

Our results do not indicate effects of AT on quality of life or overall satisfaction with hospital care. Previous findings have been inconsistent, showing positive [26] or no impact [25,27]. We believe that the intervention period in our study might have been too short to significantly improve quality of life and that satisfaction with hospital care did not differ between groups because of the host of alternative therapeutic offers in the TAU condition.

### 4.4. Limitations and recommendations for further reasearch

During the course of this pilot study, results of the largest RCT of AT in schizophrenia, the MATISSE trial, were published [27]. Along with negative findings regarding the effects of AT in psychoses, the authors mentioned a number of practical problems that might hamper interpretability of this trial. We therefore tried to address problems of feasibility in an inpatient setting, but also decided not to refrain from hypothesis-testing and to tentatively report first results, intending to motivate a continuation of research on AT for patients with psychoses.

Besides sample sizes, our small study suffers a number of limitations. There was no standardised active comparison condition to control for the unspecific effects of therapeutic contact and group dynamics. However, patients receiving TAU were engaged in other therapies and did not nessessarily suffer from less therapeutic attention. The total amount of (psycho-)therapeutic interventions in both groups should be recorded in future trials.

Even when focusing on patients with acute psychotic episodes, the follow-up period of 12 weeks was rather short, and the benefits of AT might have vanished in the longer run. A possible solution in a larger trial could be to start the intervention during a phase of hospitalisation and to continue the study without interruption in the familiar setting for a longer intervention and follow-up period.

It has also to be mentioned that AT might have "selected" patients who profited from this intervention. AT completers were more often female and of higher verbal intelligence. Although we statistically controlled for gender and IQ, creative activity might have particularly appealed to a subgroup of patients with a better a priori prognosis. A substantial share of excluded participants did not receive the allocated intervention. Three patients of the control group withdrew consent because they were not happy with the result of randomisation and the need to abstain from creative therapies. As psychotherapy research always has to consider personal preferences and setting, a larger RCT might include a run-in period of both AT and the control condition before randomisation to avoid selection effects [74]. However, similar to the exclusion of subjects who never received the intervention after randomisation, this will limit generalisability of findings [75].

Higher attrition rates might not be avoidable in patients with severe mental disorders, but for a sound intention-to-treat analysis outcome data should be collected from all participants regardless of whether they received the intervention. This might be achieved by closely involving outpatient services, telephone reminders, provision of transportation costs and financial incentives. A higher frequency of study visits might not only allow for registering short term changes, but also enhance motivation of patients. Reasons for drop-out and missing of visits and the respective patient characteristics should be systematically analysed as these might not occur completely at random. The problem of missing data, mainly of dropped out individuals, impeded intention-to-treat analysis which had to rely on substitution by multiple imputation. Moreover, multiple imputation methods might also lead to biased results if high amounts of missing values are substituted. Future research should try to minimise missing data and allow for sensitivity analysis [76,77].

Our findings are based on small case numbers, and we are aware of the fact that data on efficacy from such a small trial are biased and might overestimate the impact of the intervention. Moreover, patients in the per-protocol sample differed - though not significantly - in SANS and SAPS ratings, so that significant effects might be a result of regression to the mean. We accounted for this problem by using ANCOVA including baseline scores as covariates. For the purpose of a pilot study four primary outcome measures were tested, only two of which remained significant after alpha-level adjustment. Results may therefore only give a very rough indication of the direction of the treatment effect but cannot serve to confirm or reject our hypotheses, and even results on feasibility might not generalise [78].

### 4.5. Conclusion

Evidence on the efficacy and effectiveness of AT in patients with schizophrenia is far from being conclusive and benefits might be limited to a subgroup of patients. Results of this pilot study suggest that RCTs of AT can be implemented in routine hospital settings for patients experiencing acute psychotic states. With all due caution, findings from this first European pilot RCT of psychodynamic AT in acutely psychotic inpatients prove the feasibility of similar projects and point to a possible positive effect of the intervention on psychotic symptoms, psychosocial functioning and the ability to mentalise emotions. These preliminary results must be substantiated by further independent research.

## Acknowledgments

We gratefully acknowledge the commitment and trust of our patients who participated in the study and the invaluable assistance of hospital physicians and staff in implementing this project. Moreover, we would like to thank the reviewers of this manuscript for their valuable comments.

## Author Contributions

Conceived and designed the experiments: CM MB LH DS UH KD JG. Performed the experiments: LH CM MB. Analyzed the data: CM. Contributed reagents/materials/analysis tools: DS UH KD MB. Wrote the paper: CM LH DS KD. Performed art therapy: DS. Supervised art therapist: UH KD.

## References

1. Prinzhorn H (1922) Die Bildnerei der Geisteskranken. Berlin: Springer.
2. Navratil L (1965) Schizophrenie und Kunst. München: Deutscher Taschenbuchverlag.
3. Killick K, Schaverien J (1997) Art, Psychotherapy and Psychosis. London: Routledge.
4. Dannecker K. (2010) Psyche und Ästhetik. Die Transformationen der Kunsttherapie. Berlin: Medizinisch Wissenschaftliche Verlagsgesellschaft.
5. Patterson S, Debate J, Anju S, Waller D, Crawford MJ (2011) Provision and practice of art therapy for people with schizophrenia: results of a national survey. J Ment Health 20: 328–335.
6. Waller D, Gilroy A, eds. (1992) Art therapy: A handbook. Open University Press.
7. Spaniol S (2001) Art and mental illness: Where is the link? The Arts in Psychotherapy 28: 221–231.
8. Ruddy R, Milnes D (2005) Art therapy for schizophrenia or schizophrenia-like illnesses. Cochrane Database Syst Rev CD003728. 10.1002/14651858.CD003728.pub2 [doi].
9. Patterson S, Crawford MJ, Ainsworth E, Waller D (2011) Art therapy for people diagnosed with schizophrenia: Therapists' views about what changes, how and for whom. International Journal of Art Therapy 16: 70–80.
10. van 't Wout M, Aleman A, Bermond B, Kahn RS (2007) No words for feelings: alexithymia in schizophrenia patients and first-degree relatives. Compr Psychiatry 48: 27–33.
11. Sarra N (1998) Connection and disconnection in the art therapy group. Working with forensic patients on the locked ward. In: Skaife S, Huet V, editors. Art psychotherapy groups. Between pictures and words. London: Routledge.
12. Green BL, Wehling C, Talsky GJ (1987) Group art therapy as an adjunct to treatment for chronic outpatients. Hosp Community Psychiatry 38: 988–991.
13. Springham N, Findlay D, Woods A, Harris J (2012) How can art therapy contribute to mentalization in borderline personality disorder? International Journal of Art Therapy 17: 115–129.
14. Harrow M, Hansford BG, Astrachan-Fletcher EB (2009) Locus of control: relation to schizophrenia, to recovery, and to depression and psychosis – A 15-year longitudinal study. Psychiatry Res 168: 186–192.
15. Brüne M (2005) "Theory of mind" in schizophrenia: a review of the literature. Schizophr Bull 31: 21–42.
16. Mo S, Su Y, Chan RC, Liu J (2008) Comprehension of metaphor and irony in schizophrenia during remission: the role of theory of mind and IQ. Psychiatry Res 157: 21–29.
17. Sprong M, Schothorst P, Vos E, Hox J, van Engeland H (2007) Theory of mind in schizophrenia: meta-analysis. Br J Psychiatry 191: 5–13.
18. Kircher TT, Leube DT, Erb M, Grodd W, Rapp AM (2007) Neural correlates of metaphor processing in schizophrenia. Neuroimage 34: 281–289.
19. Montag C, Dziobek I, Richter IS, Neuhaus K, Lehmann A, et al. (2010) Different aspects of theory of mind in paranoid schizophrenia: Evidence from a video-based assessment. Psychiatry Res 186: 203–209.
20. Bora E, Yücel M, Pantelis C (2009) Theory of mind impairment: a distinct trait-marker for schizophrenia spectrum disorders and bipolar disorder? Acta Psychiatr Scand 120: 253–264.
21. National Institute for Clinical Excellence (2009) Schizophrenia: Core Interventions in the Treatment and Management of Schizophrenia in Adults in Primary and Secondary Care. NICE clinical guideline 82. London: NICE.
22. Riedel-Heller SG, Gühne U, Weinmann S, Becker T (2012) [Psychosocial therapies in severe mental illness: DGPPN-S3-guideline: evidence, recommendations and challenges for mental health service research]. Psychother Psychosom Med Psychol 62: 425–428.
23. Gühne U, Weinmann S, Arnold K, Ay ES, Becker T, et al. (2012) [Arts therapies in severe mental illness: are they effective?]. Nervenarzt 83: 855–860.
24. Crawford MJ, Patterson S (2007) Arts therapies for people with schizophrenia: an emerging evidence base. Evid Based Ment Health 10: 69–70.
25. Richardson P, Jones K, Evans C, Stevens P, Rowe A (2007) Exploratory RCT of art therapy as an adjunctive treatment in schizophrenia. Journal of Mental Health 16: 483–491.
26. Meng P, Zheng R, Cai Z, Cao D, Ma L, et al. (2005) Group intervention for schizophrenia inpatient with art as medium. Acta Psychologica Sinica 37: 403–412.
27. Crawford MJ, Killaspy H, Barnes TR, Barrett B, Byford S, et al. (2012) Group art therapy as an adjunctive treatment for people with schizophrenia: multicentre pragmatic randomised trial. BMJ 344: e846.
28. Helmchen H, Lauter H (1995) [Ethical problems in biomedical research with cognitively impaired elderly patients]. Nervenarzt 66: 231–238.
29. First MB, Spitzer RL, Gibbon M, Williams JBW (1995) Structured Clinical Interview for DSM-IV Axis I Disorders. New York, NY: Biometrics Research, New York State Psychiatric Institute.
30. Andreasen NC (1983) Scale for the assessment of negative Symptoms (SANS). Iowa City, IA: The University of Iowa.
31. Andreasen NC (1984) Scale for the assessment of positive Symptoms (SAPS). Iowa City, IA: The University of Iowa.
32. Müller MJ, Marx-Dannigkeit P, Schlosser R, Wetzel H, Addington D, et al. (1999) The Calgary Depression Rating Scale for Schizophrenia: development and interrater reliability of a German version (CDSS-G). J Psychiatr Res 33: 433–443.
33. Saß H, Wittchen HU, Zaudig M, Houben I (2003) Diagnostisches und Statistisches. Manual Psychischer Störungen - Textrevision- DSM-IV-TR. Göttingen: Hogrefe.
34. Baron-Cohen S, Wheelwright S, Hill J, Raste Y, Plumb I (2001) The "Reading the Mind in the Eyes" Test revised version: a study with normal adults, and adults with Asperger syndrome or high-functioning autism. J Child Psychol Psychiatry 42: 241–251.
35. Boelte S (2009) Reading Mind in the Eyes Test. Erwachsenenversion. Von Simon Baron-Cohen (2001). Deutsche Bearbeitung von Sven Boelte.
36. Lane RD, Quinlan DM, Schwartz GE, Walker PA, Zeitlin SB (1990) The Levels of Emotional Awareness Scale: a cognitive-developmental measure of emotion. J Pers Assess 55: 124–134.
37. Subic-Wrana C, Thomas W, Huber M, Köhle K (2001) Levels of Emotional Awareness Scale (LEAS). Die deutsche Version eines neuen Alexithymietests. Psychotherapeut 46: 176–181.
38. Lane RD, Schwartz GE (1987) Levels of emotional awareness: a cognitive-developmental theory and its application to psychopathology. Am J Psychiatry 144: 133–143.
39. Subic-Wrana C, Bruder S, Thomas W, Lane RD, Kohle K (2005) Emotional awareness deficits in inpatients of a psychosomatic ward: a comparison of two different measures of alexithymia. Psychosom Med 67: 483–489.
40. Subic-Wrana C, Beutel ME, Knebel A, Lane RD (2010) Theory of mind and emotional awareness deficits in patients with somatoform disorders. Psychosom Med 72: 404–411.
41. Baslet G, Termini L, Herbener E (2009) Deficits in emotional awareness in schizophrenia and their relationship with other measures of functioning. J Nerv Ment Dis 197: 655–660.
42. Krampen G (1991) Fragebogen zu Kompetenz- und Kontrollüberzeugungen (FKK). Göttingen: Verlag für Psychologie Dr. C. J. Hogrefe.
43. Levenson H (1981) Differentiating among internality, powerful others and chance. In: Lefcourt HM, editors. Research with the locus of control construct. New York: Academic Press. pp. 15–63.
44. Pukrop R, Möller HJ, Sass H, Sauer H, Klosterkötter J, et al. (1999) [Quality of life. Construct validation and the development of a modular system]. Nervenarzt 70: 41–53.
45. Schmidt J, Lamprecht F, Wittmann WW (1989) Zufriedenheit mit der stationären Versorgung. Entwicklung eines Fragebogens und erste Validitätsuntersuchungen. Psychother Psychosom Med Psychol 39: 248–255.
46. Lehrl S, Triebig G, Fischer B (1995) Multiple choice vocabulary test MWT as a valid and short test to estimate premorbid intelligence. Acta Neurol Scand 91: 335–345.
47. Heubrock D (1992) Der Auditiv-Verbale Lerntest (AVLT) in der klinischen und experimentellen Neuropsychologie. Durchführung, Auswertung und Forschungsergebnisse. Zeitschrift für Differentielle und Diagnostische Psychologie 13: 161–174.
48. Leech NL, Barrett KC and Morgan GA (2005) SPSS for intermediate statistics: Use and interpretation. Mahwah (New Jersey), London: Lawrence Erlbaum Associates.
49. van Ginkel JR, Kroonenberg PM (2014) Analysis of variance of multiply imputed data. Multivariate Behavioral Research 49: 78–91.

50. van Ginkel JR (2014 April) SPSS syntax for applying rules for combining multivariate estimates in multiple imputation. http://socialsciences.leiden.edu/educationandchildstudies/childandfamilystudies/organisation/staffcfs/van-ginkel.html.
51. Gold C, Heldal TO, Dahle T, Wigram T (2005) Music therapy for schizophrenia or schizophrenia-like illnesses. Cochrane Database Syst Rev CD004025. 10.1002/14651858.CD004025.pub2 [doi].
52. Ulrich G, Houtmans T, Gold C (2007) The additional therapeutic effect of group music therapy for schizophrenic patients: a randomized study. Acta Psychiatr Scand 116: 362–370.
53. Röhricht F, Priebe S (2006) Effect of body-oriented psychological therapy on negative symptoms in schizophrenia: a randomized controlled trial. Psychol Med 36: 669–678.
54. Mueser KT, Berenbaum H (1990) Psychodynamic treatment of schizophrenia: is there a future? Psychol Med 20: 253–262.
55. Brooker J, Cullum M, Gilroy A, McCombe B, Mahony J, et al. (2007) The Use of Art Work in Art Psychotherapy with People Who are Prone to Psychotic States. AN Evidence-Based Clinical Practice Guideline. London: Goldsmiths, University of London.
56. Teglbjaerg HS (2011) Art therapy may reduce psychopathology in schizophrenia by strengthening the patients' sense of self: a qualitative extended case report. Psychopathology 44: 314–318.
57. Heenan D (2006) Art as therapy: an effective way of promoting positive mental health? Disability & Society 21: 179–191.
58. Franklin M (1992) Art therapy and self-esteem. Art Therapy: Journal of the American Art Therapy Association 9: 78–84.
59. Brüne M, Abdel-Hamid M, Lehmkämper C, Sonntag C (2007) Mental state attribution, neurocognitive functioning, and psychopathology: what predicts poor social competence in schizophrenia best? Schizophr Res 92: 151–159.
60. Vauth R, Rusch N, Wirtz M, Corrigan PW (2004) Does social cognition influence the relation between neurocognitive deficits and vocational functioning in schizophrenia? Psychiatry Res 128: 155–165.
61. Fonagy P, Gergely G, Jurist E, Target M (2002) Affektregulierung, Mentalisierung und die Entwicklung des Selbst. Stuttgart: Klett-Cotta.
62. Macbeth A, Gumley A, Schwannauer M, Fisher R (2011) Attachment states of mind, mentalization, and their correlates in a first-episode psychosis sample. Psychol Psychother 84: 42–57.
63. Korver-Nieberg N, Berry K, Meijer CJ, de Haan L. (2013) Adult attachment and psychotic phenomenology in clinical and non-clinical samples: A systematic review. Psychol Psychother. 10.1111/papt.12010 [doi].
64. Greenwood H (2012) What aspects of an art therapy group aid recovery for people diagnosed with psychosis? http://eprints-gojo.gold.ac.uk/458/1/Greenwood.pdf.
65. Moritz S, Woodward TS (2007) Metacognitive training in schizophrenia: from basic research to knowledge translation and intervention. Curr Opin Psychiatry 20: 619–625.
66. Lysaker PH, Buck KD, Carcione A, Procacci M, Salvatore G, et al. (2011) Addressing metacognitive capacity for self reflection in the psychotherapy for schizophrenia: a conceptual model of the key tasks and processes. Psychol Psychother 84: 58–69.
67. Brent B (2009) Mentalization-Based Psychodynamic Psychotherapy for Psychosis. Journal of Clinical Psychology: In Session 65: 803–814.
68. Franks M, Whitaker R (2007) The image, mentalisation and group art psychotherapy. International Journal of Art Therapy: Formerly Inscape 12: 3–16.
69. Subic-Wrana C, Beutel ME, Garfield DA, Lane RD (2011) Levels of Emotional Awareness: a model for conceptualizing and measuring emotion-centered structural change. Int J Psychoanal 92: 289–310.
70. Karterud S, Pedersen G (2004) Short-term day-treatment for personality disorders: Benefits of the therapeutic components. Therapeutic Communities 25: 43–54.
71. Persons RW (2014) Art therapy with serious juvenile offenders. A phenomenological analysis. International Journal of Offender Therapy and Comparative Criminology 53: 433–453.
72. Bat Or M (2010) Clay sculpting of mother and child figures encourages mentalization. The Arts in Psychotherapy 37: 319–327.
73. Kidd DC, Castano E (2013) Reading literary fiction improves theory of mind. Science 342: 377–380.
74. Little RJ, Cohen ML, Dickersin K, Emerson SS, Farrar JT, et al. (2012) The design and conduct of clinical trials to limit missing data. Statistics in Medicine 31: 3433–3443.
75. Fergusson D, Aaron SD, Guyatt G, Hebert P (2002) Post-randomisation exclusions: the intention to treat principle and excluding patients from analysis. BMJ 325: 652–654.
76. Wright CC, Sim J (2003) Intention-to-treat approach to data from randomized controlled trials: a sensitivity analysis. J Clin Epidemiol 56: 833–842. S0895435603001550 [pii].
77. National Research Council (2010) The Prevention and Treatment of Missing Data in Clinical Trials. Washington, DC: The National Academies Press.
78. Leon AC, Davis LL, Kraemer HC (2011) The role and interpretation of pilot studies in clinical research. Psychiatry Research 45: 626–629.

# 14

# Effect of a One-Off Educational Session about Enterobiasis on Knowledge, Preventative Practices, and Infection Rates among Schoolchildren in South Korea

**Dong-Hee Kim[1], Hak Sun Yu[2,3]***

1 Department of Nursing, College of Nursing, Pusan National University, Yangsan, Gyeongsangnamdo, South Korea, 2 Department of Parasitology, School of Medicine, Pusan National University, Yangsan, Gyeongsangnamdo, South Korea, 3 Immunoregulatory therapeutics group in Brain Busan 21 project, Busan, South Korea

## Abstract

Although health education has proven to be cost-effective in slowing the spread of enterobiasis, assessments of the effectiveness of health education to reduce infectious diseases specifically in children are rare. To evaluate the effect of health education on knowledge, preventative practices, and the prevalence of enterobiasis, 319 children from 16 classes were divided into experimental and control groups. Data were collected from May 2012 to March 2013. A 40-minute in-class talk was given once in the experimental group. There were significant differences over the time in the mean scores for children's knowledge of *Enterobius vermicularis* infection in the intervention group compared to the control group ($p<0.001$). After the educational session, the score for knowledge about *E. vermicularis* infection increased from 60.2±2.32 to 92.7±1.19 in the experimental group; this gain was partially lost 3 months later, decreasing to 83.6±1.77 ($p<0.001$). Children's enterobiasis infection prevention practice scores also increased, from 3.23±0.27 to 3.73±0.25, 1 week after the educational session, a gain that was partially lost at 3 months, decreasing to 3.46±0.36 ($p<0.001$). The overall *E. vermicularis* egg detection rate was 4.4%; the rates for each school ranged from 0% to 12.9% at screening. The infection rate at 3 months after the treatment sharply decreased from 12.3% to 0.8% in the experimental group, compared to a decrease from 8.5% to 3.7% in the control group during the same period. We recommend that health education on enterobiasis be provided to children to increase their knowledge about enterobiasis and improve prevention practices.

**Editor:** David Joseph Diemert, The George Washington University Medical Center, United States of America

**Funding:** This research was supported by Basic Science Research Program through the National Research Foundation of Korea funded by the Ministry of Education, Science and Technology (NRF-2013R1A1A1A05012615). The funders had no role in study design, data collection and analysis, decision to publish, or preparation of the manuscript.

**Competing Interests:** The authors have declared that no competing interests exist.

* Email: hsyu@pusan.ac.kr

## Introduction

Although most parasitic infectious diseases have disappeared in developed countries, enterobiasis (pinworm infection) has still often been reported in many developed countries [1–3]. In South Korea, the prevalence of total intestinal helminthic parasitic infection rates has sharply decreased from 84.3% in 1971 to 2.4% in 1997 [4,5]. However, a relatively high egg positive rate of *Enterobius vermicularis* ranging from 4% to 10% has been reported in Korean children during the last decade [6–9].

Enterobiasis is transmitted through direct contact with infected (or egg-contaminated) persons or objects. Transmission of *E. vermicularis* commonly occurs by ingesting infectious pinworm eggs. Eggs are transmitted from the anus to the finger, fingernails, or hands when an individual scratches the perianal area where the gravid female worms emerge and deposit eggs. Eggs are spread to underwear and night-clothing and further transmitted to other objects including food and books, desks, and chairs [10]. When dislodged from such objects, the eggs can enter another individual's mouth and nose, thereby being ingested [10,11]. As a result of this transmission process, children's personal and hygiene habits, such as thumb sucking, overcrowded conditions, and inadequate sanitation, contribute to the spread of enterobiasis in primary schools, where close contact between children occurs [2,7,9].

Medication against *E. vermicularis*, such as albendazole, is very effective in treating enterobiasis [12]. However, reinfection is also common in spite of treatment, as the medication only kills the adult worm but not the worm larvae [10]. An important aspect in the failure of single-dose chemotherapy is the continuing presence of infectious eggs in the environment, which facilitate rapid reinfection. Therefore, individuals with enterobiasis require repeated doses of medication to cover the time taken for the eggs to become adult worms. Importantly, most parents in South Korea believe that antihelminthic medications can easily cure every helminthic infection, including those by *E. vermicularis*, by just a one-time treatment [9]. In addition, most kindergarten directors and teachers have limited knowledge of *E. vermicularis* infection [2].

Knowledge of disease has successfully improved many different health outcomes [13]. However, there has been little emphasis on the impact of health education on the prevalence of enterobiasis, despite the incidence of enterobiasis being reduced by encouraging habits of cleanliness in children. Health education promoting knowledge of enterobiasis has proven to be cost-effective in decreasing reinfection rates in schoolchildren [14]. Previously, we evaluated the impact of a health education among pre-school children [2]. We provided brochures on prevention, transmission, and treatment of enterobiasis to parents, as they are in charge of their child's personal hygiene since children younger than 6 years of age are not old enough to be responsible for self-care [2].

In the present study, we conducted an experimental health education session on enterobiasis at primary schools in South Korea and assessed its effect on knowledge about *E. vermicularis* infection, enterobiasis infection prevention practices, and the incidence rate of enterobiasis among primary school children in Korea.

## Subjects and Methods

### Subject recruitment and screening evaluation

Participants were Grade 1 and Grade 2 primary school students (aged 7–9 years) from separate school districts in three distinct regions: an industrial city, an urban site, and a suburban area of South Korea. Recruitment was conducted through the Office of Education websites at each of these sites with a letter informing about the nature, significance, and objectives of the study. Schools were approached with the help of an assistant. Once the assistant had obtained verbal consent from the principal of a school, investigators met with the principal and class teachers of each school to describe the details of the study. The class teachers sent a consent form, a letter of information, and a questionnaire to the parents of each child. A total of 3,840 children from 183 classes in 27 schools underwent a screening for enterobiasis via the sellotape anal swab technique. The parents were each given two pieces of sellotape and written instructions showing how to swab the perianal area of their child with the sellotape and other aspects of the screening procedure. The investigators emphasized that the examinations should be done before the child washed or went to the toilet in the morning to prevent any pinworms eggs from being washed from the area. We cautioned that the chances of making an incorrect diagnosis of enterobiasis increased when the parents did not swab their child's anus first thing in the morning before the child washed. We asked the parents to do this twice, on separate days.

Sample size was determined on the basis of the primary outcome, the score in the knowledge test after education. To have an 80% chance of detecting as significant (at the two sided 5% level) a 10 point difference between the two groups in the knowledge test scores after education, with an assumed standard deviation of 15, the overall sample size required is 74 individuals (37 in each arm of the study). Since this study is cluster-randomized, the sample size had to be larger than if simple randomization had been performed, in order to take into account the design effect. Assuming that the inter-cluster correlation coefficient is 0.1, and a mean cluster size is 21 individuals, the design effect is 3. Therefore, the number of individuals required in each group is 111 ('Cochrane Consumers and Communication Review Group: cluster randomized controlled trials'. http://cccrg.cochrane.org, March 2014). Assuming the expected drop-out rate of 10%, the final sample size required is 246 (123 in each arm) with a minimum of 6 clusters per arm.

### Study design

The study was designed as a pretest-posttest experiment, with an equivalent control group. We excluded schools that had classes with an incidence rate of 0% at the screening evaluation, and then selected classes in which all students were tested at the screening evaluation. Based on a combination of similar egg positive rates and geographical locations, 10 schools in different regions were involved this study; two schools were in an industrial city, four schools were in an urban site, and four schools were in a suburban area. One or two classes participated at each school. Each school was identified as either an intervention or control group in order to control for the contamination of the control group. The schools were assigned to either the intervention (8 classes from 5 schools) or control (8 classes from 5 schools) arms through a coin toss. A total of 346 children from 16 classes were included at baseline. At post-treatment examination, 319 children (130 for the experimental and 189 for the control group) participated (Fig. 1). Blinding of investigators was not possible as the intervention was educational; however, the investigators were blinded to the exposure status of participants during data collection. In the intervention group, an educational session was given once, for 40 minutes, in a group setting for each class. In the control group, children received an *E. vermicularis* infection brochure. Knowledge of *E. vermicularis* infection and enterobiasis infection prevention practice and the *E. vermicularis* infection rate among children were evaluated at baseline and at 3 months after the intervention. Children's knowledge of *E. vermicularis* infection was assessed on the day of the educational session in order to ensure that their knowledge of *E. vermicularis* infection increased.

### Intervention

The educational program was developed based on the Dick & Carey's Systematic Design of Instruction model [15]. A comprehensive review of the literature, a pilot study, and a focus group interview were used to develop the educational session. The session was comprised of topics such as the lifecycle of *E. vermicularis*, diagnosis of enterobiasis, symptoms and signs, infection and transmission, and treatment and prevention of enterobiasis. A trained teacher provided a 30-minute lecture using visual aids to stimulate interest and support explanations of the educational contents. The lecture included an example situation, describing how one student became infected with a pinworm, and showing how enterobiasis spread to other students in the same classroom. Key messages were reinforced with an interactive quiz, and there was a 10-minute session to answer students' questions.

### Measurement

The main outcome variable is the improvement of 15 or more points in children's knowledge of *E. vermicularis* infection. As there are no currently published scales for children's knowledge on *E. vermicularis* infection and children's preventative practice against enterobiasis infection, the investigators composed a scale, which was validated by experts (including parasitologists, pediatric doctors, internal medicine doctors, school nurses, and school-teachers). Four pilot studies were conducted to assess comprehension of the questionnaire items. The instrument to measure children's knowledge of *E. vermicularis* infection included 10 dichotomous items (answered as either "correct" [1 point] or "incorrect" [0 points]).

The secondary outcome variables recorded are children's prevention practices and the infection rate 3 months later. The instrument to assess children's prevention practices consisted of 8 Likert-scale items; each Likert item ranged from 1 (never) to 4 (every time).

### Study procedure

Children in both the education and control groups who tested positive for *E. vermicularis* eggs received medical treatment with 400 mg albendazole twice, at a 15-day interval. The pre-treatment structured questionnaire on knowledge of *E. vermicularis* infection was provided to the children by a class teacher. This questionnaire

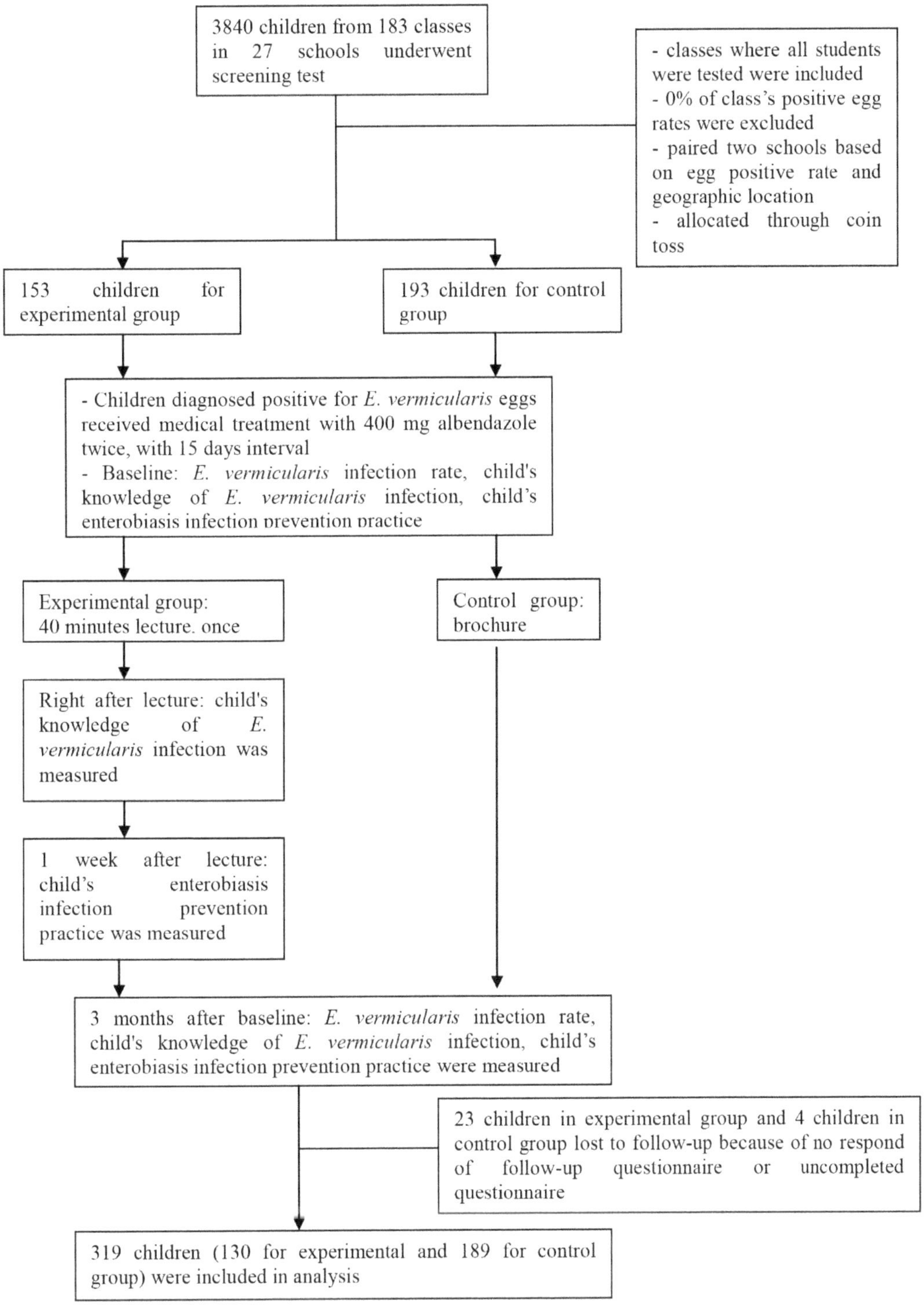


**Figure 1. Study design including screening, group allocation, and follow-up.** A total of 319 children from 16 classes were invited from among 3,840 children screened from 183 classes. The schools were assigned to either the intervention or the control arms by simple randomization using a coin toss.

was also provided to the parents of each child, enquiring about demographics and socioeconomic status, the child's enterobiasis infection prevention practices at home, and the parents' knowledge of enterobiasis. Children's knowledge of *E. vermicularis* infection was assessed the day they learned about enterobiasis and 3 months later. One week and three months after the intervention, parents were asked to complete another questionnaire on the children's enterobiasis infection prevention practices at home. *E. vermicularis* egg detection and the reinfection rates were evaluated using a sellotape anal swab 3 months after the intervention.

## Ethics statement

The study was performed after receiving approval from the Ethical Review Committee of Yangsan Pusan National University Hospital, and after informed written consent was obtained from each participant before enrollment. Participation was entirely voluntary. Participants, including principals and teachers of schools, parents, and their children, were free to refuse to participate or withdraw from the study at any time, and were informed that only the aggregate data would be reported. Informed consent for the children in this study was provided by their parents or guardians and by the children. Once we obtained written consent from the parents or guardians to contact their children, the class teacher informed the children that permission to conduct the study had been granted. We briefed the individual children about the study and what they were being asked to do. Children who diagnosed positive for *E. vermicularis* eggs at screening received medical treatment with 400 mg albendazole twice, at a 15-day interval.

## Statistical analysis

We report descriptive statistics for the characteristics of study sites and individual participants. To test the effectiveness of the education program in changing children's knowledge and prevention practices (continuous variables), we used multivariable mixed-effects analysis allowing random effects for clusters and controlling for gender and age. Each estimator was presented with its 95% confidence interval (95% CI). The prevalence of *E. vermicularis* eggs at baseline and after treatment in each group was compared using proportions and the McNemar test.

To examine the effectiveness of the education program in reducing infection (yes: 1; no: 0, binary response), we used multivariable logistic regression allowing random effects for clusters. All statistical analyses were performed using SAS 9.2 (SAS Institute, Inc., Cary, NC) statistical package and $p$ values less than 0.05 were considered as statistically significant.

# Results

Participant characteristics were compared between the experimental and control groups, most of which were similar. The small differences observed between groups were not statistically significant. Several characteristics of the participants are shown in Table S1. The overall *E. vermicularis* egg detection rate was 4.4%; the rate for each school ranged from 0% to 12.9% at screening (Table 1). Characteristics of study sites and individual participants are summarized in Table 2. Experimental and control groups enrolled 130 and 189 children, respectively. There were no statistically significant differences in children's baseline characteristics ($p>0.05$).

Between-group comparisons of knowledge of and prevention practices for *E. vermicularis* infection, as well as the prevalence of *E. vermicularis* egg positive rates, are show in Table 3. There were significant time effects in the mean scores for children's knowledge of *E. vermicularis* infection in the intervention group compared to the control group ($p<0.001$). Regarding *E. vermicularis* infection prevention practices, the experimental group increased from 3.22 to 3.45 (a difference of 0.23), whereas the control group increased from 3.19 to 3.23 (a difference of 0.04) between baseline and 3 months after treatment ($p<0.001$). The experimental group had a higher increase in knowledge test scores than the control group (adjusted difference = 1.95 [95% CI, 1.57–2.34]; $p<0.001$). The experimental group also had a higher increase in prevention practices than the control group (adjusted difference = 0.19 [95% CI, 0.13–0.25]; $p<0.001$). Clustering was considered in all logistic and multivariate regression models.

The incidence rate was lower in the experimental group, although this finding was not significant after adjustment for the clusters as random effects (adjusted odds ratio = 0.20, 95% CI = 0.02–2.41, $p = 0.175$). The infection rate at 3 months after treatment sharply decreased from 12.3% to 0.8% in the experimental group ($p<0.001$), while that in the control group decreased from 8.5% to 3.7% ($p = 0.049$) during the same period. Some children were diagnosed with new infections at 3 months after treatment; however, the number of new infections in the experimental group was lower than that in the control group. Moreover, although children who tested positive for *E. vermicularis* eggs were treated with antihelminthic drugs at baseline, *E. vermicularis* reinfection was observed in the control group.

We also jointly compared baseline, post-education, and 3-month changes in the experimental group. Correct answer rates on the *E. vermicularis* infection knowledge test in the experimental group are shown in Table 4. After the educational session, the score for knowledge about *E. vermicularis* infection increased from 60.2±2.32 to 92.7±1.19 in the experimental group; this gain was partially lost 3 months after the educational session, decreasing to 83.6±1.77 ($p<0.001$). The correct answer rate was 34.6% to 78.5% at baseline, 80.0% to 99.2% at post-education, and 75.4% to 93.1% 3 months after the intervention. At baseline, the item "Proper teeth brushing can prevent *E. vermicularis* infection" (34.6%) had the lowest rate of correct answers, followed by "Weekly change of underwear is important for preventing *E. vermicularis* infection" (36.9%), "*E. vermicularis* is not transmitted to other humans via hand contact" (47.7%), and "*E. vermicularis* infection can be treated by taking antihelminthic medication once" (50.0%); the rates for these items increased to over 80% correct responses at post-education, and over 75% correct 3 months later.

Results for children's practices for the prevention of *E. vermicularis* infection are shown in Table 5. Children's enterobiasis infection prevention practice scores also increased, from 3.23±0.27 to 3.73±0.25, 1 week after the educational session, and then partially decreased to 3.46±0.36 after 3 months ($p<0.001$). Items related to hand washing had lower scores than other items, such as keeping nails short and cleaning underwear. After 3 months, the item "My child does not bite his/her nails" had the lowest score of all items at both 1 week and 3 months after the health education session.

# Discussion

Mass drug administration is the most effective means to control enterobiasis, but this method also has some limitations in that it does not prevent reinfections. In a previous study, we found new infection cases in the mass drug administration treatment group at both 3 and 6 months after treatment [2]. Moreover, reinfection increases the financial burden placed on preventative medicine programs. Consensus among government health employees and social workers might be necessary, because part of the cost of group treatment must be covered by the government. Furthermore, there is concern that mass drug administration might lead to the development of drug-resistant parasites [16]. The development of drug resistance in nematodes that infect humans is considered inevitable, given the number of species infecting livestock that are now resistant to antihelminthic agents due to continuous and extensive drug use [17,18]. Strategies to reduce the overall incidence of enterobiasis infection are likely to require an integrated approach, including pharmacological treatment to

**Table 1.** Egg positive rates of *E. vermicularis* infection among children in South Korea (n = 3840).

| School | No. class | No. examined/total No. student (compliance %) | No. positive (%) |
|---|---|---|---|
| 1 | 2 | 31/37 (83.8) | 4(12.9) |
| 2 | 11 | 260/287 (90.6) | 21(8.1) |
| 3 | 6 | 97/133 (72.9) | 7(7.2) |
| 4 | 2 | 15/19 (78.9) | 1(6.7) |
| 5 | 6 | 139/152 (91.4) | 9(6.5) |
| 6 | 6 | 122/136 (89.7) | 7(5.7) |
| 7 | 4 | 57/57 (100.0) | 3(5.3) |
| 8 | 13 | 317/361 (87.8) | 16(5.0) |
| 9 | 6 | 142/155 (91.6) | 7(4.9) |
| 10 | 10 | 238/256 (93.0) | 11(4.6) |
| 11 | 9 | 160/203 (78.8) | 7(4.4) |
| 12 | 6 | 115/149 (77.2) | 5(4.3) |
| 13 | 8 | 189/242 (78.1) | 8(4.2) |
| 14 | 10 | 288/309 (93.2) | 12(4.2) |
| 15 | 9 | 135/220 (61.4) | 5(3.7) |
| 16 | 10 | 202/259 (78.0) | 7(3.5) |
| 17 | 8 | 145/182 (79.7) | 5(3.4) |
| 18 | 8 | 134/189 (70.9) | 4(3.0) |
| 19 | 12 | 277/316 (87.7) | 8(2.9) |
| 20 | 9 | 272/272 (100.0) | 8(2.9) |
| 21 | 4 | 82/100 (82.0) | 2(2.4) |
| 22 | 6 | 127/158 (80.4) | 3(2.4) |
| 23 | 4 | 84/89 (94.4) | 2(2.4) |
| 24 | 7 | 134/169 (79.3) | 1(0.7) |
| 25 | 2 | 33/33 (100.0) | 0(0.0) |
| 26 | 2 | 17/17 (100.0) | 0(0.0) |
| 27 | 3 | 28/59 (47.5) | 0(0.0) |
| Total | 183 | 3840/4559 (84.2) | 163 |
| Mean positive rate | | | 4.4% |

reduce the infection rate and health education for prevention and sustainable control.

Our results showed that health-education increased students' knowledge about enterobiasis transmission and changed their behavior. Notably, students washed their hands more frequently and sucked their fingers or toys less after the health education session (Tables 4 and 5). Most instances of infection transmission could be effectively prevented by repeated hand washes; therefore, behavioral changes might contribute to a reduction in enterobiasis rates. Interestingly, most students remembered general facts about enterobiasis (life cycle, transmission route, prevention, etc.) 3 months after receiving an educational lecture (Table 4).

In Korea, over 80% of people were infected with intestinal helminthic parasites in the 1960s [19]. Most people at the time lived in poor environments in which parasitic infections were easily transmitted [20]. Additionally, farmers at the time used "Night-soil" (human feces and urine) as fertilizer on food crops. Furthermore, underground water was easily contaminated by parasite eggs found in human and animal feces; therefore, parasites were not easily eradicated in humans by mass drug administration. However, after the South Korean government launched a life environmental improvement project ("Saemaeul" [new village] Movement) and established the Korean Parasite Eradiation Association (KPEA), parasitic infection rates rapidly decreased. The Saemaeul Movement improved the drinking water supply system and sewage treatment system. The KPEA (now, Korea Association of Health Promotion) strived to eradicate parasite infections by conducting periodic examinations of the parasite infection rate, treating infected people, and providing preventative education for inhabitants in endemic areas. After the 1990s, most intestinal parasitic infection rates decreased to less than 3.0% in South Korea, with soil-transmitted helminthic infection rates decreasing to less than 1.0% [2,9].

However, in spite of the struggles of the government, enterobiasis has yet to be eliminated. One of the reasons for this is that there are misconceptions about enterobiasis in South Korea [2,9]. The first is the belief that parasitic infections, including enterobiasis, have already disappeared in South Korea; due to this belief, approximately half of children have not taken medication against helminthic parasites, including pinworms. The second misconception is that enterobiasis can easily be cured by a one-time anti-helminthic medication, as is the case for other intestinal nematodes. It was recently shown that the numbers of young children being cared for in group facilities, including private

**Table 2.** Characteristics of study sites and individual participants (n = 319).

| Characteristic | | Experimental (n = 130) | Control (n = 189) | P value |
|---|---|---|---|---|
| Site's characteristic | | | | |
| Cluster size | | | | |
| | mean ± SD | 19.13±3.94 | 24.25±2.25 | |
| No. of Conforming Requests/Total | | | | |
| | | 11/14(78.6%) | 25/26 (96.2%) | |
| | | 21/23 (91.3%) | 21/21 (100.0%) | |
| | | 18/21 (85.7%) | 27/27 (100.0%) | |
| | | 18/21 (85.7%) | 21/21 (100.0%) | |
| | | 16/20 (80.0%) | 23/24 (95.8%) | |
| | | 19/24 (79.2%) | 23/24 (95.8%) | |
| | | 14/16 (87.5%) | 26/26 (100.0%) | |
| | | 13/14 (92.9%) | 23/25 (92.0%) | |
| Total | | 130/153 (85.0%) | 189/194 (97.4%) | |
| Children's characteristics | | | | |
| Sex | | | | |
| | Male | 69 (53.9%) | 104 (57.1%) | 0.581 |
| | Female | 59 (46.1%) | 78 (42.9%) | |
| Age | | | | |
| | Mean ± SD | 8.22±0.70 | 8.24±0.67 | 0.827 |
| House type | | | | |
| | Apartment | 109 (85.2%) | 158 (86.8%) | 0.823 |
| | Non-apartment | 19 (14.8%) | 24 (13.2%) | |
| Job of parents | | | | |
| | Single | 71 (55.5%) | 99 (54.4%) | 0.261 |
| | Both | 57 (44.5%) | 83 (45.6%) | |
| Family size | | | | |
| | ≤3 persons | 96 (76.8%) | 142 (78.5%) | 0.583 |
| | >4 persons | 29 (23.2%) | 39 (21.5%) | |

educational institutes, have increased, and the employees and teachers of these facilities have such misconceptions [2]. Therefore, opportunities for infection and transmission from child to child have increased as a result. These misconceptions should be rectified through health education providing the correct information, which would be expected to result in a rapid decrease in infection rates [2,9].

Visual educational materials targeting schoolchildren have been shown to have a positive effect on knowledge and attitudes [18,21,22]. In this study, the educational information on enterobiasis included cartoon materials and real-life visual representations, such as microscopic images of pinworms, sellotape used for the diagnosis of enterobiasis, and the medications used to treat it. Most students who participated in this study were interested and immersed in the example situation as if he/she was the infected student. We believe that storytelling using cartoon materials was effective in helping children to focus on the educational contents. Moreover, descriptions of other aspects, such as the sellotape anal swab technique for diagnosis, elicited a response from the students, as they had themselves experienced this during the baseline data collection period. Finally, the interactive quiz emphasized the major educational content. This interactive health education session might lead to behavioral changes that result in decreasing the risk of *E. vermicularis* infection.

The health education session increased knowledge about enterobiasis. We were worried that at the 3-month follow-up assessment children would not remember the information acquired earlier. However, interestingly, the majority of children remembered most of the information they had learned on the subject. In addition, their prevention practices against *E. vermicularis* infection were maintained in their daily lives. Some children were administered the antihelminthic drug (albendazole) at the same time as their family members (personal communication), indicating that educating children may also have an indirect influence on their family members. These results could provide substantial gains in the elimination of enterobiasis in Korea, since Grade 1 and 2 primary school students are the most commonly infected population [6,23].

The prevalence of the *E. vermicularis* egg positive rate was not significant after adjusting for clusters as a random effect in this study, although the infection rates in the experimental group showed larger changes than in the control group. In a previous study, Gai et al. reported the negative relationship between the rate of parasitic infection and knowledge of prevention [24]. Enterobiasis was successfully treated with an anthelminthic agent.

**Table 3.** Comparison of the prevalence of *E. vermicularis* egg positive rates, knowledge, and prevention practices for *E. vermicularis* infection between groups (n = 319).

| | Time | Experimental (n = 130) | Control (n = 189) | P value of Difference | Treatment Difference |
|---|---|---|---|---|---|
| | | n (%)/mean ± SD | n (%)/mean ± SD | | (95% CI) |
| Knowledge | | | | | |
| Baseline | | 6.02±2.32 | 6.12±2.09 | | |
| 3 months after | | 8.36±1.77 | 6.45±2.04 | | |
| Difference | | 2.35±2.43 | 0.33±0.97 | <0.001 | 1.96‡ (1.57–2.34) |
| Preventing Practice | | | | | |
| Baseline | | 3.22±0.28 | 3.19±0.43 | | |
| 3 months after | | 3.45±0.36 | 3.23±0.40 | | |
| Difference | | 0.23±0.37 | 0.04±0.18 | <0.001 | 0.19‡ (0.13–0.25) |
| Infection rate | | | | | |
| Baseline | Positive | 16(12.3%) | 16 (8.5%) | 0.263 | |
| 3 months after | Positive | 1(0.8%)* | 7 (3.7%)* | 0.175 | 0.20†(0.02–2.41) |
| Baseline - 3 months after | Positive – positive (re-infection case) | 0(0.0%) | 3(1.6%) | | |
| | Negative – positive (New infected case) | 1(0.8%) | 4(2.1%) | | |

*Statistically significant between baseline and 3 months in experimental group (p<0.001) and control group ($p$ = 0.049), based on the McNemar test.
†OR was adjusted for clusters as a random effect.
‡Mean difference was adjusted for clusters as a random effect, as well as gender and age.

Children in both the education and control groups who tested positive for *E. vermicularis* eggs received medical treatment with albendazole at baseline according to ethical considerations. Moreover, we evaluated the effect of the intervention for 3 months since participants changed classes as they advanced into the next grade. Future long-term evaluation studies need to assess whether health education increasing students' knowledge about enterobiasis transmission impacts infection rates.

Our study has a few limitations. First, there was potential confounding effect due to interaction between teachers in the experimental and control groups, despite our attempts to maintain a distance between groups by selecting them from different districts. Second, we asked the parents to assess their children's enterobiasis infection prevention practices, that is an indirect measure and might not be accurate. In addition, we asked the parents to do the Sellotape swab of their child's anus first thing in the morning, before the child had washed. There is a possibility that the children's parents decided to wash their child first, before preparing the swab, to show that their child had not become reinfected. This would influence the infection rates 3 months after the educational session. Third, as the study could not be double-blinded, other factors may have affected the results. Furthermore,

**Table 4.** Assessment of children's correct answer rates on *E. vermicularis* infection knowledge test (Experimental group: n = 130).

| Items | Correct answer rate (%) | | |
|---|---|---|---|
| | Baseline | After education | 3 month after |
| *E. vermicularis* is parasitic worm that can live inside the human | 74.6 | 99.2 | 88.5 |
| *E. vermicularis* is not transmitted to other human via hands | 47.7 | 86.9 | 88.5 |
| *Enterobius vermicularis* infection can be diagnosed by using sellotape anal technique | 68.5 | 98.5 | 83.1 |
| Child with *E. vermicularis* may have anal itching | 71.5 | 98.5 | 93.1 |
| The habits of sucking fingers or biting nails is associated with *E. vermicularis* infection | 63.4 | 93.1 | 89.2 |
| Good hand hygiene can help prevent the spread of *E. vermicularis* infection | 78.5 | 95.4 | 91.5 |
| Proper brushing teeth can be preventive *E. vermicularis* infection | 34.6 | 91.5 | 79.2 |
| Anal cleansing can help prevent *E. vermicularis* infection | 73.8 | 95.4 | 86.2 |
| Weekly change of underwear is good for preventing *E. vermicularis* infection | 36.9 | 80.0 | 75.4 |
| *E. vermicularis* infection can be treated by taking antihelminthic medication once | 50.0 | 88.5 | 80.0 |
| Over all M± SD | 60.2±2.32 | 92.7±1.19 | 83.6±1.77 |
| Generalized linear mixed model test statistic ($p$) | 157.230 (<0.001) | | |

**Table 5.** Children's prevention practices for *E. vermicularis* infection (Experimental group: n = 130).

| Items | Baseline | 1 week after | 3 month after |
|---|---|---|---|
| My child practices hand washing after defecation | 3.00±0.29 | 3.71±0.47 | 3.32±0.60 |
| My child practices hand washing before eating | 2.72±0.51 | 3.57±0.53 | 3.32±0.61 |
| My child practices hand washing after coming in from outside | 2.89±0.44 | 3.77±0.48 | 3.51±0.59 |
| My child does not sucking fingers or toys | 3.30±0.86 | 3.68±0.62 | 3.50±0.79 |
| My child does not biting nails | 3.12±0.97 | 3.45±0.82 | 3.28±0.96 |
| My child keeps the nails short | 3.58±0.75 | 3.78±0.54 | 3.40±0.55 |
| My child practices proper anal cleansing | 3.49±0.61 | 3.96±0.20 | 3.59±0.55 |
| My child wears clean underwear | 3.63±0.60 | 3.96±0.20 | 3.65±0.48 |
| Over all M± SD | 3.23±0.27 | 3.73±0.25 | 3.46±0.36 |
| Generalized linear mixed model test statistic (*p*) | | 149.486 (<0.001) | |

it was not clear whether the educational session would have an impact on infection rates due to lack of previous studies. That is why we tested children's knowledge as a primary outcome. To detect the infection rate difference of 2.9 derived in this study, the total number of clusters required is 117. Due to the lack of statistical power, the result regarding infection rates need to be interpreted with caution and future studies with large sample sizes are required.

In spite of these limitations, we believe that health education can be a cost-effective and safe strategy to decrease enterobiasis and other childhood diseases through to adulthood, as behaviors obtained early in life can result in long-term favorable sanitary habits later in life.

## Acknowledgments

We would like to thank J. M. Choi at ACE statistical consulting for his valuable recommendations on statistical aspects of this paper.

## Author Contributions

Conceived and designed the experiments: DHK HSY. Performed the experiments: DHK HSY. Analyzed the data: DHK HSY. Contributed reagents/materials/analysis tools: DHK HSY. Wrote the paper: DHK HSY.

## References


1. Degerli S, Malatyali E, Ozcelik S, Celiksoz A (2009) Enterobiosis in Sivas, Turkey from past to present, effects on primary school children and potential risk factors. Turkiye Parazitol Derg 33: 95–100.
2. Kang IS, Kim DH, An HG, Son HM, Cho MK, et al. (2012) Impact of health education on the prevalence of enterobiasis in Korean preschool students. Acta Trop 122: 59–63.
3. Bager P, Vinkel Hansen A, Wohlfahrt J, Melbye M (2012) Helminth infection does not reduce risk for chronic inflammatory disease in a population-based cohort study. Gastroenterology 142: 55–62.
4. Report of Ministry of Health and Welfare of Republic of Korea and the Korea Association of Health (1971) Prevalence of intestinal parasitic infections in Korea—1st report. Ministry of Health and Welfare of Republic of Korea and the Korea Association of Health.
5. Report of Ministry of Health and Welfare of Republic of Korea and the Korea Association of Health (1997) Prevalence of intestinal parasitic infections in Korea -6th report. Ministry of Health and Welfare of Republic of Korea and the Korea Association of Health.
6. Kim BJ, Lee BY, Chung HK, Lee YS, Lee KH, et al. (2003) Egg positive rate of Enterobius vermicularis of primary school children in Geoje island. The Korean J Parasitol 41: 75–77.
7. Song HJ, Cho CH, Kim JS, Choi MH, Hong ST (2003) Prevalence and risk factors for enterobiasis among preschool children in a metropolitan city in Korea. Parasitol Res 91: 46–50.
8. Kang S, Jeon HK, Eom KS, Park JK (2006) Egg positive rate of Enterobius vermicularis among preschool children in Cheongju, Chungcheongbuk-do, Korea. Korean J Parasitol 44: 247–249.
9. Kim DH, Son HM, Kim JY, Cho MK, Park MK, et al. (2010) Parents' knowledge about enterobiasis might be one of the most important risk factors for enterobiasis in children. Korean J Parasitol 48: 121–126.
10. Roberts LS, Schmidt GD, Janovy J (2009) Foundations of parasitology. Boston: McGraw-Hill Higher Education. xvii, 701 p.
11. Cook GC (1994) Enterobius vermicularis infection. Gut 35: 1159–1162.
12. St Georgiev V (2001) Chemotherapy of enterobiasis (oxyuriasis). Expert Opin pharmacother 2: 267–275.
13. Owais A, Hanif B, Siddiqui AR, Agha A, Zaidi AK (2011) Does improving maternal knowledge of vaccines impact infant immunization rates? A community-based randomized-controlled trial in Karachi, Pakistan. BMC Public Health 11: 239.
14. Nithikathkul C, Akarachantachote N, Wannapinyosheep S, Pumdonming W, Brodsky M, et al. (2005) Impact of health educational programmes on the prevalence of enterobiasis in schoolchildren in Thailand. J Helminthol 79: 61–65.
15. Dick W, Carey L, Carey JO (2005) The systematic design of instruction. Boston; London: Pearson/Allyn & Bacon. xx, 376 p.
16. Keiser J, Utzinger J (2010) The drugs we have and the drugs we need against major helminth infections. Adv Parasitol 73: 197–230.
17. Albonico M (2003) Methods to sustain drug efficacy in helminth control programmes. Acta Trop 86: 233–242.
18. Bieri FA, Gray DJ, Williams GM, Raso G, Li YS, et al. (2013) Health-education package to prevent worm infections in Chinese schoolchildren. N Engl J Med 368: 1603–1612.
19. Seo BS, Rim HJ, Loh IK, Lee SH, Cho SY, et al. (1969) [Study On The Status Of Helminthic Infections In Koreans]. Kisaengchunghak chapchi 7: 53–70.
20. Kim CH, Park CH, Kim HJ, Chun HB, Min HK, et al. (1971) [Prevalence Of Intestinal Parasites In Korea]. Kisaengchunghak chapchi 9: 25–38.
21. Myint UA, Bull S, Greenwood GL, Patterson J, Rietmeijer CA, et al. (2010) Safe in the city: developing an effective video-based intervention for STD clinic waiting rooms. Health Promot Pract 11: 408–417.
22. Naldi L, Chatenoud L, Bertuccio P, Zinetti C, Di Landro A, et al. (2007) Improving sun-protection behavior among children: results of a cluster-randomized trial in Italian elementary schools. The "SoleSi SoleNo-GISED" Project. J Invest Dermatol 127: 1871–1877.
23. Lee KJ, Ahn YK, Ryang YS (2001) *Enterobius vermicularis* egg positive rates in primary school children in Gangwon-do (province), Korea. Korean J Parasitol 39: 327–328.
24. Gai L, Ma X, Fu Y, Huang D (1995) [Relationship between the rate of parasitic infection and the knowledge of prevention]. Zhongguo ji sheng chong xue yu ji sheng chong bing za zhi 13: 269–272.

15

# Coverage and Quality of Antenatal Care Provided at Primary Health Care Facilities in the 'Punjab' Province of 'Pakistan'

**Muhammad Ashraf Majrooh[1]*, Seema Hasnain[1], Javaid Akram[1], Arif Siddiqui[1], Zahid Ali Memon[2]**

**1** Allama Iqbal Medical College, Lahore, Pakistan, **2** Population Survives International - Greenstar, Karachi, Pakistan

## Abstract

***Background:*** Antenatal care is a very important component of maternal health services. It provides the opportunity to learn about risks associated with pregnancy and guides to plan the place of deliveries thereby preventing maternal and infant morbidity and mortality. In 'Pakistan' antenatal services to rural population are being provided through a network of primary health care facilities designated as 'Basic Health Units and Rural Health Centers. Pakistan is a developing country, consisting of four provinces and federally administered areas. Each province is administratively subdivided in to 'Divisions' and 'Districts'. By population 'Punjab' is the largest province of Pakistan having 36 districts. This study was conducted to assess the coverage and quality antenatal care in the primary health care facilities in 'Punjab' province of 'Pakistan'.

***Methods:*** Quantitative and Qualitative methods were used to collect data. Using multistage sampling technique nine out of thirty six districts were selected and 19 primary health care facilities of public sector (seventeen Basic Health Units and two Rural Health Centers were randomly selected from each district. Focus group discussions and in-depth interviews were conducted with clients, providers and health managers.

***Results:*** The overall enrollment for antenatal checkup was 55.9% and drop out was 32.9% in subsequent visits. The quality of services regarding assessment, treatment and counseling was extremely poor. The reasons for low coverage and quality were the distant location of facilities, deficiency of facility resources, indifferent attitude and non availability of the staff. Moreover, lack of client awareness about importance of antenatal care and self empowerment for decision making to seek care were also responsible for low coverage.

***Conclusion:*** The coverage and quality of the antenatal care services in 'Punjab' are extremely compromised. Only half of the expected pregnancies are enrolled and out of those 1/3 drop out in follow-up visits.

**Editor:** Zulfiqar A. Bhutta, The Hospital for Sick Children, Pakistan

**Funding:** This manuscript is an output from a research funded by Maternal and Newborn Health Programme - Research and Advocacy Fund (RAF) and conducted by Research Society Allama Iqbal Medical College Lahore, Pakistan. The views expressed and the information contained is not necessarily endorsed by funding agencies DFID/AusAID. The funders had no role in study design, data collection and analysis, decision to publish, or preparation of the manuscript.

**Competing Interests:** The author have declared that no competing interests exist.

* Email: majrooh58@yahoo.com

## Introduction

Low up take of Antenatal care (ANC) is an important determinant of high maternal mortality rate in developing countries and is one of the basic components of maternal care on which the life of mothers and babies depend [1]. According to WHO, 536000 women die every year in the world from causes relating to pregnancy, childbirth or postpartum. Ninety nine percent of these deaths occur in the developing countries. The majority of these deaths could be avoided if women had access to quality medical care during pregnancy, childbirth and postpartum [2]. ANC services help pregnant women by identifying complications associated with pregnancy or diseases that might adversely affect the pregnancy [3]. The ANC coverage in the Punjab province of Pakistan is only 53% and there isinequity in provision of ANC services to rural population as depicted by some studies which is 50% in comparison to 71% of urban women. About 25% of women in rural and urban areas of Punjab consulted health care providers at a public sector health care facility [4]. Multiple reasons have been reported for low coverage of ANC services that includes the weak health systems, inadequate training [5] and inaccessibility of health facilities and ANC services in Pakistan are widely cited as being responsible for a high proportion of maternal and infant deaths [6]. However, in recent decades certain low income countries have witnessed dramatic improvements in publically funded health care delivery system. For instance in Sri Lanka maternal health care is provided free of charge to all women and in 2000, 94.5% of expected mothers had visited an antenatal care clinic at least once [7]. Social developmental factors like education markedly influence the ANC coverage in low income countries for instance in a study in Ethiopia ANC utilization increases by skilled care providers as the level of education of woman increases. Only 25% of women who had no education used skilled ANC attendants compared with 90% of those who had higher than secondary level education [8]. Introduction of group ANC sessions at public health centers in Iran showed a significant improvement in patient satisfaction and mean patient satisfaction score increased for women participating in group sessions compared to individual care. Significant improvements were seen in number of women receiving full number of ANC visits. Further, increase in birth weight and use of supplements was observed among the ladies receiving group ANC sessions [9]. An intervention in India for improvement of ANC through ensuring staff had necessary equipment, increased monitoring and supervision, focused training, re-organisation of outreach clinics and scheduling Quality of care increased as more than 60% of women received all ANC components. Significant increase in blood pressure and urine testing increased significantly. Attendance at clinics also increased by 30% [10].

In a study of expectant mothers in an urban squatter settlement of Karachi, indicated that 49% received no antenatal care, even in the presence of no cost and low cost public health sector ANC services [11]. A cross-sectional community-based study in Sudan reported that out of 900 pregnant women, 811 (90%) had at least one visit. Only 11% of the women had ≥ four antenatal visits [12]. In another study conducted in North West of Pakistan about the utilization of prenatal care services by the rural women, it was reported that only 28.1% (34/121) pregnant women of Sarbund village utilized prenatal care service in either private (6/121; 0.5%) or public sectors 28/121; 23.1%) [13]. Pakistan Demographic and Health Survey confirms that maternal deaths are not merely a result of treatment failure; rather they are the final outcome of a complex interplay between a myraid of social, cultural and economic factors [14].

Client satisfaction is the litmus test that enables health programs to assess the impact of their service; hence it is an integral part of the quality assurance process of health delivery. In recent years, there has been an increasing demand of accountability and productivity by consumers. It is now a global trend in health care development towards integrating subjective user satisfaction into the evaluation of medical service quality [15]. Patients' voice must begin to play a greater role in the design of health care service delivery process in the developing countries [16]. The satisfaction of female clients of ANC has been studied in the past in other countries [17]. A study in India reported that the overall summative index for clinical quality using a scale of 0–5 was 2.1% in the North and 4.1 in the South [18]. Similarly in another studyin Oman the overall satisfaction for antenatal care was excellent in 49 (CI 48.5–69.6) respondents. Out of 89 women, 67 (81%) were satisfied with the services because of the attitude of the doctors and nurses. The main causes of dissatisfaction were the laboratory services and overcrowding in the morning hours [19]. However in a study conducted at a Hyderabad, Sindh, half of the women in study sample were satisfied with the overall care provided to them. The routine antenatal investigations were provided to majority of women like urine, blood, antenatal examination and blood pressure. About 86.2% women said that they have to wait for more than two hours for checkups. Regarding satisfaction with getting medicine 63% were found dissatisfied, 75% of women did not have complete tetanus vaccine. Only 31% received instructions about perinatal care, 46% received information about exercise and 36% were reassured about discussing fear and anxiety [20].

In 'Punjab' province of Pakistan, there is network of PHC health facilities named as Rural Health Centers (RHCs) and Basic Health Units (BHUs). RHCs are relatively larger PHC facilities serving 10–50 thousands rural population while BHUs are relatively smaller health facilities providing PHC services to 5000 to 10,000 rural populations. One BHU is available up to almost each 'Union Council' level. There is uniform package of health services, infrastructure, physical and human resources. Medical Officers are in-charge of RHCs/BHUs and ANC services are supposed to be provided by the Lady Health Visitors (LHVs) at these facilities. This study is an attempt to evaluate the coverage and quality of antenatal care being provided to the rural population of this province. Although the study was focused on antenatal care but it will reflect the overall gaps in the health system of Pakistan to be bridged through appropriate interventions. The objectives of the study were:

1. To assess the proportion of expected pregnancies enrolled for ANC services in the catchment areas of PHC health facilities.
2. To assess the proportion of the enrolled clients coming for follow-up ANC visits.
3. To assess the quality ANC services delivery process in terms of assessment, treatment and counseling of the clients.
4. To explore and identify the causes of low coverage and quality of services at managerial, provider and client level.

## Methods

A cross-sectional study was conducted to assess the coverage and quality of ANC services in first-level health care facilities. Both quantitative and qualitative research methods were used to undertake this study. The study proposal was approved by National Bioethics Committee (NBC) Pakistan vide Ref No.4-87/09/NBC-36/RDC/7451 and the inception of the study was undertaken after the approval. A multi-stage sampling procedure was adopted to select the districts and primary level health facilities from each district. In first stage all the districts of Punjab were ranked from 1 to 36 on the basis of a composite indicator which was developed from eight socio-demographic indicators [21]. Total nine out of thirty six districts were selected from the Punjab province so that three district from each high, medium and low social stratum could be included in the study. In the second stage of sampling, 19 health facilities (17 BHUs and 2 RHCs) were randomly selected from each district. Initially a total 171 health facilities BHUs/RHCs were accessed for completion of facility performance data. Approval for health facility assessment and interviews for health care providers was taken from Punjab Health Department. A consent form was developed in the local language that was approved by National Bioethics Committee (NBC) Pakistan. Informed verbal consent was taken from the clients and health care providers for interviews. The Consent form for each interview was filled and signed by a witness at health facilities and its record was maintained along with other data forms. Written consent was not possible for the reason that majority of the clients were illiterate (unable to read or write). During the survey in the first attempt, data collection from 151 health care facilities was completed and an additional 20 alternate health facilities were visited by teams in second attempt due to non-availability of providers or clients to complete the target sample. Client exit interviews were conducted after each client-provider interaction to assess the client satisfaction. The client exit interviews included the questions about the behavior of provider, ANC examination, time spent and the overall perception of satisfaction for the services provided.

Focal Group Discussions (FGDs) and in-depth interviews were conducted in qualitative part of assessment. Nine FGDs for clients and nine for providers were conducted in each of the nine sampled districts. The criteria for the selection of the clients was pregnant women who had already experienced at least one pregnancy and birth process, belonged to lower or middle social class and these clients came from the catchment area of health facility. There were 12 clients in each FGD session who were identified by the 'Lady Health Workers (LHW) in the catchment areas of the health facilities. LHWs enroll the pregnant ladies keep the records and refer them to the BHUs and RHCs for ANC services. The selection criterion for health care providers (Lady Health Visitor) was that their duration of working in these facilities was more than six months. The participation of health care providers was voluntary and the invitations were extended to them with permission of management of provincial health department. A total of 12 LHVs were included in each FGD. One FGD was conducted for Medical Officers/Women Medical Officers at the provincial level. In-depth interviews were conducted with district health managers (Executive District Officers for Health/District Officers for Health) and the provincial managers (Director General Health, Director MNCH Program and Director MIS Cell.

The data was collected on objectively developed semi-structured questionnaire from October-November 2010. Total eight teams were engaged for data collection and each team consisted of one team leader/supervisor and two surveyors/interviewers. A qualitative assessment team comprised of two sociologists and one public health consultant. All teams were provided extensive training in two separate 3-day workshops, one for qualitative and other for quantitative assessment teams. Field monitoring was carried out by two Regional Coordinators, a Public Health Consultant and the Principal investigator. Qualitative data was collected from December 2010 to February 2011.

Univariate analysis was done to describe the frequency and percentage by type of facility and by districts. ANC coverage was evaluated by examining the record of services provided to ANC clients at health facilities. For this purpose, annual ANC first enrolment and ANC follow-up visits were used as indictors. The percentage of the annual expected [22] pregnancies in the catchment area of health facility who reported first time for ANC services during the year before survey (2010) was operationally defined as ANC Enrollment. Percentage of the annual expected pregnancies in the catchment area of health facility reported for follow-up ANC services during the year before survey (2010) was defined as ANC-follow-up visits [19]. It was not possible to calculate the number of visits of a particular client from this data source. The revisits reported from this column are also termed as revisits in the reporting tools of Punjab MIS. The quality of ANC services was based on the steps followed by the health care-providers. A standard check list of steps to be followed health care provider, was developed by consultation of WHO criteria and Minimum Service Delivery Standards (MSDS) adopted by Maternal and Newborn and Child Health Program (MNCH) of the Punjab. This check list was used to observe the client provider interaction during ANC service provision. The providers that follow more than 80% of the steps enlisted in the checklist of assessment, treatment and counseling of the clients were ranked as good, between 60–80% as average and less than 60% as poor to measure the quality of ANC.

The qualitative data processing was initiated in the field with development of field transcripts by the interviewers/facilitator. A qualitative analysis framework was prepared for each target group e.g. clients, providers, facility in-charges, district health managers and provincial stakeholders. The findings were categorized under the main titles of the themes included in qualitative tools relevant to specific participants in FGDs. Findings were analyzed by inductive reasoning approach and qualitative assessment report was compiled under the supervision of a senior sociologist by consulting the individual session reports, transcripts/notes of FGDs and transcripts/notes of all in-depth interviews. Broadly, the analysis of data was arranged by the objectives of the study as stipulated in the research proposal.

## Results

### ANC coverage

The overall enrollment was 51.6% in sampled districts of the Punjab province including the 17 redundant health facilities where no services being provided. Wide range of variations was observed among districts in ANC enrollment. Maximum coverage was observed in district Gujranwala at 79.6% followed by district Toba Tek Singh with 79.1% ANC-1 coverage annually. Minimum coverage was reported from district Sahiwal as 24.9% followed by district Multan as 33.8%. Out of the whole sample, five districts – Multan, Vehari, Bahawalnagar, Sahiwal and Sargodha – had coverage below overall mean and four districts – Gujranwala, Rawalpindi, Toba Tek Singh and Kasur – had ANC coverage above overall mean. (Fig. 1) The regression analysis indicates that there was 1.347% decrease in ANC coverage with one digit rise in ranking of the districts with constant value at base line of 71.7%. The Pearson Product Correlation coefficient, r = 0.64 and r2 = 0.41. All the districts in the Punjab were ranked from 1 to 36 according to a composite indicator based on adult literacy, primary school enrolment, under-five mortality, prevalence of under-nutrition, adequate water and sanitation, the percentage of deliveries with a skilled birth attendant, and use of contraceptive. The rank 1 mean most developed district and rank 36 mean least developed district. The higher ranks number are indicating lower social developmental index and low coverage. In other words with one degree increase rank mean decrease in social development and there is decrease in 1.347% ANC coverage and 71.7% is the highest base line coverage on the line of best fit of regression line. (Fig. 2).

ANC-enrollment percentage was increased from 51.6% to 55.9% when the data from 17 alternative non-redundant facilities was added to the analysis. The overall dropout was 32.8% in subsequent visits after the ANC visit in the health facilities. The drop was observed in all the districts except 'Rawalpindi' where there was a 29.1% increase in the number of follow-up visits. The reason for increase follow-up visits in this district was the availability of WMOs, free ultrasound services and accessible locations of some of the RHC health facilities.

Health facilities were ranked according to monthly percentage of expected pregnancies enrolled for ANC in the catchment area of health facilities. Health facilities enrolling more than 80% of expected pregnancies were ranked as good, 60–80% as average and less than 60% as poor. ANC coverage facility ranking revealed that overall only 24% facilities achieved a good ranking, 13.5% had average and 62.6% facilities had poor ranking in monthly ANC-1 coverage. ANC-follow-up/revisits followed a similar trend. (See Table 1).

The inferential analysis shows that <80% coverage was observed in 76% of facilities with 95% confidence limits from 69% to 82%. In comparison by type of facility, 56% of RHCs were providing good coverage compared to only 20% of BHUs. Thus more than half of RHCs had a good ranking for coverage while 80% BHUs had poor or average ranking.

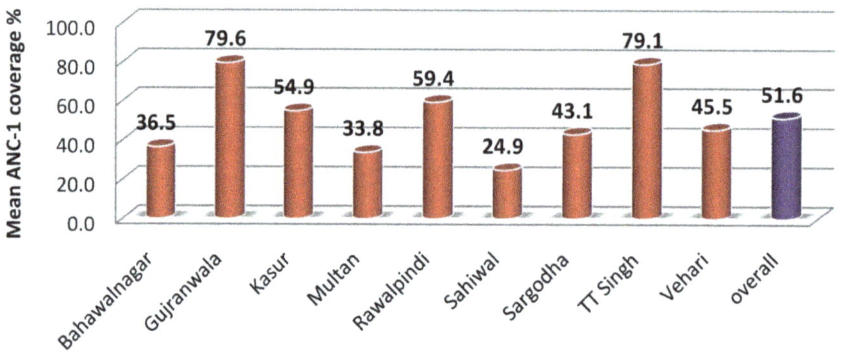


**Figure 1. District-wise and overall mean annual ANC-1 coverage in PHC health facilities.**

## Service quality

The appropriate history taking was followed by less 30% of providers in the context of asking about previous still births, bleeding, assisted deliveries, abortions, headache/blurring of vision, swelling and fever. Feeling of baby movement was enquired from only 9% of the clients. Most of the history steps were falling less than 50% range. The standard protocols for clinical examination were not being fulfilled in most of the cases. The breast examination was practiced in 10%, looked for edema 25%, test advised 21%, heard fetal heart sound in 51%, abdomen was palpated in 76% and BP was recorded in 74% of the services provided. The overall ranking of quality of clinical assessment was poor in 72%, average in 23% and good in only 5% of the services provided. (Fig. 3, Table 2).

The standard protocol steps for counseling were at lowest level that extremely compromised the quality of the ANC services. Counseling for breast feeding was 6%, talked about contraception 6%, asked about place of delivery 31%, transport arrangement 20% and discussed about cost of delivery by 5% providers. TT was advised by 57% and next date of visits was advised by the 80% of the health care providers. The overall ranking of quality of counseling was poor in 92%, average in 6% and good in only 2% of the services provided.

Service delivery protocols practice for the treatment were relatively better than assessment and counseling but the large gaps were identified in treatment practices of the health care providers that includes Tetanus Toxoide (TT) vaccination, prescription for antimalarials, iron and folic acid tablets. Iron and folic acid and TT were prescribed by 69, 64 and 62% respectively but anti-malarial was advised by only by 2% of the health care providers in suspected malaria cases. The overall ranking of quality of treatment was poor in 32%, average in 23% and good in 44% of the services provided. Inferential statistical analysis showed that the overall gap to achieve above 80% level of counseling quality was 48 to 63% at 95% confidence limits. In response to questions in the client exit interview overall 46% clients perceived that they were satisfied with the provided ANC services. The proportion of clients who were satisfied with the services was almost similar in RHCs (50%) and BHUs (46%). (See detail in Table 2).

## Qualitative findings

The underlying factors for low coverage and quality explored from the clients, providers and managers. The translated views of each stakeholder are given in the Box-1. Distant location of facilities and lack of functional equipment, medicines and supplies was perceived by the clients, providers as well as health managers. Indifferent attitude and uncertainty in availability of the staff was complained by most of the clients. Community based indigenous ANC providers (Dais) are negatively influencing the ANC services enrollment due to affordability, availability 24/7 at door steps, providing massage, helping for household work and attending the deliveries at home. All these services can't be taken as substitute of the ANC services that needs examination from skilled persons and needs some lab diagnostic services from the health facility set-up.

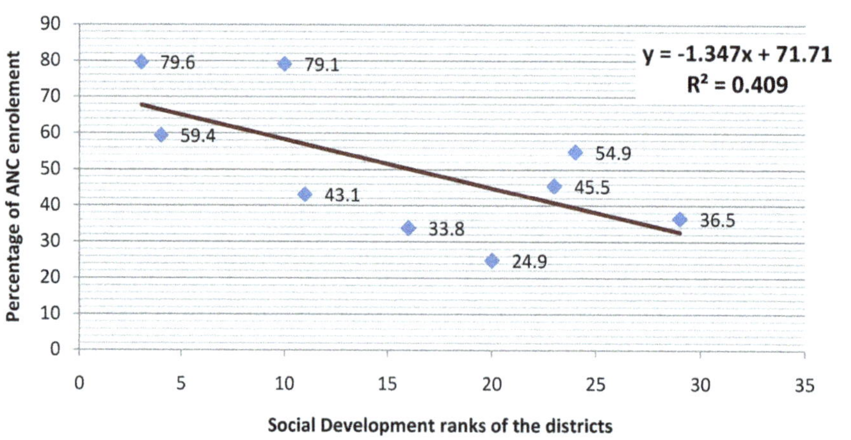


**Figure 2. Association of Social Development Ranking with the District ANC coverage.**

**Table 1.** Ranking of health facility by ANC-enrolment and follow-up visits in the catchment areas.

| | Overall | | RHCs | | BHUs | |
|---|---|---|---|---|---|---|
| **Number of facilities** | **171** | | **18** | | **153** | |
| | n | % | n | % | n | % |
| **Ranking of facilities by monthly ANC enrolment** | | | | | | |
| Good coverage >80% | 41 | 24 | 10 | 56 | 31 | 20 |
| Average coverage ≥60% ≤80% | 23 | 13 | 3 | 17 | 20 | 13 |
| Poor coverage <60 | 107 | 63 | 5 | 28 | 102 | 67 |
| **Ranking of facilities by monthly ANC-follow-up/revisits** | | | | | | |
| Good coverage >80% | 27 | 16 | 6 | 33 | 21 | 14 |
| Average coverage ≥60% ≤80% | 19 | 11 | 3 | 17 | 16 | 10 |
| Poor coverage <60 | 125 | 73 | 9 | 50 | 116 | 76 |

Lack of awareness and self decision power to visit the health facilities are also contributory factors for low coverage of ANC services in the rural area. Most of clients are visiting health facilities with expectation of being examined by ultrasound machine (USG) with hope to determine the sex of the fetus. The specific problems pointed out by providers were lack of guidance and supervision from the WMOs and facility in-charges and managers pointed out the deficiencies in district target setting, periodic monitoring systems, cumbersome purchase process and lack of training and skills.

## Discussion

Antenatal care is a very important component of maternal health services. It gives women and their families an opportunity to learn about the risks associated with pregnancy and guides their health seeking practices and decision making thereby preventing maternal and infant morbidity and mortality. Counseling during ANC provides a critical opportunity for women to learn when to seek help and where to give birth. It also helps prepare women for the mental and physical challenges they may face during pregnancy and childbirth. This study was focused on the current situation of coverage and quality of ANC services being provided to the rural mothers in the Punjab. ANC services are being offered by the government in rural areas of the Punjab through a network of PHC health facilities designated as 'RHCs' and 'BHUs'. The private clinics/maternity homes and community health care providers are mainly providing delivery services because they are unable to provide the essential laboratory services package included in the standard ANC protocol. The rural women are mainly dependent on government's PHC health facilities for ANC services. The study finding revealed that overall 51.6% of the expected pregnancies first time reported for the ANC and out of those 33% didn't return back for follow-up. These findings straight way revealed that there is a gap of about 50% in the coverage of ANC services in the Punjab. The dropout in follow-up indicates the poor quality of the services that are annoying the clients not to return back for follow-up services. The overall coverage indicated in this study is very closer to that (57%) claimed by the HMIS cell Punjab [19] in DHIS report of 2010 and MICS 2007–2008, that is about (53%) [23]. This study was focused on rural areas and there was no opportunity for urban comparison but inequity in provision of ANC services to rural population have been reported in the literature [4]. The variation in coverage is associated with the number of standard ANC visits in assessment criteria e.g. in a study conducted in Alwar district of Rajasthan state, India, the practices of 3 or more ANC visits were lower in rural (36.1%) as compared to (71.4%) in urban areas [24].

Fifty percent ANC-1 registration of clients does not mean that the services are fulfilling quality of ANC services. It is just a registration figures. Although WHO recommends four ANC visits for every pregnant woman but the facility register contains only two columns one for the first visit and the other for revisits. Since all revisits are recorded in the same column, it is impossible to know how many of the registered cases completed four ANC visits. On the other hand, revisit/follow-up data indicates that about one third of the clients dropped out after the first visit, which means that a majority of the clients did not even complete two visits. Generally there were dropouts in revisits, in majority of the districts but in Rawalpindi there was an increase in revisits after

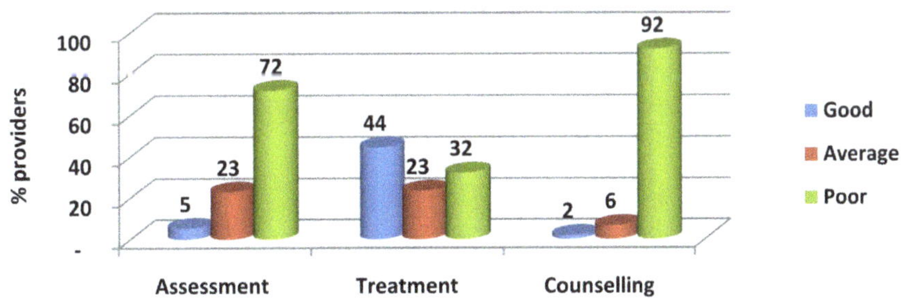


**Figure 3. Ranking of ANC Services for Assessment Treatment and Counselling.**

**Table 2.** Quality of ANC services and client satisfaction (Overall and by types of facilities).

| | Overall | | RHCs | | BHUs | |
|---|---|---|---|---|---|---|
| **Number of facilities** | **171** | | **18** | | **153** | |
| | n | % | n | % | n | % |
| **Areas of client assessment by history** | | | | | | |
| Age of client | 139 | 81 | 15 | 83 | 124 | 81 |
| Use of medication by client | 77 | 45 | 8 | 44 | 69 | 45 |
| Date of LMP asked | 103 | 60 | 10 | 56 | 93 | 61 |
| Previous pregnancies | 111 | 65 | 11 | 61 | 100 | 65 |
| Previous still births/neonatal deaths | 45 | 26 | 6 | 33 | 39 | 25 |
| Heavy bleeding | 23 | 13 | 5 | 28 | 18 | 12 |
| Assisted deliveries | 30 | 18 | 4 | 22 | 26 | 17 |
| Abortions | 42 | 25 | 5 | 28 | 37 | 24 |
| Asked about bleeding | 47 | 27 | 6 | 33 | 41 | 27 |
| Fever | 57 | 33 | 6 | 33 | 51 | 33 |
| Headache/blurred vision | 45 | 26 | 5 | 28 | 40 | 26 |
| Swelling | 59 | 35 | 6 | 33 | 53 | 35 |
| Tiredness/breathlessness | 56 | 33 | 6 | 33 | 50 | 33 |
| Felt fetal movement | 105 | 61 | 12 | 67 | 93 | 61 |
| Mentioned bleeding | 16 | 9 | 4 | 22 | 12 | 8 |
| Mentioned fever | 35 | 20 | 4 | 22 | 31 | 20 |
| Mentioned headache/blurred vision | 30 | 18 | 3 | 17 | 27 | 18 |
| Mentioned swelling | 36 | 21 | 5 | 28 | 31 | 20 |
| Mentioned tiredness/breathlessness | 52 | 30 | 6 | 33 | 46 | 30 |
| Mentioned Fetal Movements | 79 | 46 | 9 | 50 | 70 | 46 |
| **Areas of client assessment by examination** | | | | | | |
| Record BP | 127 | 74 | 9 | 50 | 118 | 77 |
| Recorded weight | 102 | 60 | 7 | 39 | 95 | 62 |
| Palpated abdomen | 130 | 76 | 16 | 89 | 114 | 75 |
| Foetal heart sounds heard | 88 | 51 | 12 | 67 | 76 | 50 |
| Looked for oedema | 42 | 25 | 5 | 28 | 37 | 24 |
| Breast exam done | 17 | 10 | 3 | 17 | 14 | 9 |
| Tests advised | 36 | 21 | 9 | 50 | 27 | 18 |
| ANC card filled | 73 | 43 | 10 | 56 | 63 | 41 |
| Talked about TT | 109 | 64 | 11 | 61 | 98 | 64 |
| **Areas of client counselling** | | | | | | |
| Advice about food | 108 | 63 | 10 | 56 | 98 | 64 |
| Importance of TT vaccination told | 48 | 28 | 6 | 33 | 42 | 27 |
| Advised TT | 97 | 57 | 7 | 39 | 90 | 59 |
| Talked about Contraception | 10 | 6 | 2 | 11 | 8 | 5 |
| Talked about breast feeding | 10 | 6 | 2 | 11 | 8 | 5 |
| Place of delivery | 53 | 31 | 7 | 39 | 46 | 30 |
| Arrangement for transport | 35 | 20 | 4 | 22 | 31 | 20 |
| Who will accompany her | 9 | 5 | 1 | 6 | 8 | 5 |
| Time to reach place of delivery | 9 | 5 | 1 | 6 | 8 | 5 |
| Cost of delivery | 11 | 6 | 1 | 6 | 10 | 7 |
| Give next visit date | 136 | 80 | 12 | 67 | 124 | 81 |
| **Ranking of client counselling** | | | | | | |
| Adequate counselling practices >80% | 3 | 2 | 1 | 6 | 2 | 1 |
| Average counselling practices ≥60% ≤80% | 11 | 6 | 2 | 11 | 9 | 6 |
| Poor counselling practices <60% | 157 | 92 | 15 | 83 | 142 | 93 |

**Table 2.** Cont.

| Number of facilities | Overall | | RHCs | | BHUs | |
|---|---|---|---|---|---|---|
| | 171 | | 18 | | 153 | |
| | n | % | n | % | n | % |
| **Areas of client treatment** | | | | | | |
| Iron pills prescribed | 118 | 69 | 12 | 67 | 106 | 69 |
| Folic acid tablets prescribed | 109 | 64 | 10 | 56 | 99 | 65 |
| TT injection prescribed | 106 | 62 | 11 | 61 | 95 | 62 |
| Anti-malarial prescribed | 4 | 2 | | – | 4 | 3 |
| **Ranking of client treatment** | | | | | | |
| Good quality of treatment >80% | 76 | 44 | 9 | 50 | 67 | 44 |
| Average quality of treatment ≥60% ≤80% | 40 | 23 | 2 | 11 | 38 | 25 |
| Poor quality of treatment <60% | 55 | 32 | 7 | 39 | 48 | 31 |
| **Areas of client satisfaction** | | | | | | |
| Respectful behavior | 113 | 66 | 13 | 72 | 100 | 65 |
| Physical examination done | 166 | 97 | 18 | 100 | 148 | 97 |
| Satisfied with exam time | 94 | 55 | 11 | 61 | 83 | 54 |
| Satisfied with answers | 155 | 91 | 16 | 89 | 139 | 91 |
| Respectful behaviour of the facility staff | 98 | 57 | 11 | 61 | 87 | 57 |
| Client was satisfied | 79 | 46 | 9 | 50 | 70 | 46 |

the first visit. The reasons for this increase in revisits were the availability of Women Medical Officers, free facility of ultrasound, accessible locations, and availability of resources and awareness of the clients in these areas.

The ANC coverage was linearly increasing with better social developmental ranking a. composite proxy indicator [18]. The social factors have 'push' factor and quality of services have 'pull' factor for availing ANC services by the clients. Regarding quality of services the healthcare providers are not following the standard services delivery protocols during the history taking, clinical examination, treatment and counseling of the clients. Although about half of the clients were satisfied but that was their subjective perception that does not mean that quality services are being provided. Normative quality needs were not being met in more than 90% of the services being provided. The ultimate outcome of poor quality was reflected in the form of loss of follow-up for ANC. The loss of follow-up in about one 3rd of the enrolled clients raised a serious question on the quality of the services being provided. The evidence from another study supported that there was a significant association between satisfaction (outcome) and type of care, attitude of care provider, assessment of weight of women and waiting time [25]. The reasons identified for dissatisfaction among pregnant women in a public sector hospital of Hyderabad, Sindh were long waiting time, inadequate medicine supply and incomplete tetanus vaccination which were reported by 50% clients [19]. It is evident from a study conducted in Oman that short waiting time and positive behavior providers were the most satisfying aspects of the services [26]. Another study in India revealed that, the quality is a more significant predictor of utilization antenatal care services [17].

Reasons for low coverage at managerial level were distant location of health facilities, lack of functional equipment, medicine and supplies. Although government is providing services free or on nominal user charges, but the cost become unaffordable to marginralized clients due to unauthorized over changing for services in the PHC health facilities. Social factor effecting the coverage and drop-out at client level were lack of awareness and self decision power to visit the health facilities. The decisions about availing of ANC culturally endowed to the mother in law or husband. One of the factors responsible for the drop outs were indifferent attitude and uncertainty in availability of the staff.

Community based indigenous maternal care providers (Dais) are negatively influencing the ANC services enrolment due to affordability and availability 24/7 at door steps. The objective of ANC is to detect the high risk pregnancies and deliveries and if any services fail to do so can't be labeled as ANC whether provided at health facility or at home.

## Conclusion

The study revealed that both coverage and quality of the ANC services in Punjab are extremely inadequate. For coverage, only half of the expected pregnancies in the catchment areas of PHC health facilities are enrolled for ANC and out of those 1/3 never returned for follow-up visits. The quality of ANC is extremely compromised as perceived by clients and observed during the study. More than 50% of the clients are not satisfied with the ANC services they receive.

The major factors contributing for low coverage and quality at managerial and provider levels were distant location of health facilities, lack of functional equipment, insufficient supplies, inconvenient facility working hours and uncertainty in availability of staff. The social factors include lack of awareness, self decision power for seeking ANC, indifferent attitude of facility staff, affordability and availability of transport services. The miscellaneous home services provided by indigenous birth attendants are mistakenly considered as substitute of quality ANC, able to detect high risk pregnancies and deliveries.

Interventions are recommended to address the both coverage and quality issues depicted in the study findings. Health mangers can address the quality issues training, motivation and monitoring of health facility staff for client friendly behavior. Facility working hours must be extended and adjusted according to the convenience of clients in PHC health facilities. Removing transport barriers through sustainable public private partnerships or community development programs and retention of health care providers through incentivized package and facilities. Client awareness and self empowerment should be improved through involvement of local NGOs and social workers. For ANC client referral, the community based service health workers such as LHWs and CMWs must be targeted for advocacy and motivation for referring the clients to the public health facilities for ANC services.

To improve the quality of services health care providers should be trained to improve their technical skills for assessment, treatment and counseling of clients. Providers should get motivation and training to encourage them to follow the standard protocols for provision of quality ANC services.

## Acknowledgments

We acknowledge the efforts of Research and Advocacy Fund (RAF) team members for their financial assistance in logistic and field work of both quantitative and qualitative data collection and provision of technical assistance. We are grateful for the cooperation of Director General Health Punjab Dr. Muhammad Aslam, Director MNCH programme Dr. Sabiha Khurshid and Director MIS Dr. Muhammad Anwar Janjua. We also acknowledge with thanks the efforts of consultants, Dr. Muhammad Anwar, Head of Sociology Department, University of Central Punjab, Irum Bukhari, Saima Aslam and Sabahat Mushtaq for their contributions in the qualitative and quantitative interviews. We appreciate the efforts of the regional Coordinators Inam-ul-Haq and Fayyaz Ahmed Butt, team supervisors and field enumerators (both male and female) made it possible to complete this assignment on schedule. Particular gratitude is due to the entire field team. All district health managers (EDOH/DOH, district coordinators for MNCH programme) provided valuable support by contributing the services of their staff. Special thanks are owed to the communities, local leadership and clients of sampled districts who devoted their time and resources to enable the survey teams to complete their assignment and focus group discussions.

## Author Contributions

Conceived and designed the experiments: AM SH. Performed the experiments: AM SH JA AS. Analyzed the data: AM SH ZM. Contributed reagents/materials/analysis tools: JA AS ZM. Wrote the paper: AM SH JA AS ZM. Developed proposal and supervised all the steps from development of data collection tools to completion of draft of the manuscript: AM. Remained actively involved in pre-testing, review of tools and monitoring the quality of data collection, entry and analysis: AM. Involved in the preparation of manuscript: AM SH JA AS. Involved in the process development of study proposal, qualitative themes, qualitative data collection: SH JA AS. Provided technical assistance in analysis and interpretation of focal group discussions and in depth interviews: SH JA AS. Drafted qualitative findings, discussion, field monitoring and involved in data entry and analysis: ZM.

## References


1. McCarthy J, Maine D (1992) A framework for analyzing the determinants of maternal mortality. Stud FamPlann 23(1): 23–33.
2. World Health Organization (2008) Maternal mortality in 2005: estimates developed by WHO, UNICEF, UNFPA, and the World Bank. Geneva: World Health Organization: 48.
3. Abou-Zahr CL, Wardlaw TM (2003) *Antenatal care in developing countries: promise, achievements and missed opportunity: an analysis of trends, levels and differentials, 1990–2001*. Geneva: World Health Organization.
4. Pakistan Statistical Year Book (2007) Federal Bureau of Statistic Government of Pakistan.
5. Raisa BG, Paul P, Oslon JK (2009) Strengths and challenges of the first pre-licensure Baccalaureate of Science in Nursing Program of Pakistan. Journal of Professional Nursing 25(4): 240–248.
6. Jabeen M, Gul F, Rehman M (2005) Maternal Mortality ratio and its causes in a District Headquarter Hospital of NWFP. Journal of Postgraduate Medical Institute 19(4): 377–381.
7. Millenium Development Goals Country Report Sri Lanka (2005) Improve Maternal Health. NewYork: United Nations Development Programme: 1–6.
8. Tarekegn SM, Lieberman LS, Giedraitis V (2014) Determinants of maternal health service utilization in Ethiopia: analysis of the 2011 Ethiopian Demographic and Health Survey. BMC Pregnancy and Childbirth. 2014; 14: 161.
9. Jafari F, Eftekhar H, Fotouhi A, Mohammad K, Hantoushzadeh S (2010) Comparison of maternal and neonatal outcomes of group versus individual prenatal care: a new experience in Iran. Health Care for Women International 31: 571–584.
10. Barua A, Waghmare R, Venkiteswaran S (2003) Implementing reproductive and child health services in rural Maharashtra, India: a pragmatic approach. Reproductive Health Matters 11: 140–149.
11. Nisar N, White F (2003) Factors affecting utilization of Antenatal Care among reproductive age group (15–49years) in an urban squatter settlement of Karachi. JPMA 53(2): 1–10.
12. Ali AA, Osman MM, Abbaker AO, Adam I (2010) Use of antenatal care services in Kassala, eastern Sudan. BMC Pregnancy and Childbirth 10: 67 doi:10.1186/1471-2393-10-67.
13. Hasan Z, Zia S, Maracy M (2007) Prenatal care service uptake by rural women in North West of Pakistan. JPMI vol 21(1): 29–35.
14. National Institute of Population Sciences (NIPS), Macro International Ltd. (2008) Pakistan. Demographic and Health Survey 2006–2007. Islamabad: National Institute of Population Studies & Macro International Ltd.
15. Hudak PL, Wright JG (2000) The characteristics of patient satisfaction measures. Spine 25: 3167–3177.
16. Andaleeb SS (2001) Service quality perceptions and patient satisfaction: a study of hospitals in developing countries. Social Science and Medicine 52(90): 1359–1370.
17. Luyben AG, Fleming VE (2005) Women needs from ANC in three European countries. Midwifery 21: 212–223.
18. Rani M, BonuSekhar, Harvey S (2008) Differentials in the quality of antenatal care in India. International Journal for Quality in Health Care 20(1): 62–71.
19. Ghobashi M, Khandekar R (2008) Satisfaction among expectant mothers with antenatal care services in the Musandam region of Oman. Sultan QaboosUniv Med J 8(3): 325–332.
20. Nisar N, Amjad R (2007) Pattern of antenatal care provided at a public sector hospital Hyderabad Sindh. J Ayub Med Coll Abbottabad 19(4): 11–13.
21. District –Based Multiple Indicators Cluster Survey 2003–2004. Lahore: Government of Punjab. Planning & Development. Department: 12–13.
22. District Health Information System (DHIS) Repot 2010. Lahore. Health Department, Government of Punjab.
23. Multiple Indicator Cluster Survey (MICS) Punjab 2007–2008. Provincial Report. Government of the Punjab Planning and Development Bureau of Statistics.
24. Gupta RS, Gupta A, Gupta HO, Venkatesh S, Shiv Lal (2006). Mother and Child Service Coverage: Reproductive and Child Health Prgramme in Alwar District, Rajasthan state. J. Commun. Dis 38(1): 79–87.
25. Zeidan ZA, Idris AM, Bhairy M (2011) Satisfaction among pregnant women towards antenatal care in public and private care clinics in Khartoum. Khartoum Medical Journal Vol. 04, No. 02, 590–595.
26. Ghobashi M, Khandekar R (2008) Satisfaction among expectant mothers with antenatal care services in the Musandam Region of Oman. Sultan QaboosUniv Med J 8(3): 325–332.

# 16

# A Time Series Evaluation of the FAST National Stroke Awareness Campaign in England

**Darren Flynn[1]*, Gary A. Ford[2], Helen Rodgers[2], Christopher Price[3], Nick Steen[1], Richard G. Thomson[1]**

**1** Institute of Health and Society, Newcastle University, Newcastle upon Tyne, United Kingdom, **2** Institute for Ageing and Health (Stroke Research Group), Faculty of Medical Sciences, Newcastle University, Newcastle upon Tyne, United Kingdom, **3** Wansbeck General Hospital, Northumbria Healthcare NHS Foundation Trust, Ashington, United Kingdom

## Abstract

***Objective:*** In February 2009, the Department of Health in England launched the Face, Arm, Speech, and Time (FAST) mass media campaign, to raise public awareness of stroke symptoms and the need for an emergency response. We aimed to evaluate the impact of three consecutive phases of FAST using population-level measures of behaviour in England.

***Methods:*** Interrupted time series (May 2007 to February 2011) assessed the impact of the campaign on: access to a national stroke charity's information resources (Stroke Association [SA]); emergency hospital admissions with a primary diagnosis of stroke (Hospital Episode Statistics for England); and thrombolysis activity from centres in England contributing data to the Safe Implementation of Thrombolysis in Stroke UK database.

***Results:*** Before the campaign, emergency admissions (and patients admitted via accident and emergency [A&E]) and thrombolysis activity was increasing significantly over time, whereas emergency admissions via general practitioners (GPs) were decreasing significantly. SA webpage views, calls to their helpline and information materials dispatched increased significantly after phase one. Website hits/views, and information materials dispatched decreased after phase one; these outcomes increased significantly during phases two and three. After phase one there were significant increases in overall emergency admissions (505, 95% CI = 75 to 935) and patients admitted via A&E (451, 95% CI = 26 to 875). Significantly fewer monthly emergency admissions via GPs were reported after phase three (−19, 95% CI = −29 to −9). Thrombolysis activity per month significantly increased after phases one (3, 95% CI = 1 to 6), and three (3, 95% CI = 1 to 4).

***Conclusions:*** Phase one had a statistically significant impact on information seeking behaviour and emergency admissions, with additional impact that may be attributable to subsequent phases on information seeking behaviour, emergency admissions via GPs, and thrombolysis activity. Future campaigns should be a0ccompanied by evaluation of impact on clinical outcomes such as reduced stroke-related morbidity and mortality.

**Editor:** C. Mary Schooling, CUNY, United States of America

**Funding:** These authors have no support or funding to report.

**Competing Interests:** The authors have read the journal's policy and have the following conflicts - DF, GAF, HR, CP and RGT have been involved in developing a computerised decision aid for thrombolytic treatment in acute stroke care. GAF has received personal remuneration for educational and advisory work from Boehringer Ingelheim (manufacturer of Alteplase) and Lundbeck. GAF's previous institution has received research grants from Boehringer Ingelheim, and honoraria from Lundbeck for stroke-related activities. GAF developed the Face Arm Speech Test for use by ambulance paramedics in England.

* Email: darren.flynn@ncl.ac.uk

## Introduction

Stroke is the third leading cause of death worldwide and a major cause of severe adult disability in developed countries [1,2]. For acute ischaemic stroke, rapid thrombolysis within 4.5 hours can improve the prognosis, with greater benefit from earlier treatment [3,4]. An expeditious response to stroke symptoms is critical [5]. Many patients present too late to hospital due to a failure, for a variety of reasons, or inability to call emergency services rapidly [5–7].

Mass media interventions are promoted as an effective method of improving awareness of health issues and changing behaviour, including encouraging appropriate use of services [8]. A systematic review of 20 evaluations of mass media interventions for a range of conditions reported a positive effect on health services utilisation [8]. Such interventions targeted at stroke have a positive impact on knowledge, including awareness of the need for an emergency response, but with little impact on public behaviour [9].

In February 2009, the Department of Health in England launched the Face, Arm, Speech, and Time (FAST) mass media campaign, to raise public awareness of stroke, specifically its symptoms and the need for an emergency response [10,11]. An adapted version of the FAST mnemonic (used to screen for the presence of stroke in clinical practice) was used to convey information on three typical stroke symptoms (F = facial weakness, A = arm weakness and S = speech disturbance) and the desired behavioural response (T = time to call emergency services if you recognise any of one of the stroke symptoms). The damage to the brain from stroke was illustrated with an evocative image of a fire rapidly spreading in the head of an older adult depicted. The need for an expeditious response was further emphasised with the aphorism 'ACT FAST' along with the key message "The faster you act the more of the person you save".

Phase one was launched on 9th February 2009 and ran until end of March 2009 with television, press, and radio advertisements. A second phase ran from November 2009 to December 2009; a third phase during February 2010 to March 2010; with a fourth phase during March 2011. Fifth and sixth phases ran from February 2012 to March 2012, and during March 2013. The most recent phase took place during March 2014. Whilst the overall cost of the campaign to date is unclear, and unlikely to be the figure of £105 million in funding over three years quoted in a Wellcome Trust article [12], the costs are not insignificant; the Department of Health stated that the more restricted three month advertising campaign in phase 4 cost £740,000 [13].

Few studies have evaluated the impact of the campaign on behaviour, although face-to-face structured interviews with members of the public in England conducted immediately before and after the first phase identified increases in awareness of stroke signs, the FAST mnemonic, and behavioural intentions to seek emergency medical care for stroke symptoms [7,14]. A questionnaire survey administered in one mixed urban/rural population in England also reported high-levels of awareness of the campaign (70%) and FAST symptoms (other symptoms, leg weakness and visual loss that were not highlighted in the FAST campaign, were poorly recognised as signs of stroke) [15]. An audit of ambulance trusts in England reportedly attributed an average increase of 50% in absolute numbers of emergency calls categorised as stroke according to paramedics between April to June 2008 (N = 2020) and April to June 2009 (N = 3040) to the campaign [16]. No effect of the campaign on speed of presentation or numbers of patients thrombolysed were reported by single site studies in England [17,18].

An evaluation (using observational data and modelling) commissioned by the Department of Health attributed a range of impacts on public and professional behaviour to the FAST campaign within the first year: (i) increased numbers of stroke-related emergency calls (55% over the first four months); (ii) increased numbers of patients presenting earlier to hospital (9900) and receiving specialist treatment (2500); (iii) reduced stroke-related morbidity and mortality (640 patients); (iv) gains in quality adjusted life years (2200); and (v) a return on marketing investment of £3.20 for every £1 spent on the campaign [19]. However the time frame and assumptions of the modelling process have not been clearly described.

Attributing these findings to the campaign is difficult since they are cross-sectional surveys [15], clinical outcomes are based on modelling as opposed to objective data [19], or only report changes in summary statistics between pre- and post-intervention periods [14,16–18]. Consequently, they fail to provide an estimate of effect that takes into account the influence of time trend [8]; for example thrombolytic treatment rates in England were already increasing rapidly before the FAST campaign due to service developments [20].

In order to account for the influence of the campaign over and above background time trend, we aimed to evaluate the impact of three consecutive phases of the FAST campaign using objective measures of behaviour at the population level in England with a time series evaluation.

## Methods

### Data sources

An interrupted time series design was used as it is the optimal research design for retrospectively evaluating the impact of the FAST campaign, which also takes into account the influence of background time trend. Three data sources covering the period May 2007 to February 2011 were used to assess the impact of the first, second, and third phases of the FAST campaign: data from the Stroke Association (SA – a registered national charity that provides support and information to stroke survivors and funds research on prevention and treatment of stroke) on resource utilisation [21]; Hospital Episode Statistics (HES) for England (routinely collected information on all patients who receive care from the National Health Service - publicly-funded primary and secondary care services, the majority of which are free to anyone who is legally residing in England) [22]; and data from a monitoring registry set up to audit the safety and efficacy of thrombolysis in the treatment of acute ischaemic stroke in routine settings - the Safe Implementation of Thrombolysis in Stroke UK (SITS-UK) database [23]. The number of SITS-UK hospital sites in England that contributed data to the reported analysis throughout the study period (2007, 2008, 2009, 2010 and up to Feb 2011) was 27.

Data provided by the SA were used to establish the impact of the campaign on information seeking behaviour for stroke: calls to their helpline; visits to their website, including page views; and information materials on stroke dispatched.

HES data for England (finished admission episodes) were used to determine the proportion of overall emergency admissions with a primary diagnosis of stroke admitted via (i) Accident and Emergency (A&E) services – emergency 999 calls, (ii) general practitioner (primary care practitioner) - where members of public contacted a primary care practitioner as the first response to stroke symptoms, rather than initiated an immediate 999 call).; (iii) Bed Bureau, including the Central Bureau (service that collates information on care homes in the UK); (iv) consultant outpatient clinics; and (v) other means, including patients who arrive via the A&E department of another healthcare provider. The following ICD diagnosis codes were aggregated to determine a primary diagnosis of stroke: G45, G46, I61, I63, I64, and I67. Sub-group analyses of emergency admissions via A&E services and emergency admissions via general practitioners were also conducted.

Data from the SITS-UK database [23] from hospitals in England that submitted data to the register throughout the study period (n = 27) were used to assess the impact of the campaign on numbers of patients receiving thrombolytic treatment.

### Statistical analyses

Segmented regression analyses [24] were conducted to establish the following parameters with 95% confidence intervals (CIs): (i) time trends (monthly changes) for data before the campaign (May 2007 to February 2009); (ii) predicted value for outcomes at March 2009 if phase one had not occurred; (iii) any step change in levels for data immediately after phase one (between February 2009 and March 2009); and (iv) magnitude of time trends (monthly changes) for data across March 2009 to October 2009 (corresponding to the period with no campaign activity after phase one), November 2009 to February 2010 (corresponding to the period during the second and third phases), and March 2010 to February 2011 (corresponding to the period of no campaign activity following phase three).

This approach differs to a standard segmented regression analysis where it would be typical to allow for step changes in level for data between October 2009/November 2009 to December 2009, and between January 2010/February 2010 to March 2010. However, in view of the intense compact nature of the initial campaign (and due to the measurement interval of our data we could not model changes during the February 2009 and March 2009) we assumed that the maximum impact on outcomes would occur at the end of March 2009; therefore, it was more appropriate to fit a step change in level only for data between February 2009 and March 2009. The second and third phases occurred over a sufficiently long period to be included as separate segments in our analyses.

The Durbin-Watson statistic ($d$) with lower ($dl$) and upper ($du$) bounds for critical values at 1% level of significance for regression models with an intercept term [25] was used to establish the presence of autocorrelation of error terms in the regression analyses (i.e. whether consecutive monthly time points were correlated). If $d>du$, or $4\text{-}d>du$ then there is no statistical evidence of positive or negative autocorrelation respectively. The inclusion of dummy variables for calendar month into the regression models was undertaken to adjust for seasonality in the datasets. These were conducted as sensitivity analyses, as opposed to main analyses for the following reasons: (i) they constituted 11 of 45 degrees of freedom that may increase the standard errors associated with estimates of effects; and (ii) some variation between months is likely due to FAST activity and thus controlling for calendar months may produce conservative estimates of campaign effects. All analyses were conducted using SPSS version 19.

## Results

There was no evidence of autocorrelation in the regression models for the main analyses. The results are presented graphically in figures 1 and 2 and summarised in tables 1 and 2. Regression models adjusted for seasonality are shown in Tables S1 and S2.

### The Stroke Association (SA)

Figure 1 (panels A and B) shows data on resource utilisation for the SA: website hits (N = 3104722), website page views (N = 17668701), calls to their helpline (N = 74428) and information materials dispatched (N = 4463983). There were no statistically significant changes in trends for these outcomes before the campaign.

With the exception of website visits, significant changes in level between February 2009 and March 2009 were identified for webpage views (82144, 95% CI = 13845 to 150384), information materials dispatched (101081, 95% CI = 43530 to 158632), and calls to the SA helpline (339, 95% CI = 26 to 652). Significant monthly decreases in website visits (−2550, 95% CI = −5014 to −85), webpage views (−13875, 95% CI = −25582 to −2167), and information materials dispatched (−20970, 95% CI = −30840 to −11101) occurred during the period of no campaign activity following phase one. These outcomes increased significantly during the second and third phases of the campaign. Changes in numbers of calls to the SA helpline across subsequent phases of the campaign were not statistically significant.

### HES for England

Figure 2 (panel A) shows HES data (N = 353305) for overall emergency admissions for stroke, and for emergency admissions via A&E (n = 280338) and general practitioners (n = 48019). Statistically significant increases over 22 months before the campaign were identified for overall emergency admissions (26 patients per month; 95% CI = 7 to 45) and A&E admissions (35 patients per month, 95% CI = 16 to 54), with significant increases in levels between February 2009 and March 2009 (FAST Phase one) for both overall (505 patients, 95% CI = 75 to 935) and A&E admissions (451 patients, 95% CI = 26 to 875). Subsequent increases for these outcomes immediately after the first phase, during the second and third phases, and after the third phase were not significant.

Emergency admissions via general practitioners were declining during the period before the campaign (−14 patients per month; 95% CI = −19 to −10). Changes for this mode of emergency admission between February 2009 and March 2009, after the first phase, and during the second and third phases were not significant. However, a significant decrease was identified during the period of no campaign activity after phase three (−19 patients per month, 95% CI = −29 to −9).

### SITS-England

Figure 2 (panel B) shows the number of patients in England receiving thrombolysis from 27 participating hospitals in England that submitted data to the SITS-UK database throughout the observation period (N = 3450). There was a significant monthly increase in thrombolysis activity before the campaign (2 patients per month; 95% CI = 2 to 3), with a non-significant increase in level between February 2009 and March 2009. During the period of no campaign activity after phase one, there was a significant increase in thrombolysis activity (3 patients per month, 95% CI = 1 to 6), followed by a monthly non-significant decline during the second and third phases. A significant increase in thrombolysis was also identified during the period of no campaign activity after phase three (3 patients per month, 95% CI = 1 to 4).

### Results adjusted for seasonality

Adjusting for variation between calendar months in regression models (Tables S1 and S2) resulted in the change in levels between February 2009 and March 2009 for information materials dispatched by the SA and calls to their helpline no longer being statistically significant. There were no longer significant changes in trends for webpage views and information materials dispatched by the SA after phase one and during the second and third phases. Decreased hits on the SA website were also no longer significant after phase one.

Adjusted regression models did not alter the pattern of statistically significant results for emergency admissions or thrombolysis activity; although the magnitudes of effects were decreased (trends before the campaign for emergency admissions) or increased (emergency admissions and webpage views between February 2009 and March 2009, and thrombolysis activity after the first phase).

## Discussion

Statistically significant time trends (monthly increases) before the campaign were reported for emergency hospital admissions for stroke (overall and A&E) and thrombolysis activity from hospitals in England that submitted data to the SITS-UK database, but not for access to information about stroke from the SA. There was also a significant monthly decline before the campaign in numbers of emergency hospital admissions for stroke via general practitioners (GPs) - where the public contacted a primary care practitioner as the first response to stroke symptoms, rather than initiated an immediate 999 call. These underlying trends may in part be explained by (i) the publication of the National Stroke Strategy in December 2007 [10], with subsequent national media attention; (ii) discussions and preparation pertaining to implementation of

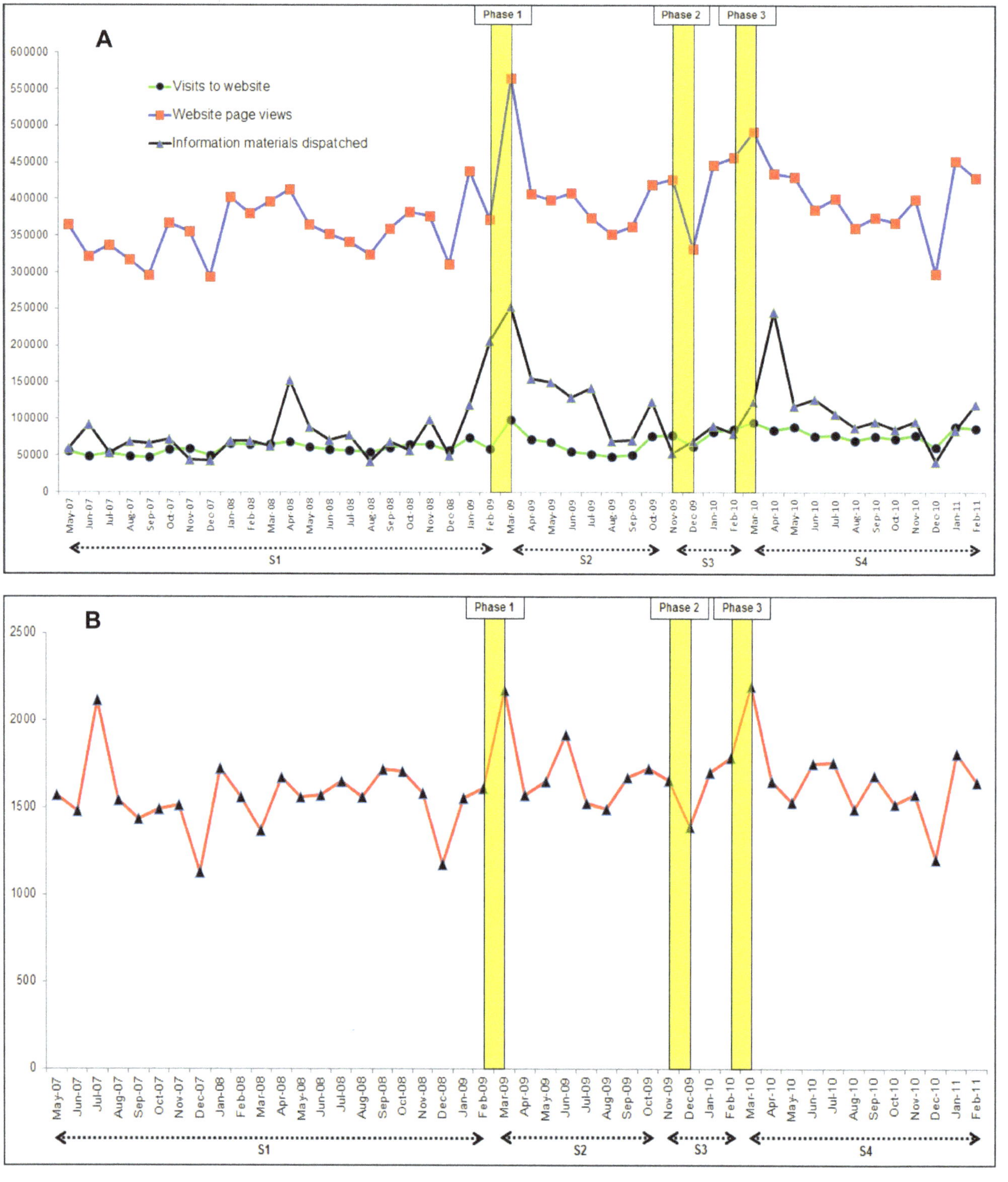


**Figure 1. Time series graphs of monthly resource utilisation by the Stroke Association over the study period (May 2007 to February 2011).** A: Absolute numbers of website page views, website hits and information materials dispatched by the Stroke Association. B: Absolute numbers of telephone calls received by the Stroke Association helpline. S1: period before the campaign (May 2007 to Feb 2009). S2: period of no campaign activity after phase one of the campaign (Mar 2009 to Oct 2009). S3: period during phases two and three of the campaign (Nov 2009 to Feb 2010). S4: subsequent period with no campaign activity after phase three (Mar 2010 to Feb 2011). Yellow vertical bars represent the time periods for the different phases of campaign activity.

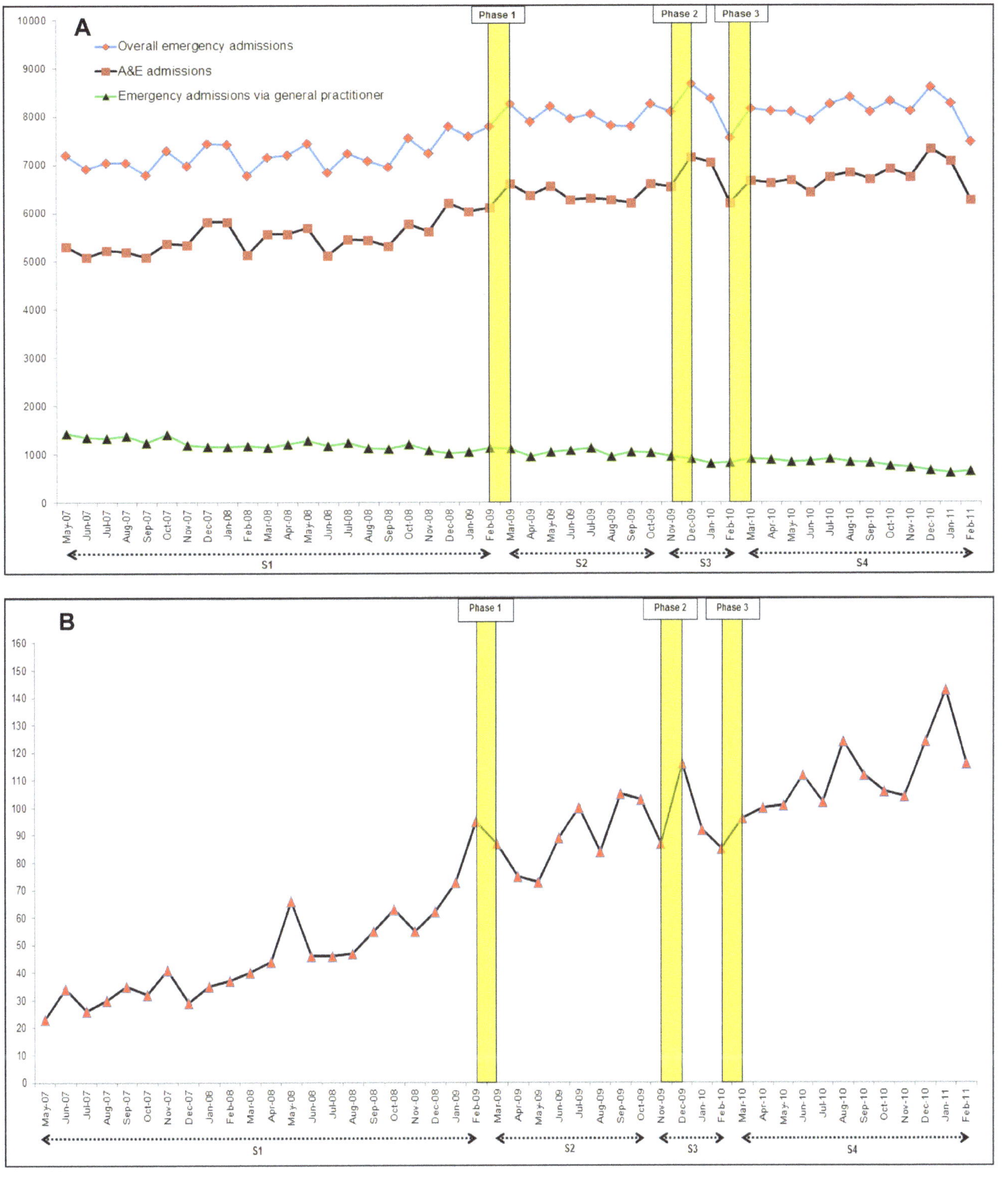


**Figure 2. Time series graphs of monthly emergency admissions for stroke and thrombolysis activity over the study period (May 2007 to February 2011).** A: Absolute numbers of emergency admissions with a primary diagnosis of stroke in England. B: Absolute numbers of patients receiving thrombolytic treatment in England (centres that submitted data to the SITS register throughout the study period). S1: period before the campaign (May 2007 to Feb 2009). S2: period of no campaign activity after phase one of the campaign (Mar 2009 to Oct 2009). S3: period during phases two and three of the campaign (Nov 2009 to Feb 2010). S4: subsequent period with no campaign activity after phase three (Mar 2010 to Feb 2011). Yellow vertical bars represent the time periods for the different phases of campaign activity.

**Table 1.** Interval estimates of segmented regression coefficients for changes in data for different time periods.

| | S1: before the campaign (May 07 to Feb 09) | | | Predicted mean at March 2009 | | | Change in level immediately after phase one (Feb 09 to Mar 09) | | | S2: period of no campaign activity after phase one (Mar 09 to Oct 09) | | | S3: period during phases two and three of the campaign (Nov 09 to Feb 10) | | | S4: period with no campaign activity after phase three (Mar 10 to Feb 11) | | |
|---|---|---|---|---|---|---|---|---|---|---|---|---|---|---|---|---|---|---|
| **Measure** | **Trend** | **95% CI** | | **Mean** | **95% CI** | | **Mean** | **95% CI** | | **Trend** | **95% CI** | | **Trend** | **95% CI** | | **Trend** | **95% CI** | |
| SA: website hits | 613 | −22 | 1248 | 66387 | 58051 | 74722 | 10030 | −4341 | 24401 | −2550 | −5014 | −85 | 7553 | 3729 | 11378 | −1116 | −2518 | 287 |
| SA: webpage views | 2043 | −972 | 5058 | 381589 | 341991 | 421188 | 82114 | 13845 | 150384 | −13875 | −25582 | −2167 | 20946 | 2779 | 39113 | −6357 | −13020 | 305 |
| SA: information materials | 2372 | −170 | 4913 | 106099 | 72717 | 139480 | 101081 | 43530 | 158632 | −20970 | −30840 | −11101 | 22362 | 7048 | 37677 | −5433 | −11050 | 183 |
| SA: calls to helpline | −2 | −16 | 12 | 1538 | 1356 | 1719 | 339 | 26 | 652 | −48 | −101 | 6 | 72 | −11 | 155 | −27 | −57 | 4 |
| HES: overall admissions | 26 | 7 | 45 | 7510 | 7260 | 7759 | 505 | 75 | 935 | 13 | −60 | 87 | 4 | −111 | 118 | 1 | −41 | 43 |
| HES: A&E admissions | 35 | 16 | 54 | 5916 | 5669 | 6162 | 451 | 26 | 875 | 23 | −49 | 96 | 27 | −86 | 140 | 18 | −23 | 60 |
| HES: admissions via GP | −14 | −19 | −10 | 1046 | 986 | 1106 | 35 | −68 | 138 | −13 | −31 | 4 | −21 | −49 | 6 | −19 | −29 | −9 |
| SITS England: Thrombolysis activity | 2 | 2 | 3 | 73 | 65 | 82 | 5 | −10 | 19 | 3 | 1 | 6 | −2 | −6 | 2 | 3 | 1 | 4 |

Figures are absolute numbers.
Predicted mean at March 2009 are predicted values for data if phase 1 had not occurred.
Change in level - step change in levels for data immediately after phase one (between February 2009 and March 2009).
Trends refer to monthly changes in data.
SA: Stroke Association; HES (Hospital Episode Statistics); A&E (accident and emergency); SITS (Safe Implementation of Thrombolysis in Stroke).

**Table 2.** Summary of statistically significant (p<0.5) changes in data for different time periods.

| Data Source/Measure | S1: Trend before the campaign (May 07 to Feb 09) | Predicted mean at March 2009 | Change in level immediately after phase one (Feb 09 to Mar 09) | S2: Trend for period of no campaign activity after phase one (Mar 09 to Oct 09) | S3: Trend for period during phases two and three of the campaign (Nov 09 to Feb 10) | S4: Trend for period with no campaign activity after phase three (Mar 10 to Feb 11) |
|---|---|---|---|---|---|---|
| SA: Website hits | NS increase | 66387 | NS increase | Significant decline | Significant increase | NS decline |
| SA: Website page views | NS increase | 381589 | Significant increase | Significant decline | Significant increase | NS decline |
| SA: Information materials | NS increase | 106099 | Significant increase | Significant decline | Significant increase | NS decline |
| SA: Calls to helpline | NS decline | 1538 | Significant increase | NS decline | NS increase | NS decline |
| HES: Overall emergency admissions | Significant increase | 7510 | Significant increase | NS increase | NS increase | NS increase |
| HES: A&E admissions | Significant increase | 5916 | Significant increase | NS increase | NS increase | NS increase |
| HES: Emergency admission via GP | Significant decline | 1046 | NS increase | NS decline | NS decline | Significant decline |
| SITS England: Thrombolysis activity | Significant increase | 54 | NS increase | Significant increase | NS decline | Significant increase |

Figures for predicted mean at March 2009 are absolute numbers – predicted values if phase 1 had not occurred.
Change in level - step change in levels for data immediately after phase one (between February 2009 and March 2009).
Trends refer to monthly changes in data.
SA: Stroke Association; HES (Hospital Episode Statistics); A&E (accident and emergency); SITS (Safe Implementation of Thrombolysis in Stroke).
NS = non-significant at $p<0.05$.

the National Stroke Strategy within stroke services at the regional level across England; (iii) additional factors influencing the screening of patients for stroke by paramedics (ambulance service national Care Quality Commission audit, and the proposal for emergency response times for suspected stroke occurring less than three hours prior to a 999 call to be changed from category B [serious, but not immediately life-threatening – response time 20 minutes] to a category A [life threatening – response time 8 minutes]) connected with the National Stroke Strategy [26,27]); and (iv) service development with regards to thrombolytic treatment [20].

We found evidence of increased public access to stroke-related information (website hits, webpage views, information materials dispatched by the SA, and calls to their helpline), increased overall/A&E emergency admissions, decreased emergency admissions via GPs, and increased thrombolysis activity that were attributable to the FAST campaign over and above underlying trends. Although adjusted analyses indicated that the SA datasets may have been influenced by seasonality, emergency hospital admissions for stroke (overall and via A&E) increased significantly immediately after the initial phase, whereas emergency hospital admissions via GPs and thrombolysis activity showed statistically significant decreases and increases respectively after the third phase of the campaign. In contrast to a retrospective audit of stroke patients presenting to a single hospital in England [17], we found a statistically significant increase in thrombolysis activity.

Our findings provide evidence of an enduring impact of the campaign in England on public behaviour (i.e. increased awareness of stroke and more people arriving at secondary care, due to fewer people contacting GPs as the first response to stroke symptoms) and greater numbers of appropriate patients with stroke symptoms arriving at specialist centres within the stroke onset time to treatment window for evidence-based treatments such as thrombolysis.

In contrast to our findings, a time series evaluation of a similar FAST campaign rolled out in Ireland during 2010 was not shown to have a sustained impact on emergency department attendance [28]. Mass media campaigns targeting stroke in the Czech Republic [29] and the USA [30] have also met with limited success.

The reasons for the differences between our findings, and evaluations of other campaigns are complex and multi-factorial, and as previously noted their dual nature (public and professional) makes it difficult to elucidate active components that might explain any reported impact [9]. It has been posited that effectiveness of mass media campaigns targeting stroke may be enhanced by spend on media, media mix, and key messages [14]. Message content (e.g. possibility of acute treatments such as thrombolysis [31]) and the type of language (used by patients/bystanders versus professional) used to describe common stroke symptoms [31] may also impact on effectiveness. Furthermore, failure to present details of theoretically grounded development and piloting of the interventions [9] further compounds identification of the optimal active ingredients of effective campaigns.

The message content of FAST in England did not focus on overcoming barriers to performing the desired response (call an ambulance) or adequately address response efficacy (i.e., beliefs associated with executing the desired response by explicitly referring to the availability of an effective emergency treatment such as thrombolysis). Additional impact may be observed with the addition of these components to the message content.

The measures of emergency admissions and thrombolysis activity directly relate to impact on patients with incident stroke and subsequent outcomes, whereas measures of information seeking (access to information resources from the SA) is more indicative of behaviour of people who wish to know if they (or their services) should have done something different when they (or others) experienced a stroke.

These findings are important, but should also be interpreted with some caution. Time series designs increase the confidence that estimates of effect can be attributed to the intervention [32]. Nevertheless, there is always a chance that patterns in these observational data were due to unobserved confounding variables; not all sites in England enter data onto the SITS database and it is possible that thrombolysis activity at these sites had different trends. The number of hospital sites in England that contributed data to the SITS-UK database during 2007, 2008, 2009, 2010 and 2011 were 50, 84, 112, 124 and 89 respectively. However, analyses based on 27 centres contributing thrombolysis activity data throughout the observation period enable a more accurate estimate of an effect of the campaign on public behaviour (changes in thrombolysis activity in other centres might have been due to internal hospital factors). Furthermore, in line with national guidelines [27] the proposed change in emergency 999 response times for suspected stroke was implemented in March/April 2009 (stroke occurring less than three hours prior to a 999 call was changed to a category A (life threatening – response time 8 minutes), which may have led to increased screening of patients for stroke by 999 dispatchers and paramedics, which resulted in more patients reaching hospital within the timeframe for thrombolysis.

Overall, our analyses show a statistically significant impact of phase one of the FAST campaign over and above underlying time trends on information seeking behaviour on stroke (via the SA data) and emergency admissions for stroke (overall and cases admitted via A&E). Our analyses also provide evidence that subsequent phases supported the maintenance and augmented the impact of the initial phase on information seeking behaviour, emergency hospital admissions via GPs and thrombolysis activity. The statistically significant impact on the latter two outcomes after the third phase is likely due to the close proximity of the second and third phases, in effect a 'double-dose' of the intervention.

Nevertheless, our findings for magnitudes of the direct effects for phase one and subsequent phases in terms of their clinical significance are at best modest, indicating that the clinical significance and cost-effectiveness of the campaign was substantially less than that modelled by a previous evaluation [19].

Analyses exploring the impact of time from onset of stroke symptoms to time to arrival at hospital would be important (as earlier treatment with thrombolysis increases likelihood of a good outcome), but data on onset time of the stroke are not available in any routine system. Similarly, data reporting on changes in time from arrival to hospital to time of receipt of thrombolysis (door to needle times) are also not routinely available; however door to needle time is not relevant to the aim of the campaign, which targeted emergency response to symptoms of stroke by members of the public.

The underlying assumption is that if more people with stroke symptoms arrive rapidly at secondary care that outcomes will improve through the increased use of evidence-based treatment such as thrombolysis (as identified by our analysis of emergency admissions and thrombolysis activity, although as stated above not all sites in England enter data onto the SITS database). Using the figures for the statistically significant step change increase (FAST Phase one) between February 2009 and March 2009 for overall emergency stroke admissions in England (505 patients, 95% CI = 75 to 935) as an exemplar allows a very conservative estimate (that takes no account of patients arriving at hospital more rapidly and being treated earlier within the 4.5 hour time window for thrombolysis and the resultant increased likelihood of benefit from treatment) of clinical impact on the campaign. Assuming 85% of these cases will be acute ischaemic stroke ($505 \times 0.85 = 429$ patients), and further assuming a thrombolysis rate of 12% [33] ($429 \times 0.12$) then 51 additional patients may have received thrombolysis. The mean number needed to treat for a good outcome (independence) is 8 [3], which equates to an additional (51/8) 6 patients in England who may have had good outcomes from treatment. Applying the confidence interval ranges for the step change between February 2009 and March 2009 results in a lower and upper conservative estimate of 1 and 12 additional patients who may have received a good outcome from treatment with thrombolysis.

The conclusions are strengthened by the inclusion of three independent data sources. Segmented regression analyses enabled us to estimate the effect of FAST on multiple objective measures of behaviour, which further highlights the importance of robust evaluation of mass media interventions [8,9]. Reliance on findings from evaluative studies reporting on awareness and behavioural intentions, small single site studies, and modelling techniques can lead to false confidence in the effectiveness of this type of complex intervention on health outcome benefits and cost-effectiveness. The findings from our study emphasise the importance of robust evaluation and this should extend to all mass media campaigns that represent significant investment of resources.

The need for continuous advertising to sustain public stroke awareness has been highlighted previously [34,35]. Additional evaluation studies of subsequent phases of the FAST campaign (phase four during March 2011, with fifth, sixth and seventh phases rolled out during February and March 2012, March 2013 and March 2014 respectively) would be helpful to establish if subsequent phases yielded any additional statistically significant impact or sustain the impact of previous phases on public behaviour.

Theory-based interventions targeting the entire range of stroke symptoms, barriers to calling an ambulance, and specific information on the availability of effective secondary care treatments such as thrombolysis, may be warranted to further augment the impact of the campaign message on clinical outcomes [36].

In order to elucidate causal mechanisms that sustain the impact of mass media interventions on public behaviour, designers, policy makers, clinicians and researchers in the field of stroke (and other disciplines where the design of mass media interventions are planned) should utilise appropriate theory and adhere to a structured development process, and undertake robust evaluation before, during and after the roll-out phases using objective measures of behaviour at the population level.

## Conclusions

We used the optimal research design to retrospectively evaluate the impact of the FAST campaign, which enables analysis of impact over and above any underlying time trend (interrupted time series evaluation of appropriately available behavioural data at the population level in England). There was an initial statistically significant impact of phase one on information seeking behaviour of the public about stroke and emergency admissions for incident stroke, with additional statistically significant impact on information seeking behaviour, emergency hospital admissions (reduction in inappropriate care seeking behaviour of the public, i.e. contacting a primary care practitioner as the first response to stroke symptoms), and thrombolysis activity (arguably the most important measure of impact directly related to clinical outcomes). The FAST campaign has been promoted internationally as a great success [19,37]; although our analysis suggests more modest effects in terms of its clinical impact. Consequently, the clinical impact and cost-effectiveness of the FAST campaign in England remains unclear and future campaigns should be accompanied by formal evaluation of impact on clinical outcomes.

## Supporting Information

**Table S1 Interval estimates of segmented regression coefficients for changes in data for different time periods (adjusted for seasonality).** Figures are absolute numbers. Predicted mean at March 2009 are predicted values for data if phase 1 had not occurred. Change in level - step change in levels for data immediately after phase one (between February 2009 and March 2009). Trends refer to monthly changes in data. SA: Stroke Association; HES (Hospital Episode Statistics); A&E (accident and emergency); SITS (Safe Implementation of Thrombolysis in Stroke).

**Table S2 Summary of statistically significant ($p<0.5$) changes in data for different time periods (adjusted for seasonality).** Figures for predicted mean at March 2009 are absolute numbers – predicted values if phase 1 had not occurred. Change in level - step change in levels for data immediately after phase one (between February 2009 and March 2009). Trends refer to monthly changes in data. SA: Stroke Association; HES (Hospital Episode Statistics); A&E (accident and emergency); SITS (Safe Implementation of Thrombolysis in Stroke). NS = non-significant at $p<0.05$.

## Acknowledgments

We would like to express our thanks to: Nikki Hill (Deputy Director Communications, The Stroke Association); Kennedy R Lees (Professor of Cerebrovascular Medicine, Acute Stroke Unit, University Department of Medicine and Therapeutics, Gardiner Institute, Western Infirmary and Faculty of Medicine, University of Glasgow); Barbara Coyle (Senior Information and Research Manager, The North East Public Health Observatory); Leanne Woolmer (Administrator, Institute for Ageing and Health, Newcastle University) and Justin Presseau (Lecturer in Health Psychology, Institute of Health and Society, Newcastle University). GAF is supported by an NIHR Senior Investigator award.

## Author Contributions

Conceived and designed the experiments: GAF RGT HR DF. Analyzed the data: NS DF. Wrote the paper: DF GAF RGT CP HR NS. Prepared the figures and tables: DF NS.

## References

1. Wolfe CD, Rudd AG (2007) The burden of stroke white paper: raising awareness of the global toll of stroke-related disability and death. Available: http://www.safestroke.org/Portals/10/FINAL Burden of Stroke.pdf. Accessed 2013 Oct 31.
2. World Health Organization (2004) The atlas of heart disease and stroke. Mackay J, Mensah G (eds). Geneva: World Health Organisation.
3. Lees KR, Bluhmki E, Kummer R, Brott TG, Toni D, et al. (2010) Time to treatment with intravenous alteplase and outcome in stroke: an updated pooled analysis of ECASS, ATLANTIS, NINDS and EPITHET trials. Lancet 375: 1695–1703.
4. Hacke W, Kaste M, Bluhmki E, Brozman M, Dávalos A, et al. (2008) Thrombolysis with alteplase 3 to 4.5 hours after acute ischemic stroke. New Engl J of Med 359: 1317–1329.
5. National Audit Office (2005). Reducing brain damage: faster access to better stroke care. London: National Audit Office.
6. Lecouturier J, Murtagh MJ, Thomson RG, Ford GA, White M, et al. (2010) Response to symptoms of stroke in the UK: a systematic review. BMC Health Serv Res doi:10.1186/1472-6963-10-157.
7. Mackintosh JE, Murtagh MJ, Rodgers H, Thomson RG, Ford GA, et al. (2012) Why people do, or do not, immediately contact emergency medical services following the onset of acute stroke: qualitative interview study. PLoS One doi: 10.1371/journal.pone.0046124.
8. Grilli R, Ramsay C, Minozzi S (2002) Mass media interventions: effects on health services utilisation. Cochrane Database Syst Rev 1: CD000389. doi: 10.1002/14651858.CD000389
9. Lecouturier J, Rodgers H, Murtagh MJ, White M, Ford GA, et al. (2010) Systematic review of mass media interventions designed to improve public recognition of stroke symptoms, emergency response and early treatment. BMC Health Serv Res doi:10.1186/1471-2458-10-784.
10. Department of Health (2007) National Stroke Strategy. London: Department of Health.
11. Department of Health (2009) Stroke: Act F.A.S.T. awareness campaign. Available: http://webarchive.nationalarchives.gov.uk/20130107105354/http://www.dh.gov.uk/en/Publicationsandstatistics/Publications/PublicationsPolicyAndGuidance/DH_094239. Accessed 2014 Jan 30.
12. Wellcome Trust (2012) Focus on stroke: making a campaign out of a crisis. Available: http://blog.wellcome.ac.uk/2012/05/10/focus-on-stroke-making-a-campaign-out-of-a-crisis/. Accessed 2014 Jun 26.
13. Department of Health (2011) Act F.A.S.T. campaign relaunched to save more lives. Available: http://webarchive.nationalarchives.gov.uk/+/www.dh.gov.uk/en/MediaCentre/Pressreleases/DH_124696. Accessed 2014 Jun 28.
14. Trobbiani K, Freeman K, Arango M, Lalor E, Jenkinson D, et al (2013) Comparison of stroke warning sign campaigns in Australia, England, and Canada. Int J Stroke 8(Suppl. A100):28–31.
15. Robinson TG, Reid R, Haunton VJ, Wilson A, Naylor R (2013) The face arm speech test: does it encourage rapid recognition of important stroke warning symptoms? Emerg Med J 30: 467–471.
16. National Audit Office (2010) Progress in improving stroke care: ambulance trust feedback report. London: National Audit Office.
17. Wood E, Sykes L, Jenkinson S, David O. (2010) Impact of the FAST campaign to improve the speed of acute stroke presentation in the UK [abstract]. Cerebrovasc Dis 29.
18. Fitzsimmons PR, Cronin H, Martin H, Sharma A, Durairaj E (2010) Changes in stroke onset to presentation times before and after the UK FAST stroke awareness campaign. European Stroke Conference, Barcelona, Spain; 2010.
19. Fuel. Department of Health: Stroke Campaign Diagnosis. Available: http://www.fueldata.co.uk/case-study#department-of-health-stroke-campaign-diagnosis. Accessed 2014 Jan 30.
20. Lees KR, Ford GA, Muir KW, Ahmed N, Dyker AG, et al. (2008) Thrombolytic therapy for acute stroke in the United Kingdom: experience from the safe implementation of thrombolysis in stroke (SITS) register. QJM 101: 863–869.
21. Stroke Association (2014) Available: http://www.stroke.org.uk/. Accessed 2014 Jan 30.
22. The NHS Information Centre for Health and Social Care: Hospital Episode Statistics. Available: http://www.ic.nhs.uk/. Accessed 2014 Jan 30.
23. Safe Implementation of Treatment - International Stroke Thrombolysis Registry. Available: https://sitsinternational.org/. Accessed 2014 Jan 30.
24. Wagner AK, Soumerai SB, Zhang F, Ross-Degnan D (2002) Segmented regression analysis of interrupted time series studies in medication use research. J Clin Pharm Therapeut 27: 299–309.
25. Savin NE, White KJ (1977) The Durbin-Watson test for serial correlation with extreme sample sizes or many regressors. Econometrica 45:1989–1996.
26. Care Quality Commission (2009) Care of patients with stroke and transient ischaemic attack. Available: http://archive.cqc.org.uk/periodicreview/nationalcommitmentsandpriorities2009/10/ambulancetrusts/nationalpriorities/careofpatientswithstrokeandtransientischaemicattack.cfm. Accessed 2014 Jan 30.
27. National Collaborating Centre for Chronic Conditions (2008) Stroke: national clinical guideline for diagnosis and initial management of acute stroke and transient ischaemic attack (TIA). London: Royal College of Physicians.
28. Mellon L, Hickey A, Doyle F, Dolan E, Williams D (2013) Can a media campaign change health service use in a population with stroke symptoms? Examination of the first Irish stroke awareness campaign. Emerg Med J doi: 10.1136/emermed-2012-202280.
29. Mikulík R, Goldemund D, Reif M, Brichta J, Neumann J, et al. (2011) 911 in response to stroke: no change following a four-year educational campaign. Cerebrovasc Dis 32(4): 342–348.
30. Kleindorfer D, Khoury J, Broderick JP, Rademacher E, Woo D, et al. (2009) Temporal trends in public awareness of stroke: warning signs, risk factors, and treatment. Stroke 40(7): 2502–2506.
31. Bray JE, O'Connell B, Gilligan A, Livingston PM, Bladin C (2010) Is FAST stroke smart? Do the content and language used in awareness campaigns describe the experience of stroke symptoms? Int J Stroke 5: 440–446.
32. Grimshaw J, Campbell M, Eccles M, Steen N (2000) Experimental and quasi-experimental designs for evaluating guideline implementation strategies. Fam Pract 17: 11–18.
33. Royal College of Physicians (2013) Clinical Effectiveness and Evaluation Unit on behalf of the Intercollegiate Stroke Working Party. Sentinel Stroke National Audit Programme (SSNAP). Clinical audit first pilot public report. National results, 2013. Available: http://www.rcplondon.ac.uk/sites/default/files/ssnap_first_

pilot_national_report_january_-_march_2013_admissions_with_appendices_.pdf. Accessed 2014 Jan 12.
34. Hodgson C, Lindsay P, Rubini F. (2007) Can mass media influence emergency department visits for stroke? Stroke 38: 2115–2122.
35. Reeves MJ, Rafferty AP, Aranha AAR, Theisen V (2008) Changes in knowledge of stroke risk factors and warning signs among Michigan adults. Cerebrovasc Dis 25: 385–391.
36. Dombrowski SU, Mackintosh JE, Sniehotta FF, Araujo-Soares V, Rodgers H, et al. (2013) The impact of the UK 'Act FAST' stroke awareness campaign: content analysis of patients, witness and primary care clinicians' perceptions. BMC Public Health doi:10.1186/1471-2458-13-915.
37. NHS Networks (2014) Latest figures show that the annual "act fast" stroke campaign has had a significant impact on patients receiving stroke treatment. Available: http://www.networks.nhs.uk/news/government-claims-success-for-2018act-fast2019-stroke-campaign. Accessed 2014 Jan 30.

17

# Factors That Drive Dentists towards or Away from Dental Caries Preventive Measures: Systematic Review and Metasummary

**Uhana Seifert Guimarães Suga[1], Raquel Sano Suga Terada[1]*, Adriana Lemos Mori Ubaldini[1], Mitsue Fujimaki[1], Renata Corrêa Pascotto[1], Adelia Portero Batilana[2], Ricardo Pietrobon[2], João Ricardo N. Vissoci[2,3], Clarissa G. Rodrigues[2,4]**

1 Department of Dentistry, State University of Maringá, Maringá, Brazil, 2 Department of Surgery, Duke University Medical Center, Durham, North Carolina, United States of America, 3 Department of Medicine, Faculdade Ingá, Maringá, Brazil, 4 Instituto de Cardiologia do Rio Grande do Sul - Fundação Universitária de Cardiologia (IC-FUC), Porto Alegre, Brazil

## Abstract

*Background:* Dental caries is a serious public health concern. The high cost of dental treatment can be avoided by effective preventive measures, which are dependent on dentists' adherence. This study aimed to evaluate the factors that drive dentists towards or away from dental caries preventive measures.

*Methods and Findings:* This systematic review was registered in PROSPERO (CRD42012002235). Several databases as well as the reference lists and citations of the included publications were searched according to PRISMA guidelines, yielding 18,276 titles and abstracts, which were assessed to determine study eligibility. Seven qualitative studies and 41 surveys (36,501 participants) remained after data extraction and interpretation. A total of 43 findings were abstracted from the reports and were grouped together into 6 categories that were judged to be topically similar: education and training, personal beliefs, work conditions, remuneration, gender, place of residence and patients. The main findings for adherence based on their calculated frequency effect sizes (ES) were teamwork (21%) and post-graduation (12%), while for non-adherence were biologicism (27%), and remuneration for preventive procedures (25%). Intensity ES were also calculated and demonstrated low prevalence of the findings. Quality assessment of the studies demonstrated that the methodological quality, particularly of surveys, varied widely among studies.

*Conclusions:* Despite the questionable quality of the included reports, the evidence that emerged seems to indicate that further education and training coupled with a fairer pay scheme would be a reasonable approach to change the balance in favor of the provision of dental caries preventive measures by dentists. The results of this review could be of value in the planning and decision making processes aimed at encouraging changes in professional dental practice that could result in the improvement of the oral health care provided to the population in general.

**Editor:** Zezhang Wen, LSU Health Sciences Center School of Dentistry, United States of America

**Funding:** The authors have no support or funding to report.

**Competing Interests:** The authors have declared that no competing interests exist.

* Email: rssterada@uem.br

## Introduction

Dental caries is considered a serious public health problem with significant impact on the quality of life that causes pain and suffering, leads to the loss of school and working hours and affects social relationships [1]. Dental caries is still one of the most prevalent diseases of the oral cavity, afflicting 60 to 90% of school-age children and the vast majority of adults in industrialized countries [1], [2]. The distribution of oral diseases varies among different parts of the world and within the same country or region [3], and according to the availability and accessibility of oral health services [1]. Dental caries is a most prevalent oral disease in several Asian and Latin-American countries, while it appears to be less common and less severe in most African countries [3]. Risk factors for oral diseases include an unhealthy diet, tobacco use, harmful alcohol use and poor oral hygiene, as well as social determinants [1]. In all countries, the oral disease burden is significantly higher among poor and disadvantaged population groups [4].

The treatment of dental caries requires restorative procedures that represent a significant cost in many high-income countries, where oral health can account for 5 to 10% of all public health expenditure [4]. For the majority of low-income nations, the cost of treating caries with the traditional method of restorative dentistry is beyond their financial capabilities, as most of these countries can not finance an essential package of health care services for their children [5]. The high cost of dental treatments can be avoided and caries prevalence can be more effectively tackled by effective prevention and health promotion measures. However, although information on the various etiological factors involved in the development of caries and strategies for its prevention have become widely available, much of the population in many parts of the world is still affected by the disease [6], and the global incidence of dental caries in school-age children remains high [4].

It has already been shown that dentists have poorly contributed to the reduction in the prevalence of dental caries [7]. However, dentists have the potential to influence what their patients know and do regarding dental caries prevention [8], and are often necessary especially in individual prevention. Knowing the reasons that drive dentists away from performing prevention and those that facilitate its adoption can bring an important contribution towards the implementation of dental caries preventive programs.

Thus, the aim of this systematic review was to analyze studies that have investigated the factors that drive dentists towards or away from dental caries preventive measures and conduct a metasummary of the results found.

## Materials and Methods

### Protocol and registration

This systematic review was carried out in accordance with the Preferred Reporting Items for Systematic Review and Meta-Analyses (PRISMA) Statement [9], and was registered in the International Prospective Register of Systematic Reviews (PROSPERO) under the registration number CRD42012002235.

### Eligibility criteria

The inclusion criteria were as follows: 1) publications methodologically designed as a "qualitative study" or "survey", qualitative studies classified as those whose findings were abstracted from unstructured data, i.e., individual or group interviews, while surveys were those studies whose findings were compiled from structured questionnaires; and 2) publications reporting factors that drove dentists (public and private) towards or away from incorporating dental caries preventive measures in their practice. The following exclusion criteria were applied: 1) publications in which the research subjects were dental technicians, doctors, nurses or dental students, and 2) publications presenting factors related to preventive measures such as the use of sealants, mouthrinses, or water fluoridation investigated in isolation.

### Literature search

The following electronic databases were used for the selection of the primary studies: PubMed, EMBASE, PsycoInfo, Scielo, Scopus, Web of Science, BBO, Lilacs and York. To ensure the widest possible search, no language filters were applied [10]. The reference lists of the retrieved studies were searched for additional publications, and the citations were also analyzed using Google Scholar. The authors of included studies were contacted by email for the identification of additional studies.

### Search strategy

The following terms were used in the search strategy: "dentist", "dentists", "general dental practitioner", "general dental practitioners", "dental caries", "prevention", "oral health". MeSH terms were used along with the listed entry terms to construct a highly sensitive search strategy. Terms related to the study type were not used because the term "qualitative research" was only introduced in EMBASE in 1988 and as a MeSH term in PubMed in 2003. The complete search strategy used for the PubMed database is shown in Appendix S1.

### Study selection

Two reviewers (USGS and ALMU) independently read all retrieved titles, abstracts, and full-text articles. If one assessor regarded a publication as having met the inclusion criteria, the full

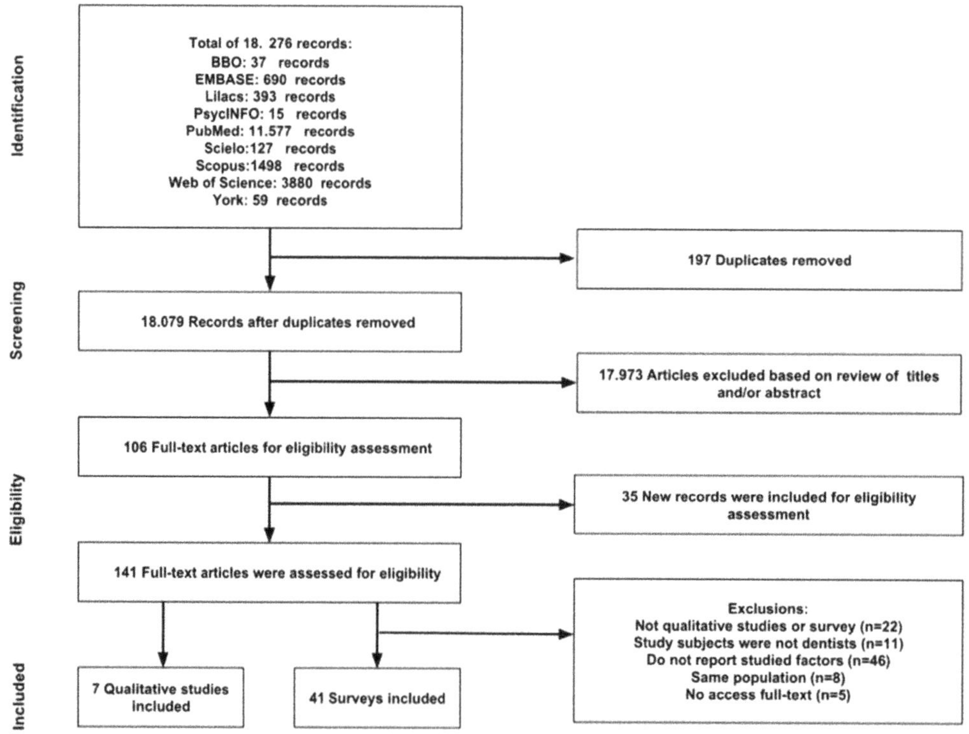


**Figure 1. Flowchart showing the number of publications identified, retrieved, extracted, and included in the final analysis.**

text was obtained. Abstracts considered as potentially eligible, as well as those that did not supply enough information, were reserved for the assessment of the full-text article. Any differences concerning eligibility after the full text was evaluated were resolved through consensus, and when differences still persisted, a third reviewer (RSST) was consulted before a final decision was reached.

## Quality assessment

The quality of the selected studies was assessed by classifying each study according to items adapted from Bennett et al., (2010) [11] for surveys, and the Joanna Briggs Institute Qualitative Assessment and Review [12] for qualitative studies.

The quality assessment of included surveys considered the inclusion of the following items: i) research question justification; ii) explicit research question; iii) clear objectives; iv) description of the methods used to analyze data; v) method used to administer the research instrument (questionnaire); vi) place and date of the study; vii) method described well enough to be replicated; viii) reliability of evidence; ix) validity of evidence; x) method used to verify data entry; xi) use of codification; xii) sample size calculation; xiii) method for selecting the sample; xiv) description of the study population; xv) description of the research instrument; xvi) description of the research instrument development; xvii) instrument pre-test; xviii) instrument reliability and validity; xix) scoring method; xx) informed consent obtained; xxi) ethics approval; and xxii) evidence of ethical treatment of research participants; and xxiii) sample representativeness.

The items analyzed in the qualitative studies were: i) correspondence between the methodology and the indicated philosophical perspective (theory); ii) correspondence between the methodology and the research question or objective; iii) correspondence between the methodology and the methods used for data collection; iv) correspondence between the methodology and data presentation and analysis; and v) correspondence between the methodology and interpretation of the results. Other considerations included statements that: vi) placed the researcher culturally or theoretically; vii) indicated researchers' influence on the study or vice-versa; viii) demonstrated the representation of participants and their voices; ix) showed the investigation was ethically performed according to current criteria or, in more recent studies, the evidence of ethical approval by recognized institutions; and x) indicated that conclusions were drawn from research reports or from data analysis or interpretation.

The items above were verified and classified as definitely present (yes), partially or unclearly present (not clear), or definitely not present (no). Studies that presented a prevalence of "yes" answers (>50%) in the quality assessment were deemed to have a low risk of bias, studies that did not clearly present many of the items assessed were classified to have a moderate risk of bias, while studies that presented a prevalence of "no" answers (>50%) were considered to have a high risk of bias.

## Data extraction

Two reviewers (USGS and ALMU) independently conducted data extraction. General information such as authors, year of publication and first author geographic region were collected from each study. Additionally, the following specific characteristics were also collected: objective, type of study, place where the research was carried out, interventions, number of participants in the sample, inclusion and exclusion criteria, participant characteristics, data collection, data analysis, main results, and authors' conclusions.

## Data analysis

Qualitative metasummary is a quantitatively oriented aggregation of qualitative findings originally developed to accommodate the different characteristics of qualitative studies and surveys [13]. Qualitative metasummary includes the extraction, grouping, and formatting of findings and the calculation of frequency and intensity effect sizes (ES), which permits to produce mixed research syntheses and to conduct a posteriori analyses of the relationship between reports and findings [13].

After the extraction of results from the included studies and the grouping of relevant findings, categories (concise but comprehensive representations) concerning the factors that drive dentists towards or away from carrying out dental caries preventive measures were developed. The categories concerned not only dentists, but also their views of how the factors studied affected their patients. Qualitative data analysis software (ATLAS.ti 7) was used to codify the themes that emerged from the analysis.

To assess the relative magnitude of the extracted results, frequency ES was calculated by taking the number of studies containing a particular finding (minus the studies derived from a common parent study and representing a duplication of the finding) and dividing this number by the total number of included studies (minus the reports derived from a common parent study and representing a duplication of the finding), and expressed as a percentage.

After that, to ascertain which findings reports contributed to the final set of abstracted themes, intensity ES of each report was also calculated. This information is useful for various a posteriori analyses: for example, to determine whether any findings were derived from largely "weaker" studies, which reports contributed most of the findings with the largest frequency effect sizes across reports, and which reports contained findings no other reports contained. Intensity ES calculation was performed by: i) dividing the number of findings contained in the study by the total number of findings across all studies; and ii) by dividing the number of findings with effect sizes >25% contained in that study by the number of findings with effect sizes >25% across all studies.

# Results

## Study selection

The search of electronic databases yielded 18,276 references. After removing duplicates and assessing titles and abstracts, 106 publications were considered potentially eligible. Full texts were retrieved and analyzed for eligibility. After analysis of the reference lists and Google Scholar citation, 35 additional publications were selected and their full text retrieved and analyzed. Ninety-two publications were excluded for the following reasons: 1) the design of 22 publications did not meet the criteria of a "qualitative study" or "survey"; 2) the research subjects in 11 publications were not dentists; 3) 46 publications did not report the factors that drive dentists towards or away from dental caries preventive measures; 4) the full text of five publications could not be retrieved; and 5) eight publications presented the same sample population. A total of 48 publications were selected comprising seven qualitative studies [14–20] and 41 surveys [8], [21–60]. The electronic contact with authors of included publications did not result in any additional studies. Figure 1 summarizes the process of literature identification and selection.

## Study characteristics

Information on the included studies (sampling, intervention, objectives, outcome and risk of bias) is presented in Table 1 (qualitative studies) and Table 2 (surveys). The total number of

**Table 1.** Publication characteristics of the qualitative studies included in the analysis.

| Study | Sampling | Intervention | Objectives | Outcome | Risk of bias |
|---|---|---|---|---|---|
| Cashmore AW et al, 2011 (Australia) [14] | 8 program dental staff and 2 co-ordinating staff | Focus group interviews and semi structured interviews | To explore the attitudes and beliefs of dental staff about the factors that helped or hindered the establishment and implementation of a hospital-based parent counseling program to manage existing, and prevent new, carious lesions in children | The participants identified a number of factors that they felt influenced the establishment and implementation of the program, including the dental team's support of the initiative, the advantages of building on existing clinic infrastructure and procedures, the utility of harnessing dental assistants as a resource for oral health promotion, and the confidence of dental professionals to provide parent counseling. | Low |
| Gussy MG et al, 2006 (Australia) [15] | 22 dental professionals working in the four local government areas. | Qualitative focus group discussions and semi-structured interviews | To explore the oral health beliefs and practices of primary health care professionals which may act as barriers to the development of a model of shared care for the oral health of pre-school children. | Dental professionals did not believe that they had a primary role in the oral health of pre-school aged children but those others particularly maternal and child health nurses did. However other health care professionals were not confident in assuming this role. | Low |
| Humphreys RE et al, 2010 (Wales) [16] | 19 First year foundation dentits in South wales | Focus group discussions | To explore the perceptions of first year foundation dentists (FD1s) regarding oral health education (OHE) and its role in general dental practice. | OHE is often compartmentalized and a simplistic approach to its delivery is taken. Against a backdrop of commissioning to improve health this has implications in developing organizational processes within general dental practice and training in order to achieve this. | Low |
| Nettleton S et al, 1989 (England) [17] | 28 Community dentists | --- | To describe the perceived problems and difficulties of 28 community dentists when carrying out dental health education | Before enthusiastically endorsing dental health education in the dental surgery it is necessary to clarify what the people involved understand by it, and the extent to which they are willing and able to adopt new practices | Moderate |
| Sbaraini A et al, 2012 (Australia) [18] | 8 General dental practices in Australia | Participants were interviewed for approximately one hour in locations convenient to them. | What factors influence a general dental practitioner to offer preventive care to patients? | The key conditions needed for practices to reorient to preventive care included the presence of a committed leader with a prevention-supportive peer network, and the reorientation of space, routines and fee schedules to support preventive practice. | Low |
| Threlfall AG et al, 2007 (England) [19] | 93* general dental practitioners practicing within the general dental service in North West of England | Semi-structured interviews | To increase understanding about how and to whom general dental practitioners provide preventive advice to reduce caries in young children. | Children with caries were more likely to be questioned about diet and oral hygiene and if dentists believed parents to be motivated they were more inclined to spend time providing advice. Most dentists seemed to believe that education was the key to preventing caries and gave preventive advice in the form of a short educative talk. There was little use of visual aids or material for parents to take home. | Low |
| Threlfall AG et al, 2007 (England) [20] | 93* (see above) | Semi-structured interviews | To increaseunderstanding about the content of preventive advice and care offered by general dental practitioners to young children | Preventive advice given to parents of young children is usually about sugar consumption and tooth brushing behavior but the emphasis and specific messages provided varies among general dental practitioners. Use of fluorides varied considerably, suggesting that some dentists either have reservations or are unclear about the appropriate use of fluorides. | Low |

*Same population. Number of participants counted only once.

**Table 2.** Publication characteristics of the surveys included in the analysis.

| Study | Sampling | Intervention | Objectives | Outcome | Risk of bias |
|---|---|---|---|---|---|
| ADAHF, 1984, (USA) [21] | 4000 Dentists identified in the American Dental Associations master file as actively in private practice, including specialists | mailed survey questionnaire | To present the results of a preventive dentistry survey. | The current thinking of dentists regarding caries prevention, as reflected by attitudes toward and use of procedures, is not entirely consistent with the state-of-the-art or consensus positions of the academic and research communities. Although practitioners are aware of the primacy of community water fluoridation for caries prevention, they do not appear to fully appreciate the values of other fluoride modalities, including topical fluorides, dentifrices, and mouthrinses. They especially undervalue pit and fissure sealants. Conversely, practitioners emphasize oral hygiene and diet counseling procedures for caries prevention despite scientific reports questioning their worth in this regard. | High |
| Ananaba N et al, 2010 (USA) [22] | 137 general and 45 pediatric dentists in Michigan and 2, 112 pediatric dentists outside Michigan | questionnaire | To explore attitudes and behavior concerning IOHE among general and pediatric dentists in Michigan and pediatric dentists in the remaining 49 U.S. states. | General dentists had more negative attitudes towards IOHE than pediatric dentists in Michigan and other U.S. states. Only 41% of general dentists vs. 84% and 89% of pediatric dentists in Michigan and other states performed IOHE. While general dentists who performed IOHE had better attitudes towards IOHE than their non-IOHE-performing colleagues, they engaged less in prevention directed activities compared to pediatric dentists. | High |
| Anderson R et al, 2002 (Wales) [23] | 1160 identified dental professionals working in Wales | questionnaire | To provide a comprehensive profile of the current nature and scale of health promotion by dental professionals in Wales. | Acceptable and achievable goals of effective preventive practice should be informed by evidence of what practitioners currently do and currently believe as well as the evidence of what is shown to be effective. | High |
| Badan DEC et al, 2010 (Brazil) [24]* | 72 recently graduated students from UFG Dental School from 2000 to 2002. | e-mailed questionnaire | To know the perceptions and uses of the collective health knowledge in the daily practice of the dentists in the period | Dentists showed doubts about collective health actions in spite of saying that they practiced them. They reported the lack of complementary material and little valorization by the population of prevention activities. Collective health practices should be made clearer and deeper, and curriculum integration should take place during dental courses. | High |
| Brennan DS et al, 1996 (Australia) [25] | 202 private general practitioners who provided service rate data in both 1983 and 1988 | questionnaire | To establish dentist practice styles and to assess the distribution of these styles of practice between 1983 and 1988 | Net movement away from the "High restorative" " and " "Low Total Rates" " clusters toward the "High Diagnostic and Preventive" "cluster was shown, but there was movement by practitioners away from and into all clusters. | low |
| Brennan DS et al, 1998 (Australia) [26] | A random sample of Australian dentists in 1983–84, 1988–89, and 1993–94. | questionnaire | To identify trends in service provision over time. | Findings indicate changing patterns of practice over time, consistent with an increasing orientation towards prevention of disease and maintenance of a natural dentition. | High |

**Table 2.** Cont.

| Study | Sampling | Intervention | Objectives | Outcome | Risk of bias |
|---|---|---|---|---|---|
| Brennan DS, et al. 2001 (Australia) [27] | 345 from a random sample of Australian dentists | mailed questionnaire | To replicate practice belief scales in Australia and investigate associations with dentist and practice characteristics and services. | The findings confirm the factor structure of practice beliefs and demonstrate small to moderate associations with variation in service rates. | Low |
| Brennan DS et al, 2003 (australia) [28] | 489 random sample of dentists from each State/ Territory in Australia in 1998–99 | mailed questionnaire | To examine the provision of examinations, radiographs, prophylaxis and topical fluoride, and to assess whether these services varied by patient, visit and oral health characteristics. | Radiographs may often be used to confirm disease rather than in early detection, and prevention was mainly provided to asymptomatic patients in routine maintenance schedules. Many emergency patients and those with oral diseases presented missed the benefits of prevention. | High |
| Brennan DS & Spencer AJ, 2007 (Australia) [29] | NA - A random sample of dentists in 1983, 1988, 1993, 1998 and 2003 | mailed questionnaire | To investigate time trends in dental service provision by location. | While the overall content of dentist workloads has changed to include less emphasis on removal and replacement of teeth and more effort on diagnosis and prevention aimed at retention of natural dentitions, a gap by location remains, with dentist workloads outside of major city locations marked by higher rates of tooth extraction and lower rates of preventive services. | High |
| Calnan M et al, 2000 (England) [30]* | 1956 dentists with open General Dental Service contracts | questionnaire | To explain why some dentists have changed private/public mix, and why private practice appears to be increasingly attractive. | The movement toward selective NHS dentistry might be perceived as an appropriate solution by dentists, but evidence suggest that is not acceptable to the public in general or to the users of dental services | High |
| Chen M, 1990 (USA) [31] | 1000 dentists in general practice and pedodontics in Texas, USA, who were registered with the Texas Board of Dental Examiners as of 1984. | questionnaire | To present the results of a 1985 survey of 1000 Texas dentists regarding three major types of preventive measures–educational services, preventive procedures, and diagnostic services. | Among preventive procedures, most dentists removed plaque or calculus. Income, attendance of continuing education programs, and number of dental hygienists were strong, positive predictors of provision of all three types of preventive measures. Dentists who practiced in more populous areas, or had practiced for fewer years, more likely provided patients with educational services and preventive procedures. Dentists delivered more preventive procedures if they attended more professional dental meetings. Dentists who worked more hours were more likely to provide educational services and preventive procedures. | High |
| Chestnut IG et al, 2007 (Wales) [32] | 691 general dental practitioners in Wales | mailed questionnaire | This study investigated the perceptions and attitudes to the new contract, in the three months immediately prior to its implementation. | This study has established baseline perceptions of reform in state-funded dental care in Wales. As the new contract evolves, it will be interesting to determine whether the largely negative perceptions of new ways of working expressed in this study are realised. | Low |

**Table 2.** Cont.

| Study | Sampling | Intervention | Objectives | Outcome | Risk of bias |
|---|---|---|---|---|---|
| Craft M et al, 1976 (Australia) [33] | 502 practitioners who worked in 6 comparable towns, 3 from the North and 3 from the South of England | questionnaire | Five areas of practice that were likely to be affected by differing attitudes to prevention were studied: (I) fluoridation; (2) employment of ancillaries; (3) professional life and self-image; (4) prevention in patients; (5) practitioners own immediate family. | The findings tended to show that in parallel with studies of regional distribution of treatment and services, more negative attitudes to prevention are found in areas with fewer services and poorer treatment patterns, and vice-versa | High |
| Fiset L et al, 1997 (USA) [34] | 532 Washington State general dentists | questionnaire | Dentists were surveyed about their use of four caries-control services among adult patients. | Leaders in the dental community and those with a wider network of professional colleagues were likely to adopt new services more quickly than other dentists. Earlier adopters also had more correct information about these services than later or no adopters. | Low |
| Freeman R et al, 2005 (Northern Ireland) [35] | 166 General dental practices located within the region of the EHSSB (Northern Ireland Eastern Health and Social Services Board) | questionnaire | To investigate the preventive orientation of general dental practices by examining their patient-active prevention activities, practice policies for prevention and employment strategies. | The findings suggest that the employment of a hygienist is central to the reorientation of primary dental care. The Government must be encouraged to provide the financial means to allow primary care to shift from being disease-centered to health-focused. | Low |
| Ghasemi H et al, 2007 (Iran) [36] | 1033** dentists who participated in two annual dental meetings in December 2004 and in July 2005, in Tehran, Iran | self-administered questionnaire | To assess Iranian dentists' knowledge of and attitudes towards preventive dental care. | Dentists' knowledge of and attitudes towards prevention should be improved and updated to enable and encourage them to provide their patients with preventive care. | High |
| Ghasemi H et al, 2008 (Iran) [37] | 1033** (see above) | self-administered questionnaire | To study risk-based preventive practice among Iranian dentists. | To better meet each patient's need, more emphasis on a risk-based approach in preventive dental care is called for in dental school curricula and continuing education. In this process, comprehensive guidelines for preventive practice would be helpful. | High |
| Ghasemi H et al, 2009 (Iran) [38] | 1033** (see above) | self-administered questionnaire | To examine the perceived barriers to preventive dental practice among Iranian dentists. | Dentists recognized a broad range of factors as barriers to the provision of preventive dental care, the strongest addressed to the patient-related barriers. The perceived barriers to the provision of preventive care should be investigated in greater detail and tackled to enhance oral health in Iran. | Low |
| Grembowski D et al, 1990 (USA) [39] | 200 general dentists based on a homogeneous, well-educated, upper-middle-class population of patients | questionnaire | Factors influencing variation in dentist service rates | Results indicate that practice characteristics, patients' exposure to fluoridated water supplies, and the extent of no price competition in the market influence the services that patients receive. Therefore, attempts to address these issues will necessarily involve altering dentists' decisions regarding practice organization and the delivery of care. However, because these factors account for less than 30 percent of the variation in the rates, the future impact of any single intervention may be limited. | Low |

**Table 2.** Cont.

| Study | Sampling | Intervention | Objectives | Outcome | Risk of bias |
|---|---|---|---|---|---|
| Holloway P J et al 1994 (England) [40]* | 50 successful, general dental practitioners | questionnaire | To discover what preventive procedures on which patients considered were the benefits of their practices and why. | All dentists thought that prevention on selected patients was of value to their practice. They said that prevention enhances the reputation of the practice, adds to the job satisfaction of the dentist and is part of modern dental philosophy. However, only when practised selectively would it be cost-beneficial. Dentists who employed hygienists had a significantly higher 'mean preventive awareness score' than those who did not. | High |
| Kallestål C et al, 1999 [41] | Random samples of dentists, dental hygienists, and dental nurses working with children during 1995 and 1996 | questionnaire | To compare the caries-preventive methods used for children and adolescents in Denmark, Iceland, Norway, and Sweden. | Informational basis of decisions on preventive strategies varied between the different dental professionals in each country as well as between the countries, indicating that national professional cultures are being shaped differently. Despite the differences in choice of preventive methods, the dental health of children varies little across the frontiers. | High |
| Kay EJ et al, 2003 (England) [42] | 15 Fifteen general dental practices conducting a simultaneous survey of attending patients and 15 practitioners from these practices. | Mailed questionnaire | To measure the subjective impact of oral health in a group of patients attending general dental practices in the North West of England and to investigate the attributes of dentists and practices in order to examine how such attributes might relate to patients' subjective perceptions of oral health. | Fourteen percent of the differences in patients' subjectively perceived oral health can be attributed to dentist attitudes and attributes. Further research regarding the influence of dentists personality and professional beliefs on patients well-being needs to be undertaken. | High |
| Malcheff S et al, 2009 (USA) [43] | 2157 members of the AAPD | questionnaire | To: (1) determine pediatric dentists' behaviors and attitudes concerning infant oral health examinations (IOHEs); and (2) explore how respondents who do or do not perform IOHEs differ in their behavior and attitudes concerning IOHEs. | The finding that only 53% of the respondents see 1-year-old children or younger shows that efforts need to continue to increase the percentage of dentists who offer IOHEs. Most respondents held rather positive attitudes toward IOHEs. They differed in the amount of time they schedule for these exams and the issues they address. | High |
| Milgrom P et al, 1988 (USA) [44] | 521 general practitioners in Washington State. | questionnaire | To investigate dentist attitudes and activities regarding oral self care. | Though most dentists say they counsel patients about oral self care, when specific practices are reported it was found that only a small percentage actually utilize an approach that would be considered effective. | Low |
| Moon H et al 1998 (Korea) [8] | 2,047 dentists, selected by a stratified random sampling allocated proportionately | a pretested, 27-item questionnaire | To determine the level of knowledge and opinions about caries etiology and prevention among Korean dentists and to describe related factors. | The majority of dentists do not know current information concerning etiology and prevention of dental caries, mechanisms of action of fluoride, and effectiveness of preventive procedures for children and adults. Efforts to enhance the level of knowledge and practices of Korean dentists about caries prevention should focus on strategies to educate older graduates and female dentists, especially those in private practice. | Low |

**Table 2.** Cont.

| Study | Sampling | Intervention | Objectives | Outcome | Risk of bias |
|---|---|---|---|---|---|
| Murtomaa H et al 1988 (Finland) [45] | 570 dentists registered on the Finnish Dental Association | questionnaire | To investigate de attitudes of practitioners towards health dental education and their opinion about its development and difficulties related to it | Younger dentists were less in favor than their older colleagues of increasing the amount of health education. −9% considered that health education should be carried out only by auxiliaries. -Older dentists recognized more often than younger colleagues that the lack both material and individual resources were a problem in health education. | High |
| Nuca CI et al, 2011 (Romania) [46] | 348 dental practitioners registered to practice in Constanta, Braila, Galati, Tulcea, Buzau and Vrancea districts. | questionnaire | To evaluate the current working practices in preventive dentistry of dentists from six Romanian districts–the South-East Romanian Development Region. | The results of this study demonstrate the need to increase the awareness and skills of dentists from the South-East Development Region of Romania regarding the prevention of oral diseases, especially in terms of cross-infection control in dentistry, in order to meet European Union standards and to ensure health and safety at work in dentistry. | Low |
| Pine CM, et al 2004 [47] | 2,333 dentists in 14 countries (Belgium, China, Czech Republic, Denmark, Germany, Ireland, Madagascar, Mexico, Singapore, South Africa, Tanzania, Thailand and USA) and 17 sites | questionnaire | To explore whether dentists' beliefs and attitudes to providing preventive and restorative dental care for young children can form a barrier to the provision of care. | In most countries, dentists agreed that young children's coping skills limit their ability to accept dental care. Secondly, dentists with negative personal feelings, for example, that providing care can be stressful and troublesome and that they feel time constrained. Differences in dentists' beliefs can be partly explained by their work profile, with those treating children often, and those working under systems where they feel they can provide quality care being least likely to identify barriers to providing care for children. | Low |
| Pourat N, Marcus MI, 2012 (USA) [48] | 3.098 general dentists in private practice in California | questionnaire | Variations in dentists' provision of services have been documented, but information about contributing factors is limited to assess variations in service provision and its correlates. | The results show variations in services provided by general dentists in private practice. Multiple factors, including the dentist's sex, region of practice, employment of hygienists, patients' race and population income in the area of practice were significantly and independently associated with provision of services. | High |
| Razak IA & Lind, 1994 (Malaysia) [49] | 1371 Professionally trained dentists whose names appeared in the Government Gazetle of 1990 as having been granted an Annual Practicing Certificate to practice dentistry in Malaysia in I990. | questionnaire | To examine the attitudes of Malaysian dentists toward patient education and reventive dentistry and the level of preventive care adopted in Malaysian dental practice. | Generally the Malaysian dentists had positive attitudes towards patient education and preventive dentistry including fluoridation. However, a sizable proportion of them considered that preventive measures were no challenge for the dentist. The common preventive measures given to patients were scaling, dental health education, prophylaxis and instruction in correct brushing and flossing in as much as 40 to 50 percent of the queried dentist claimed that these preventive items were provided to most or all of their new patients. In spite of the fact that the majority of the dentists had good knowledge about the application and effects of sealants only about 41% of the dentists claimed to have used sealants. | High |

**Table 2.** Cont.

| Study | Sampling | Intervention | Objectives | Outcome | Risk of bias |
|---|---|---|---|---|---|
| Riley III JL et al, 2011 (USA) [50] | 393 male and 73 female general dentists who were members of The Dental Practice-Based Research Network (DPBRN) and practiced within the USA | questionnaire | A number of articles have addressed differences in productivity between male and female dentists, but little is known about differences between the sexes in practice patterns regarding caries management. | Female dentists recommended at-home fluoride to a significantly larger number of their patients than did male dentists, whereas male dentists had a preference for using in-office fluoride treatments with pediatric patients. Female dentists also chose to use preventive therapy more often at earlier stages of dental caries. There were few differences between the sexes in terms of methods, time spent on or charges for restorative dentistry, and business of the practice. The practice patterns of female dentists suggest a treatment philosophy with a greater focus on caries prevention. | Low |
| Riley III JL et al, 2010 (USA) [51] | 467 general dentists in the DPBRN who practice within the United States and treat both pediatric and adult patients | questionnaire | To test the frequency of dentists' recommendations for and use of caries-preventive agents for children as compared with adults. | General dentists use in-office caries-preventive agents more commonly with their pediatric patients than with their adult patients. General dentists should consider providing additional in-office caries-preventive agents for their adult patients who are at increased risk of experiencing dental caries. | Low |
| Riley III JL et al, 2010 (USA) [52] | 564 practitioners in DPBRN, a multi-region consortium of participating practices and dental organizations. | questionnaire | To identify factors that are significantly associated with dentists' use of specific caries preventive agents in adult patients. | Caries prevention is commonly used with adult patients. However, the results suggest that only a subset of dentists base preventive treatments on caries risk at the individual patient level. | Low |
| Rock WP & Bradnockl, 1976 (Wales and England) [53] | 885 dentists - Every 10th name on each list of dental practioners who had undertaken to provide general dental services in England and Wales. | mailed questionnaire | To discover the numbers of dentists who were using preventive methods and also to gather information about the attitude of the profession towards a suggested inclusion of fees for preventive therapy on the National Health Service scale | The majority of dentists were in favor of fees for preventive treatment. It may be argued that use of preventive measures on a large scale would be an investment for the future since the need for conservative treatment would be reduced. Cost of application could be reduced by employment of dental hygienists. | Low |
| Serrano AG et al, 1990 (Spain) [54] | 1019 dental professionals in western and eastern Andalucía, and members of the Spanish Society of Preventive and communitary Odontoestomatogy | questionnaire | To understand the attitudes, knowledge and behavior of 3 groups of Spanish dentists on methods of caries prevention. | Dental professionals should elaborate and participate more in preventive and educational for the population. | High |
| Sesma N et al, 2006 (Brazil) [55] | 400 dentists of São Paulo city | questionnaire | To identify dentists profile in the prevention of dental caries and gingival diseases | 1– The vast majority (97.6%) confirm the practice of some caries and giginval disease, but only 0.3% employ the six methods analysed in this study. 2–Time since graduation influenced the practice of prevention. Those graduated in the previous 5 years employ prevention method less often. 3– Women dentits employ prevention methods more often than men dentits. 4– Dentits that received specific traning on prevention are more likely to employ it. | High |

**Table 2.** Cont.

| Study | Sampling | Intervention | Objectives | Outcome | Risk of bias |
|---|---|---|---|---|---|
| Silva RP et al, 2006 (Brazil) [56] | 233 Dental Surgeons who was registered with CROMG (June/2002) and resident in the municipality of Lavras (Minas Gerais, Brazil) | questionnaire | To evaluate the level of Dental Surgeons' (DSs) knowledge and clinical application of scientific evidence in Dentistry, in the city of Lavras (Minas Gerais, Brazil) | 1- men, graduated from state universities were shown to be confident about prescribing and applying fluoride gel in children as a result of the diagnosed risk of dental caries; 2- those graduated up to 10 years before and attended in private dental office, were shown to be confident about prescribing and applying sealants to pit and fissure for the prevention of dental caries; 3- those that have post-graduation courses were shown to be confident to prescribe and apply chlorhexidine with a view to preventing dental caries; 4- those that graduated from state universities were shown to be more confident of monitoring white spot lesions with a view to the non-progression of dental caries; 5- men were shown to be confident about prescribing and applying ART in children for the treatment of cavitated dental caries lesions. | Low |
| Tomlinson P & Treasure E, 2006 (Wales) [57] | 400 dentists currently practising in Wales | mailed questionnaire. | To identify the attitudes of practitioners to the use of three adult preventive codes. | Few dentists provide preventive care to adults under the existing remuneration system. Work is necessary to enable dentists to use effective preventive techniques for adult patients. These results can be considered to show the baseline provision of prevention and could facilitate the evaluation of any changes to the current system. | Low |
| Tryon AM et al, 1974 (USA) [58] | 1020 actively practicing dentists in Connecticut (General practice) | questionnaire | To report on additional data on the quantity and quality of preventive services provided indental practice. | The present study only provided fragmentary evidence on the distribution of practice effort for prevention. Future studies may cast more light on some of the factors that influences dentists' decisions to change from a curative to preventive orientation. | High |
| Tseveenjav B et al, 2004 (Mongolia) [59] | 250** All dentists practising in Ulaanbaatar, in May 2000. | questionnaire | To investigate caries-preventive measures (CPMs) applied by dentists in Mongolia to their own children in relation to the dentist-parents' professional and preventive care-related backgrounds and the children's dental health. | Caries-preventive measures applied to dentists' children should be improved, especially in regard to sugar consumption. Comprehensive efforts are called for, stressing modern CPMs. Both the undergraduate curriculum and the continuing education program need to emphasize the use of modern methods of caries prevention. | High |
| Tseveenjav B et al, 2005 (Mongolia) [60] | 250** All dentists practising in Ulaanbaatar, in May 2000. | questionnaire | To study barriers to providing oral health education (OHE) to their patients among Mongolian dentists | Despite appreciation of OHE, Mongolian dentists seem to face practical barriers to providing oral helth education activities | Low |

NA: Not available.
*Mixed methods studies: qualitative and survey
**Same population; number of participants counted only once

participants in the seven qualitative studies included in this review was 390. The studies presenting the largest number of participants (311) were Threlfall et al. 2007 [19] and Threlfall et al. [20]. Other included qualitative studies presented populations that varied between 2 and 28 participants. The total number of individuals participating in the selected surveys was 36,111. Surveys, contrary

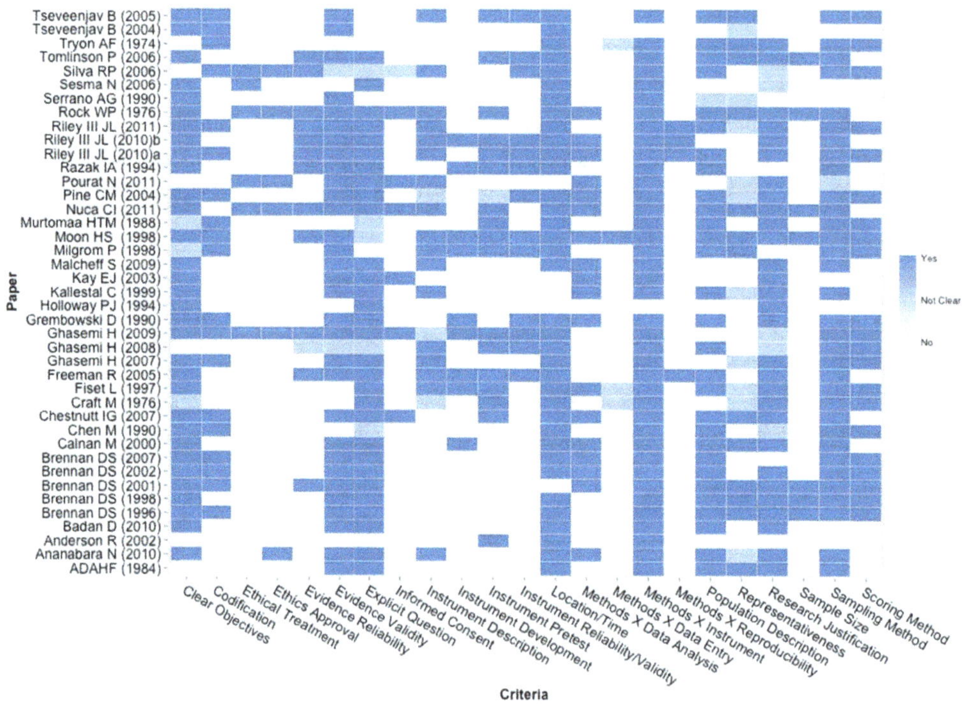


**Figure 2. Heat map showing a gradient of quality indicators for each individual survey included in the analysis.** Colors vary from white (No), light blue (Not Clear) and blue (Yes) representing the three categories used in the quality assessment.

to qualitative surveys, presented a much wider range of participants, varying from as few as 15 [42] to as many as 4,850 [22].

The included qualitative studies and surveys covered a wide geographical area with a total of 28 countries, including Australia (nine publications) [14], [15], [18], [25–29], [33], United States of America (nine publications) [21], [22], [31], [34], [39], [43], [44], [48], [58], England (six publications) [17], [19], [20], [30], [40], [42], Wales (four publications) [16], [23], [32], [57], Brazil (three publications) [24], [55], [56], Iran (three publications) [36] – [38],

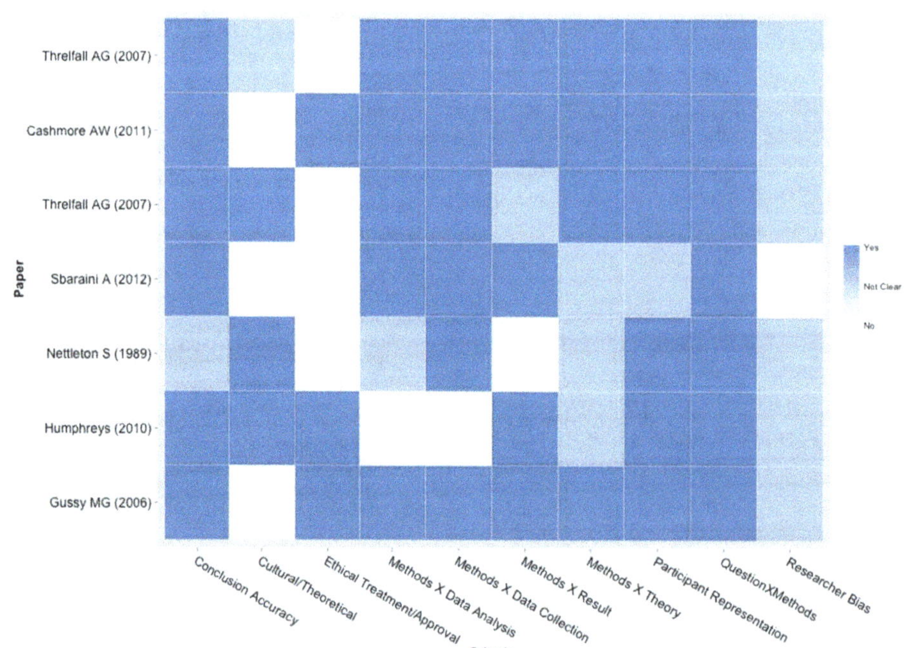


**Figure 3. Heat map showing a gradient of quality indicators for each individual qualitative study included in the analysis.** Colors vary from white (No), light blue (Not clear) and blue (Yes) representing the three categories used in the quality assessment.

**Table 3.** Abstracting, formatting, grouping in categories, and frequency effect sizes (ES) of findings.

| Driving dentists towards performing dental caries preventive measures | ES% | Driving dentists away from performing dental caries preventive measures | ES% |
|---|---|---|---|
| **Education and Training** | | | |
| Time since graduation (Tseveenjav, 2004; Ghasemi, 2007; Sesma, 2006; Razak, 1994; Murtomaa, 1988) | 10 | Time since graduation (Nettleton, 1989; Sbaraini, 2012; Tseveenjav, 2005; Riley, 2011; Riley, 2010[49]; Moon, 1988; Rock, 1974; Chen M, 1990; Riley, 2010[50]; Brennan, 1996; Brennan, 2001) | 22 |
| Communication and health education skills (Threlfall, 2007[25]; Sbaraini, 2012;Tseveenjav, 2004; Milgrom, 1988; Riley, 2010[50]) | 10 | Lack of communication and health education skills (Nettleton, 1989; Humphreys, 2010; Murtomaa, 1988) | 6 |
| Post-graduation (Tseveenjav, 2004; Ananaba, 2010; Moon, 1988; Sesma, 2006; Chen, 1990; Kay, 2003) | 12 | Lack of technical skill/knowledge (Fiset, 1997; Tseveenjav, 2005; Sesma, 2006; Murtomaa, 1988; Badan, 2006; Sbaraini, 2012) | 12 |
| Graduation from public dental schools (Silva, 2006; Badan, 2006) | 4 | Professional specialization (Humphreys, 2010; Sesma, 2006; Murtomaa, 1988) | 6 |
| Ongoing Education/Traning (Sbaraini, 2012; Ghasemi, 2007; Chen, 1990; Ghasemi, 2008; Kay, 2003) | 10 | Biologicism (Threlfall, 2007[16]; Nettleton, 1989; Humphreys, 2010; Sbaraini, 2012; Craft, 1976; Serrano, 1990; Tseveenjav, 2005; Ananaba, 2010; Malcheff, 2009; Sesma, 2006; Murtomaa, 1988; Calnan, 2000; Badan, 2006) | 27 |
| Participation in discussion groups/networks (Threlfall, 2007[17]; Sbaraini, 2012; Tryon, 1974; Tseveenjav, 2004) | 4 | Lack of educational material (Threlfall, 2007[16]; Tseveenjav, 2005; Rock, 1974; Murtomaa, 1988; Badan, 2006) | 10 |
| Complementary reading (Silva, 2006; Ghasemi, 2008) | 4 | Difficulty working with children (Pine, 2004) | 2 |
| **Personal Beliefs** | | | |
| Personal satisfaction (Holloway, 1994; Craft, 1976; Calnan, 2000) | 6 | Disbelief in fluoride effect (Threlfall, 2007[17]; Craft, 1976) | 4 |
| Professional understanding of the benefits (Holloway, 1994; Threlfall, 2007[16]; Threlfall, 2007[17]; Nettleton, 1989; Sbaraini, 2012) | 10 | Lack of professional understanding of the benefits (Sbaraini, 2012; ADAHF, 1984; Tomlinson, 2006; Murtomaa, 1988; Holloway, 1994; Calnan, 2000) | 12 |
| Positive cost/benefit ratio (Holloway, 1994; Sbaraini, 2012; Murtomaa, 1988) | 6 | Negative cost/benefit ratio (Ananaba, 2010; Malcheff, 2009; Razak, 19944; Murtomaa, 1988) | 8 |
| | | Lack of interest in the activity (Nettleton, 1989) | 2 |
| | | Depreciation of the professional image (Nettleton, 1989; Ghasemi, 2007; Murtomaa, 1988) | 6 |
| **Work conditions** | | | |
| Work in the public health system (Tseveenjav, 2004; Moon, 1988; Anderson, 2002; Chestnut, 2007) | 8 | Work in the public health system (Tseveenjav, 2005; Freeman, 2005; Riley, 2011; Badan, 2006) | 8 |
| Team work (Holloway, 1994; Threlfall, 2007[16]; Tryon, 1974; Craft, 1976; Chen, 1990; Murtomaa, 1988; Grembowsky, 1990; Freeman, 2005; Cashmore 2011) | 21 | Work should be performed by dental technicians/assistants (Threlfall, 2007[18]; Nettleton, 1989; Anderson, 2002; Murtomaa, 1988) | 8 |
| Presence of dental caries (Threlfall, 2007[16]; Humphreys, 2010) | 4 | Difficulty working with children (Pine, 2004) | 2 |
| **Remuneration** | | | |
| Coverage by private health insurance (Kay, 2003; Brennan, 2003; Riley, 2010[49]) | 6 | Lack of coverage by private health insurance (Ghasemi, 2009; Fiset, 1997; Tomlinson, 2006; Calnan, 2000) | 8 |
| | | Low pay (Threlfall, 2007[18]; Sbaraini, 2012; Fiset, 1997; Craft, 1976; Serrano, 1990; Pine, 2004; Milgrom, 1988; Ghasemi, 2007; Razak, 1994; Murtomaa, 1988; Calnan, 2000; Grembowsky, 1990) | 25 |

**Table 3.** Cont.

| Driving dentists towards performing dental caries preventive measures | ES% | Driving dentists away from performing dental caries preventive measures | ES% |
|---|---|---|---|
| **Gender** | | | |
| Male dentists (Riley, 2011; Moon, 1988; Razak, 1994; Ghasemi, 2009; Silva, 2006) | 10 | Male dentists (Nettleton, 1989; Ghasemi, 2007; Sesma, 2006; Ghasemi, 2008; Riley, 2010[49]; Riley, 2010[50]; Brennan, 2001; Pourat, 2012; Riley, 2011[51]) | 19 |
| **Residence** | | | |
| Living in the rural area (Moon, 1988) | 2 | Living in the rural area (Ghasemi, 2007; Ghasemi, 2009; Rock, 1974; Chen, 1990; Brennan, 2001; Brennan, 2003; Brennan, 2007) | 15 |
| **Patients** | | | |
| Parents' motivation (Gussy, 2006; Threlfall, 2007[16]; Threlfall, 2007[17]) | 4 | Lack of awareness (Gussy, 2006; Nettleton, 1989; Ananaba, 2010; Malcheff, 2009; Ghasemi, 2009; ADAHF, 1984; Murtomaa, 988; Badan, 2006) | 17 |
| Patients' age (Tomlinson, 2006; Threlfall, 2007[16]) | 4 | Lack of motivation (Gussy, 2006; Threlfall, 2007[16]; Nettleton, 1989; Humphreys, 2010; Murtomaa, 1988) | 8 |
| | | Fear (Gussy, 2006; Pine, 2004; Calnan, 2000) | 6 |
| | | Cost (Gussy, 2006; Murtomaa, 1988; Kay, 2003) | 6 |
| | | Age – small children (Humphreys, 2010; Pine, 2004; Milgrom, 1988; Ananaba, 2010; Malcheff, 2009; Brennan, 1996) | 12 |
| | | Embarrassment (Nettleton, 1989; Tseveenjav 2005; Murtomaa 1988) | 6 |

To conserve space, only the first author is listed.

Mongolia (two publications) [59], [60] and Spain [54], Finland [45], Korea [8], Malaysia [49], Northern Ireland [35] and Romania [46] (1 publication each). Six publications [41], [47], [50–53] were multicenter studies or surveys involving participants from Denmark, Iceland, Norway, Sweden, Belgium, China, Czech Republic, Germany, Ireland, Madagascar, México, Singapore, South Africa, Tanzania, and Thailand.

## Quality assessment

Heat maps showing the gradient of quality indicators for each individual survey and qualitative study included in the analysis are shown in Figures 2 and 3, respectively. Most surveys did not present many of the quality items assessed. A total of 24 studies were judged to present high risk of bias, while 17 studies presented low risk of bias (Table 2). All the qualitative studies, on the other hand, included in the analysis presented the majority of the quality items investigated, with 6 studies deemed to have low risk of bias and only 1 considered to have moderate risk of bias (Table 1).

## Frequency Effect size

After analysis and codification of the 48 included publications, a total of 43 relevant findings were extracted. Findings were then grouped together according to categories which were judged to be topically similar. Grouped findings and their calculated frequency ES are presented in Table 3. The categories of findings to affect dentists' motivation to perform or not preventive measures in their patients involved: dentists' dental education and training, personal beliefs on prevention, remuneration, work conditions, gender, place of residence and also the factors that dentists believed to drive patients towards or away from performing preventive measures.

The findings with the highest frequency ES to drive dentists away from performing preventive measures were "biologicism", (27%), "low pay" (25%), "time since graduation" (22%), and "male dentists" (19%). Whereas, "team work" (21%), "post-graduation" (12%), and "professional understanding of the benefits" (12%) were identified as the main reasons for dentists adherence to preventive measures. The factors for dentists' adherence or non-adherence to dental caries preventive measures are graphically shown in Figure 4.

The main factor that dentists believed keep patients from performing preventive measures were "lack of understanding of the benefits" (17%), "age/small children" (12%), and "patient lack of motivation" (8%). While "parents' motivation" and "patients' age" (4%) were the reasons to lead to patients towards the same preventive measures. Figure 5 graphically illustrates the factors that dentists believed to drive patients towards or away from performing preventive measures.

## Intensity effect sizes

Calculated intensity ES are presented in Table 4. The publication that presented the highest intensity ES, i.e., that presented the highest number of themes relative to the total number of themes, was Murtomaa [43] with a score of 40%, followed by Nettleton [14] and Sbaraini [15] with 26%, and Threlfall [16,17] with 23%. Among the 48 selected publications, 18 had scores between 8% and 22%, and 26 publications had scores below 8%. Only one finding (biologicism) presented effect size >25%, which resulted in intensity ES >25% = 100% in 13 studies, while intensity ES for the remaining studies was 0%.

# Discussion

This systematic review and metasummary of qualitative studies and surveys analyzed factors that drive dentists towards or away from dental caries preventive measures.

Surveys and qualitative research differ in how data are obtained. The minimally structured and open-ended interviewing style typically associated with qualitative studies allows an

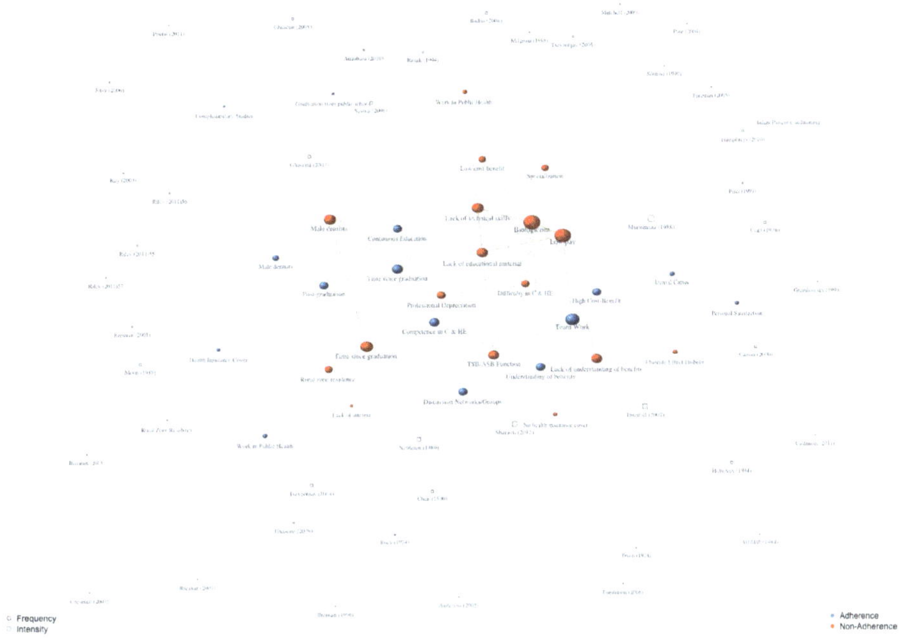


**Figure 4. Factors that drive dentists towards or away from performing preventive measures.** Graph theory-based figure showing the relation among qualitative studies and surveys included in the metasummary model. Squares represent the individual studies included, and circles the emerging factors. Size of each individual marking indicates its effect size (ES) in the model; larger markings being more recurrent. Studies presenting lower intensity ES (prevalence) appear further from the center, while studies with higher intensity ES closer to the center of the figure.

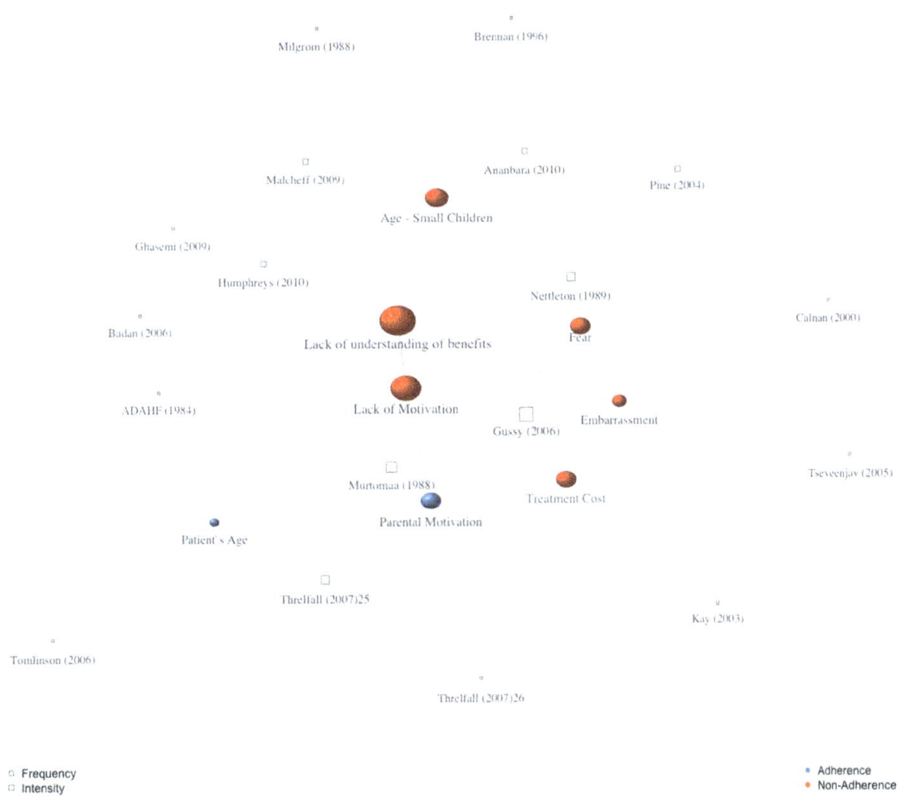


**Figure 5. Factors dentists believed to drive patients towards or away from performing preventive measures.** Graph theory-based figure showing the relation among surveys included in the metasummary model. Squares represent the individual studies included, and circles the emerging factors. Size of each individual marking indicates its effect size in the model; larger markings being more recurrent. Studies presenting lower intensity ES (prevalence) appear further from the center, while studies with higher intensity ES closer to the center of the figure.

**Table 4.** Intensity effect sizes (ES) in relation to all themes and themes with frequency effects sizes >25%.

| Report | Intensity ES (%) | Intensity ES >25% (%) | Report | Intensity ES (%) | Intensity ES >25% (%) |
|---|---|---|---|---|---|
| ADAHF (1984)[18] | 7 | * | Kay EJ (2003)[39] | 9 | * |
| Ananaba N (2010)[19] | 9 | 100 | Malcheff S (2009)[40] | 12 | 100 |
| Anderson R (2002)[20] | 5 | * | Milgrom P (1988)[41] | 7 | * |
| Badan DE (2006)[21] | 14 | 100 | Moon HS (1988)[42] | 12 | * |
| Brennan DS (1996)[22] | 2 | * | Murtomaa HTM (1988)[43] | 40 | 100 |
| Brennan DS (1998)[23] | 2 | * | Nettleton S (1989)[14] | 26 | 100 |
| Brennan DS (2001)[24] | 7 | * | Nuca CI (2011)[44] | 2 | * |
| Brennan DS (2003)[25] | 5 | * | Pine CM (2004)[45] | 9 | * |
| Brennan DS (2007)[26] | 2 | * | Pourat N (2011)[46] | 2 | * |
| Calnan M (2000)[27] | 12 | 100 | Razak I (1994)[47] | 12 | * |
| Cashmore AW (2011)[11] | 2 | * | Riley III RL (2011)[48] | 7 | * |
| Chen M (1990)[28] | 12 | * | Riley III RL (2010)[49] | 7 | * |
| Chestnut IG (2007)[29] | 2 | * | Riley III RL (2010)[50] | 3 | * |
| Craft M (1976)[30] | 14 | 100 | Rock WP (1976)[51] | 7 | * |
| Fiset L (1997)[31] | 7 | * | Sbaraini A (2012)[15] | 26 | 100 |
| Freeman R (2005)[32] | 2 | * | Serrano AG (1990)[52] | 5 | 100 |
| Ghasemi H (2007)[33] | 14 | * | Sesma N (2006)[53] | 14 | 100 |
| Ghasemi H (2008)[34] | 7 | * | Silva RP (2006)[54] | 7 | * |
| Ghasemi H (2009)[35] | 9 | * | Threlfall AG (2007)[16] | 23 | 100 |
| Grembowsky D (1990)[36] | 5 | * | Threlfall AG (2007)[17] | 7 | * |
| Gussy MG (2006)[12] | 9 | * | Tomlinson P (2006)[55] | 7 | * |
| Holloway PJ (1994)[37] | 12 | * | Tryon F (1974)[56] | 2 | * |
| Humphreys RE (2010)[13] | 14 | 100 | Tseveenjav B (2004)[57] | 7 | * |
| Kallestål C (1999)[38] | 5 | * | Tseveenjav B (2005)[58] | 14 | 100 |

*Reports that did not obtain themes with frequency effects sizes >25%.

unlimited number of responses, yielding data with a wider range of responses concerning a target event. In contrast, the highly structured and closed-ended questionnaire typically associated with surveys limits the number and specifies the nature and direction of responses, producing data with a narrower range of responses. Seeing all of the findings belonging to one topic together preserves the complexity of the findings. The methodology used in this systematic review allowed the aggregation and interpretation of descriptive findings, which were comparable among themselves [13]. A diversity of findings were abstracted from the selected studies (Table 3) that were analyzed and their potential relevance in understanding which factors drive dentists towards or away from performing preventive measures were commented.

The findings of this systematic review indicate that the reasons for dentists' adherence to providing prevention are multifactorial and dependent on how and where the study was performed. Nonetheless, it is important to point out the limitations imposed by the quality of the selected reports. The lack of standardization, together with a lack of adequate description of the study methodology, negatively affected the quality assessment, with most of the selected surveys (58%) included in this review being judged to have a high risk of bias. This clearly demonstrate that studies following well established criteria for the conduction of surveys with validated instruments are necessary to better understand dentists motivation or lack of motivation towards preventive measures.

Qualitative studies, on the other hand, were judged to present low risk of bias, with most studies presenting the items analyzed. The drawback concerning this type of study was that fact only a handful of reports were retrieved from the literature. The advantage of qualitative studies is that, due to its design, they may bring to the surface perceptions, feelings, and opinions that are sometimes impossible to be captured by surveys. The included qualitative studies covered just three countries (England, Wales and Australia), limiting the generalizability of findings. Well-designed qualitative studies performed in lower-income countries would significantly add to the understanding of this matter.

A high percentage of studies (54%) had a low intensity frequency, indicating low prevalence of the findings (Table 4). This limitation was compensated by the diversity of findings found in the studies. This multiplicity of findings accounting for dentists' attitude towards prevention abstracted from the selected reports may be explained by the methodological variability of the reports and the wide geographic area covered.

Nonetheless, despite the low calculated frequency (Table 3) and intensity (Table 4) effect sizes, two main categories of findings have emerged as being relevant to the reasons for adherence or non-adherence to preventive measures. Dental education and training has emerged as the most important category to affect dentists' attitude to their perception of how to conduct their activities. It seems clear that when dentists are continuously engaged in their professional and educational development, the more open they are to the new demands of the profession, and more likely to embrace prevention in their daily routine [31,36,55,59,60]. As a result, their education and training have a direct effect on their personal beliefs and vision of prevention as something beneficial for the patient with associated professional satisfaction. In contrast, however, the ways dentists are being remunerated for dental caries preventive measures need to be examined more carefully. The findings in this study demonstrated that low or no remuneration for preventive measures may be an important hindrance to their motivation. This is in agreement with the findings of a recent Cochrane revision, which have indicated that financial incentives within remuneration systems may produce changes to clinical activity undertaken by primary care dentists [61]. Thus, a combination of continuous education and training coupled to an acceptable pay scheme would seem to be a reasonable approach to increase dental professionals' adherence to dental caries preventive measures.

It is expected that this study may contribute to the understanding of factors that can drive dentists towards or away from performing dental caries preventive measures. Moreover, this information may then be used as a useful reference for planning and decision making aimed at changing dental practice and improving the oral health care provided to the general population.

## Author Contributions

Conceived and designed the experiments: RSST MF RCP RP CGR. Performed the experiments: USGS ALMU RSST. Analyzed the data: USGS RSST MF RCP CGR. Contributed reagents/materials/analysis tools: RSST USGS JRNV CGR APB. Wrote the paper: USGS RSST MF RCP CGR.

## References


1. World Health Organization (2012) Oral Health Fact Sheet. n. 318, April 2012. Available: http://www.who.int/mediacentre/factsheets/fs318/en/. Accessed: 2013 Mar 01.
2. Beltrán-Aguilar ED, Barker LK, Canto MT, Dye BA, Gooch BF, et al. (2005) Surveillance for dental caries, dental sealants, tooth retention, edentulism, and enamel fluorosis–United States, 1988–1994 and 1999–2002. MMWR Surveill Summ 54: 1–43.
3. World Health Organization (2014) What is the burden of oral disease? Available: http://www.who.int/oral_health/disease_burden/global/en/. Accessed: 2014 Aug 16.
4. Petersen PE, Bourgeois D, Ogawa H, Estupinan-Day S, Ndiaye C (2005) The global burden of oral diseases and risks to oral health. Bull World Health Organ [online] 83: 661–669.
5. Yee R, Sheiham A (2002) The burden of restorative dental treatment for children in Third World countries. Int Dent J 52: 1–9.
6. Petersen PE (2003) The World Oral Health Report 2003: continuous improvement of oral health in the 21st century – the approach of the WHO Global Oral Health Programme. Community Dent Oral Epidemiol 31: 3–24.
7. Nadanovsky P, Sheiham A (1995) Relative contribution of dental services to the changes in caries levels of 12-year-old children in 18 industrialized countries in the 1970s and early 1980s. Community Dent Oral Epidemiol 23: 331–339.
8. Moon HS, Paik DI, Horowitz AM, Kim JB (1998) National survey of Korean dentists' knowledge and opinions: Dental caries etiology and prevention. J Public Health Dent 58: 51–56.
9. Moher D, Liberati A, Tetzlaff J, Altman DG, The PRISMA Group (2009) Preferred reporting items for systematic reviews and meta-analyses: the PRISMA statement. PLoS Med 6(7): e1000097. doi:10.1371/journal.pmed.1000097.
10. Shea BJ, Grimshaw JM, Wells GA, Boers M, Andersson N, et al. (2009) Development of AMSTAR: A measurement tool to assess the methodological quality of systematic reviews. BMC Med Res Methodol 7: 10.
11. Bennett C, Khangura S, Brehaut JC, Graham ID, Moher D, et al. (2011) Reporting Guidelines for Survey Research: An Analysis of Published Guidance and Reporting Practices. PLoS Med 8(8): e1001069. doi:10.1371/journal.pmed.1001069.
12. The Joanna Brings Institute. Available: http://joannabriggs.org/sumari.html. Accessed: 2014 Sep 16.
13. Sandelowski M, Barroso J, Voils CI (2007) Using qualitative metasummary to synthesize qualitative and quantitative descriptive findings. Res Nurs Health 30: 99–111.
14. Cashmore AW, Noller J, Ritchie J, Johnson B, Blinkhorn AS (2011) Reorienting a paediatric oral health service towards prevention: Lessons from a qualitative study of dental professionals. Health Promot J Austr 22: 17–21.
15. Gussy MG, Waters E, Kilpatrick NM (2006) A qualitative study exploring barriers to a model of shared care for pre-school children's oral health. Br Dent J 201: 165–170.
16. Humphreys RE, Richards W, Gill P (2010) Perceptions of first year foundation dentists on oral health education and its role in general dental practice. Br Dent J 209: 601–606.
17. Nettleton S (1989) Dentists and dental health education: a study of the perceptions of 28 community dentists. Community Dent Health 6: 47–60.
18. Sbaraini A (2012) What factors influence the provision of preventive care by general dental practitioners? Br Dent J 212: 1–9.
19. Threlfall AG, Hunt CM, Milsom KM, Tickle M, Blinkhorn AS (2007) Exploring factors that influence general dental practitioners when providing advice to help prevent caries in children. Br Dent J 202: 1–4.
20. Threlfall AG, Milsom KM, Hunt CM, Tickle M, Blinkhorn AS (2007). Exploring the content of the advice provided by general dental practitioners to help prevent caries in young children. Br Dent J 202: 1–4.
21. American Dental Association Health Foundation (1984) Prevention in the dental office: results of a preventive dentistry survey. J Am Dent Assoc 108: 809, 811–812.
22. Ananaba N, Malcheff S, Briskie D, Inglehart MR (2010) Infant oral health examinations: attitudes and professional behavior of general and pediatric dentists in Michigan and pediatric dentists in the U.S. J Mich Dent Assoc 92: 38–43.
23. Anderson R, Treasure ESAS (2002) Oral health promotion practice: a survey of dental professional in Wales. Int J Health Promot Educ 40: 9–14.
24. Badan DE, Marcelo VC, Rocha DG (2010) Perceptions and use of collective health by surgeon dentists egress from Federal University of Goiás. Cien Saude Colet 15: 1811–1818.
25. Brennan DS, Spencer AJ, Szuster FS (1996) Dentist service rates and distribution of practice styles over time. Community Dent Oral Epidemiol 24: 145–51.
26. Brennan DS, Spencer AJ, Szuster FS (1998) Service provision trends between 1983–84 and 1993–94 in Australian private general practice. Aust Dent J 43: 331–336.
27. Brennan DS, Spencer AJ (2001) Practice belief scales among private general dental practitioners. Aust Dent J 46: 186–193.
28. Brennan DS, Spencer AJ (2003) Provision of diagnostic and preventive services in general dental practice. Community Dent Health 20: 5–10.
29. Brennan DS, Spencer AJ (2007) Trends in private dental service provision in major city and other Australian locations. Aust J Rural Health 15: 189–95.
30. Calnan M, Silvester S, Manley G, Taylor-Gooby P (2000) Doing business in the NHS: exploring dentists' decisions to practise in the public and private sectors. Sociol Health Illn 22: 742–764.
31. Chen M (1990) Preventive dentistry in Texas, USA. Community Dent Oral Epidemiol 18: 239–43.
32. Chestnut IG, Thomas DR, Patel R, Treasure ET (2007) Perceptions and attitudes to a fundamental reform of general dental services in Wales. Prim Dent Care 14: 13–18.
33. Craft M, Sheiham A (1976) Attitudes to prevention amongst dental practitioners. A comparison between the North and South of England. Br Dent J 141: 371–6.
34. Fiset L, Grembowski D (1997) Adoption of innovative caries-control services in dental practice: a survey of Washington state dentists. J Am Dent Assoc 128: 337–345.
35. Freeman R, Kerr G, Salmon K, Speedy P (2005) Patient-active prevention in primary dental care: a characterization of general practices in Northern Ireland. Prim Dent Care 12: 42–46.
36. Ghasemi H, Murtomaa H, Torabzadeh H, Vehkalahti MM (2007) Knowledge of and attitudes towards preventive dental care among Iranian dentists. Eur J Dent 1: 222–229.
37. Ghasemi H, Murtomaa H, Torabzadeh H, Vehkalahti MM (2008) Risk-based approach in preventive practice among Iranian dentists. Oral Health Prev Dent 6: 53–60.

38. Ghasemi H, Murtomaa H, Torabzadeh H, Vehkalahti MM (2009) Perceived barriers to the provision of preventive care among Iranian dentists. Oral Health Prev Dent 7: 339–346.
39. Grembowski D, Milgrom P, Fiset L (1990) Factors influencing variation in dentist service rates. J Public Health Dent 50: 244–250.
40. Holloway PJ, Clarkson JE (1994) Cost: benefit of prevention in practice. Int Dent J 44: 317–322.
41. Källestål C, Wang NJ, Petersen PE, Arnadottir IB (1999) Caries-preventive methods used for children and adolescents in Denmark, Iceland, Norway and Sweden. Community Dent Oral Epidemiol 27: 144–151.
42. Kay EJ, Ward N, Locker D (2003) A general dental practice research network: impact of oral health in general dental practice patients. Br Dent J 194: 621–625.
43. Malcheff S, Pink TC, Sohn W, Inglehart MR, Briskie D (2009) Infant oral health examinations: pediatric dentists' professional behavior and attitudes. Pediatr Dent 31: 202–209.
44. Milgrom P, Weinstein P, Chapko M, Grembowski D, Spadafora A (1988) Dentists' attitudes and behaviors in counseling patients about oral self-care. J Am Coll Dent 55: 48–53.
45. Murtomaa H, Telivuo M (1988) The attitudes of Finnish dentists in private practice towards dental health education. Community Dent Health 5: 369–380.
46. Nuca CI, Amariei CI, Paris SD (2011) Preventive Dentistry: current working practices of dentists from the south-eastern region of Romania. OHDM 10: 131–142.
47. Pine CM, Adair PM, Burnside G, Nicoll AD, Gillett A, et al. (2004) Barriers to the treatment of childhood caries perceived by dentists working in different countries. Community Dent Health 21: 112–120.
48. Pourat N, Marcus M (2011) Variations in self-reported provision of services by general dentists in private practice. J Am Dent Assoc 142: 1050–1060.
49. Razak I, Lind OP (1994) Patient education and preventive care in Malaysian dental practice. J Clin Pediatr Dent 18: 313–322.
50. Riley JL 3rd, Gordan VV, Rouisse KM, McClelland J, Gilbert GH (2011) Differences in male and female dentists' practice patterns regarding diagnosis and treatment of dental caries: findings from The Dental Practice-Based Research Network. J Am Dent Assoc 142: 429–440.
51. Riley JL 3rd, Richman JS, Rindal DB, Fellows JL, Qvist V, et al. (2010) Use of caries-preventive agents in children: findings from the Dental Parctice-Based Research Network. Oral Health Prev Dent 8: 351–359.
52. Riley JL 3rd, Gordan VV, Rindal DB, Fellows JL, Ajmo CT, et al. (2010) Preferences for caries prevention agents in adult patients: findings from the dental practice-based research network. Community Dent Oral Epidemiol 38: 360–370.
53. Rock WP, Bradnock G (1976) Preventive dentistry in general practice. A study of current use. Br Dent J 140: 61–64.
54. Gonzales Serrano A, Cenizo Alcaide JA, Lopez Bermejo MA (1990) Attitudes, knowledge and behavior of 3 groups of Spanish dentists on methods of caries prevention. Rev Eur Odontoestomatol 2: 107–110.
55. Sesma N, Alves AP, Telles FBA, Macedo MO, Santos PM, et al. (2006) O perfil dos cirurgiões-dentistas da cidade de São Paulo na prática da prevenção de cáries e doenças gengivais. Revista de Odontologia da Universidade Cidade de São Paulo 18: 257–263.
56. Silva RP, Loureiro CAS, Pereira CV, Flório FM (2006) Profile of the dental surgeon related to the recommendation of individual preventive strategies. Braz J Oral Sci 5: 1022–1027.
57. Tomlinson P, Treasure E (2006) Provision of prevention to adults in NHS dental practices and attitudes to prevention. Br Dent J 200: 393–397.
58. Tryon AF (1974) An analysis of preventive dental activities in general practice. J Am Soc Prev Dent 4: 20–25.
59. Tseveenjav B, Vehkalahti MM, Murtomaa H (2004) Caries-preventive measures applied by Mongolian dentists to their own children. Oral Health Prev Dent 2: 203–209.
60. Tseveenjav B, Vehkalahti MM, Murtomaa H (2005) Barriers to the provision of oral health education among Mongolian dentists. Oral Health Prev Dent 3: 183–188.
61. Brocklehurst P, Price J, Glenny AM, Tickle M, Birch S, et al. (2013) The effect of different methods of remuneration on the behaviour of primary care dentists. Cochrane Database Syst Rev 11: CD009853. doi:10.1002/14651858.CD009853.pub2.

# 18

# Engaging New Migrants in Infectious Disease Screening: A Qualitative Semi-Structured Interview Study of UK Migrant Community Health-Care Leads

**Farah Seedat¶, Sally Hargreaves*¶, Jonathan S. Friedland**

International Health Unit, Section of Infectious Diseases and Immunity, Commonwealth Building, Hammersmith Campus, Imperial College London, London, United Kingdom

## Abstract

Migration to Europe - and in particular the UK - has risen dramatically in the past decades, with implications for public health services. Migrants have increased vulnerability to infectious diseases (70% of TB cases and 60% HIV cases are in migrants) and face multiple barriers to healthcare. There is currently considerable debate as to the optimum approach to infectious disease screening in this often hard-to-reach group, and an urgent need for innovative approaches. Little research has focused on the specific experience of new migrants, nor sought their views on ways forward. We undertook a qualitative semi-structured interview study of migrant community health-care leads representing dominant new migrant groups in London, UK, to explore their views around barriers to screening, acceptability of screening, and innovative approaches to screening for four key diseases (HIV, TB, hepatitis B, and hepatitis C). Participants unanimously agreed that current screening models are not perceived to be widely accessible to new migrant communities. Dominant barriers that discourage uptake of screening include disease-related stigma present in their own communities and services being perceived as non-migrant friendly. New migrants are likely to be disproportionately affected by these barriers, with implications for health status. Screening is certainly acceptable to new migrants, however, services need to be developed to become more community-based, proactive, and to work more closely with community organisations; findings that mirror the views of migrants and health-care providers in Europe and internationally. Awareness raising about the benefits of screening within new migrant communities is critical. One innovative approach proposed by participants is a community-based package of health screening combining all key diseases into one general health check-up, to lessen the associated stigma. Further research is needed to develop evidence-based community-focused screening models - drawing on models of best practice from other countries receiving high numbers of migrants.

**Editor:** Vicki Marsh, Kilifi, Kenya

**Funding:** The study was funded by the Imperial College Healthcare Charity and the Biomedical Research Centre at Imperial College London. The funders had no role in study design, data collection, analysis, decision to publish, or preparation of the manuscript.

**Competing Interests:** The authors have declared that no competing interests exist.

* Email: s.hargreaves@imperial.ac.uk

¶ These authors are joint first authors on this work.

## Introduction

With an estimated 72.6 million migrants now residing in Europe, the region is an increasingly important recipient of approximately one third of the international migrant population [1,2]. In the past decade the UK in particular has received a sizeable and increasing number of new migrants, which has had important implications for public health services [3,4]. Infectious diseases are believed to be the key health issue for new migrants from high-prevalence countries, with asylum seekers and refugees considered to be particularly affected [5]. Migrants bear the largest burden of infectious disease in the UK; approximately 70% of newly diagnosed UK tuberculosis (TB) and 60% of new HIV cases are in migrants, with comparable trends expected for hepatitis B and C [3,5–7]. London now has the highest tuberculosis rate among all capital cities in western Europe [8]. Numerous factors contribute to the vulnerability of new migrants to infectious diseases, with migrants - and ethnic minorities more broadly - known to face barriers to healthcare, which may result in delays to screening and diagnosis [4,9]. Tackling infectious diseases may raise specific issues, including stigma and fear of discrimination [10–12]. New migrants may be particularly affected in terms of their ability to access and benefit from screening programmes for infectious disease as they attempt to navigate a new health system [13,14].

How best to screen new migrants, and what to screen for, remains an ongoing debate in the UK and Europe [15–20], with approaches varying considerably [1,21,22]. The UK Government, for example, has recently closed down its port of entry tuberculosis screening because of concerns that it was poorly run, discriminatory, and not cost-effective, opting instead for pre-entry screening. Evidence suggests that it is critical to engage new migrants from high-prevalence countries early on if they are planning to reside in

*Introductory questions*

Sex (M/F)

Date of Birth

Nationality

Years in the UK and which country did you leave to come here?

Specific role in the community organisation

Communities or nationalities representing

Demographic profile of new migrants in your community (age, sex, occupation, marital status)

Dominant citizenship statuses of the new migrants in your community?

Level of English among new migrants in your community?

Do you think that TB, HIV, and hepatitis B/C are common in your community (Y/N)?

Approximately what percentages of new migrants that you see in your community have been offered screening for TB, HIV, and hepatitis B/C?

Approximately what percentage of new migrants in your community decline screening offers?

In your opinion, what percentage of new migrants in your community would come forward for full screening of TB, HIV, and hepatitis B and C if it were on offer through a GP practice?

*Open questions*

1. What is the knowledge and perception of new migrant communities regarding infectious diseases (screening)?

Prompts: awareness of each disease and screening; perception of each disease, screening and risk; differences between diseases or migrants; sources of information

2. What is the infectious disease screening experience like for new migrants?

Prompts: Where? How? Availability? Accessibility? Views and experiences? Case studies?

3. What are the key barriers to accessing screening services for infectious diseases faced by new migrants?

Prompts: Barriers from individual, health system, community/cultural, stigma. Consequences? Vulnerable subgroups? Explore case studies.

4. How can we improve the infectious disease screening approach?

Prompts: factors that will influence success with migrants, most important factors, things to avoid, how to increase access? Best location for screening and best design?

**Figure 1. Interview topic guide.**

the UK for a period of time. TB is known to surface 3–5 years after arrival [6] and data suggests that HIV is often acquired in a migrants' home country with most unaware of their status on arrival to the UK [23]. The issue of vaccination for infectious diseases may also be important for health-care providers to address. There have been calls to strengthen primary-care-based screening programmes, and to place renewed focus on latent tuberculosis screening to tackle the rising tide of tuberculosis [17,18]. However, there remains a paucity of data on barriers to, and acceptability of, screening programmes for infectious diseases specifically in newly arrived migrants, and potential ways forward; addressing these shortfalls remains an important component in the strategy to tackle rising rates of infectious diseases.

We did a qualitative semi-structured interview study of migrant community health-care leads, who represent dominant new migrant groups in London, UK. The aim was to explore their views around barriers, accessibility, and acceptability of screening for HIV, tuberculosis, hepatitis B, and hepatitis C.

## Methods

We did a series of semi-structured face-to-face interviews to explore migrant community health-care leads' perceptions about (i) the barriers to screening for HIV, TB, and hepatitis B and C faced by new migrants; (ii) acceptability of screening; and (iii) innovative approaches to improve screening uptake in new migrants. We defined new migrants as foreign-born individuals who had resided in the UK for less than 5 years, arriving from countries outside Western Europe, North America, Australia, and New Zealand. Therefore, we sought information about new migrant groups from high prevalence disease countries. We carried out and reported this study using COREQ guidelines [24] as well as the quality guidelines of Mays and Pope (2000) [25].

**Table 1.** Characteristics of participants and the new migrants communities they represent.

| Characteristics | *N* |
|---|---|
| Participants | 20 |
| Gender of participants | F (10), M (10) |
| Mean Age (range) | 42.77 (25–64 years) |
| Mean years in the UK (range) | 21.59 (4–43 years); 4 born in the UK |
| Country of birth | Africa (8) – Kenya (1), Nigeria (3), Somalia (2), Uganda (1), Zambia (1) |
| | Asia (3) – Bangladesh (1), Iran (1), Malaysia (1) |
| | Europe (7) – Greece (1), Poland (1), Ukraine (1), United Kingdom (4) |
| | Americas (2) – Colombia (1), Jamaica (1) |
| Nationalities of new migrants represented* | Africa (13) – Algeria, Burkina Faso, Cameroon, Cote D'Ivoire, Egypt, Eritrea, Ethiopia, Ghana, Kenya, Morocco, Nigeria, Senegal, Somalia, South Africa, Tunisia, Uganda, Zambia, Zimbabwe, |
| | Americas (3) – Caribbean, Chile, Colombia, Ecuador, Venezuela, |
| | Asia (9) – Bangladesh, China, India, Iraq, Iran, Lebanon, Nepal, Pakistan, Philippines, Syria, |
| | Europe (3) – Latvia, Lithuania, Poland, Russia, Slovakia, Ukraine |
| Gender of new migrants represented | Majority female (10), Majority male (5), Equal (5) |
| Age range of new migrants represented | 20–85 years old |
| Citizenship status of new migrants represented** | Claiming citizenship (11), EC citizen (5), Indefinite resident (2), Refugee or asylum seeker (14), Spouse visa (2), Student visa (10), Tourist (1) Undocumented (3), UK citizen (5), Work permit (5), Unknown (2) |
| Level of English of new migrants represented | A few words (9), Conversational (6), Fluent (5) |

*Participants focussed on 39 different nationalities in total.
The numbers in brackets represent the number of participants who mentioned that the region is a majority that they represent.
**The numbers in brackets represent the number of participants who mention the status as one of the dominant statuses that they represent.

The study was approved by the Imperial College Research Ethics Committee.

## Participant selection and recruitment

We approached migrant community health-care leads who encompassed dominant groups of new migrants in the study site – which was a high migrant area of West London (Hammersmith and Fulham) where 42.8% of residents defined as foreign born [26]. The inclusion criteria were community leads who were expert professionals with a working knowledge of the health needs of new migrants within the communities and nationality groups they represented, who were >18 years of age, and capable of giving informed consent. This approach – of recruiting community leads rather than the new migrants themselves - is one used successfully elsewhere, and was repeated with the aim of acquiring an overview of the issues facing new migrants across a broad range of nationality groups [27].

We recruited participants using purposive sampling to enable exploration of particular aspects of behaviours relevant to the research questions. We drew up a sampling frame for the target population by carrying out internet searches of London-based community groups around the study site. This list was used as a starting point to generate a list of relevant individuals working within these community groups who would meet study inclusion criteria. Potential participants were then directly approached by telephone and invited to participate. Those who were interested in participating were emailed a Participant Information Leaflet about the study, and re-contacted to confirm participation and arrange the interview. Purposive sampling allowed us to then use our initial participants to establish subsequent contact with other relevant participants. Purposive sampling also allowed us to recruit a mix of nationality groups to represent the major new migrant community groups. We developed a topic guide (Figure 1) of both structured and open questions based on previous work conducted by the authors in collaboration with community leaders in another London-base study site [27] and pilot tested it on the first participant. Participant recruitment continued until data saturation was achieved for all categories.

## Data collection and analysis

In all but two cases, FS (female, British Asian) conducted interviews at participants' workplace in a private room where only the interviewer and participant were present. FS had previously been trained to conduct research interviews in the field of migrant health. After acquiring written informed consent, participants were reminded of the study aims and assured that all information they shared would be confidential and presented in an anonymous format, and the interview then commenced for 30–90 minutes.

The interviews were audio-recorded with permission (Sony VOR Microcassette Recorder M-740V) and transcribed verbatim for analysis by independent transcribers (anonymously) after each interview. Case memos were made after every interview in addition to theoretical memos to assist in the formulation of theories. Data were analysed using the principles of grounded theory, which involved systematically collecting and analysing data simultaneously throughout the research process. Data were managed using QSR NVivo 10 software.

Data was first coded by open coding to generate concepts. After carrying out the first three interviews a list of all the codes elicited from the transcripts were grouped into a list of categories using axial coding. To guard against selectivity, two researchers (FS/SH) independently conducted these processes and discussed the initial interpretations of the data, the reliability of the codes, explanations of particular codes, and additional areas for exploration within the subsequent interviews. This discussion combined with the research questions that shaped the topic guide formed the basis of the

**Table 2.** Barriers to screening reported.

| Level | Barrier |
|---|---|
| System and provider level barriers | Capacity/funding shortages for community organisations |
| | Lack of advocacy and promotion |
| | Lack of confidentiality |
| | Lack of psycho-social support services |
| | Low awareness of diseases amongst health professionals |
| | Poor link with community organisations |
| | Migrant unfriendly services |
| | Discrimination and stigma from health professionals |
| | Cultural insensitivity |
| | Inhospitality |
| | Time and distance to services |
| Community level barriers | Culture |
| | Cultural mentality and baggage |
| | Extra pressure for women regarding virginity and family role |
| | Lack of openness |
| | No prevention culture |
| | Faith, lack of openness, and stigma |
| | Language |
| | Stigma and misconceptions |
| Patient level barriers | Fear of a lack of confidentiality |
| | Fear of cost and eligibility (perceived or actual) |
| | Fear of disease status |
| | Isolation |
| | Lack of awareness and knowledge of diseases |
| | Lack of confidence using new health system |
| | Lack of screening services or health-system knowledge |
| | Misunderstanding between health system in current residence vs country of origin |
| | Low perception of risk |
| | Low priority on immigrant list |
| | Poorer health-seeking behaviour in men |

coding framework thereon. Transparency in the method and regular checks and discussion about the codes and categories mitigated experimenter bias.

A constant comparison approach was then used whereby transcripts were reviewed and codes were developed in an iterative process. By constantly comparing the codes and themes and using deviant case analysis to explore conflicting views, we were able to interpret the data with validity. As interviews were completed, selective coding was conducted where the most common codes and those seen as most revealing about the data were emphasised and unified around a core framework. A final re-check of all transcripts was carried out to check whether all text had been accounted for and to ensure that all initial open-codes were incorporated into each theme where appropriate. Member checking was also adopted by sending the final report to all the participants in the study for feedback.

## Results

### Sample characteristics

50 organisations working with migrants on health issues in the survey site were identified from the initial internet search, of which 34 were unable to support us in identifying participants within their own organisation (2 shut down; 5 contact details were out of date; 19 did not respond; 4 could not identify potential participants within their own organisation, 4 organisations declined). Of the four organisations that declined participation: one only dealt with more settled migrants who had been in the UK for long periods of time; two stated that they did not have a health-care lead for an interview; and one declined due to lack of experience in the field of health care specifically.

From the initial contact with the remaining 16 organisations, 20 community health leads were identified and agreed to be interviewed. By interview 20, data saturation was achieved, no new or relevant material arose, and it was highly probably that additional interviews would not have influenced results. There were an equal number of male and female participants (mean age 42.7 years). Nine participants worked in HIV & AIDS related organisations, one in a TB related organisation, and one in a hepatitis B related organisation; 16 of 20 were migrants themselves and of the remaining, 3 out of 4 were from ethnic minority groups in the UK. Five participants were Chief Executives/Directors of the organisations they represented, 5 were programme coordinators, 2 were project leaders, 3 were project managers, 2 were community development officers, 1 was a project officer, 1 was a volunteer, and 1 was a faith engager. Participants represented new migrant communities from 39 diverse nationalities across Africa, Americas, Asia and Europe (age range in these communities 20–85 years). The majority of new migrants represented were refugees and asylum seekers, followed by migrants claiming citizenship, and those on student visas; most of the population under discussion, therefore, were considered by participants to be of low socioeconomic status (Table 1).

## Key themes

Two key themes emerged from the interviews:

(i) Existing screening models are not perceived to be widely accessible to the new migrant community. The main barriers that discourage use are disease-related stigma present in their own communities and services being perceived as non-migrant friendly. New migrants may be disproportionately affected and delays to screening may impact on health status.

(ii) Screening is certainly acceptable to new migrants. Participants stressed the need for service providers to bring accessible and migrant-friendly screening into the community, strengthening collaborations with community-based organisations, and proposed a community-based package of health screening combining all of the diseases into one general health check-up with the aim of reducing stigma.

The barriers and facilitators described were points most commonly recommended or strongly recommended by participants.

## Screening is inaccessible to the new migrant community

Participants identified a range of barriers to screening for infectious diseases at the health system, community, and individual level (Table 2). There was strong agreement among participants that screening for infectious diseases was not accessible to the new migrant community in the UK. Most participants felt that although screening services do exist, they are not adequately reaching people in the community, stating that "people don't even know that these [screening services] exist" (Participant 11, age 31, male, Latin American community) and that new migrants specifically "do not easily take them up" (Participant 1, age 52, male, African community). Some participants added that the services are not well-publicised as information on them is not given to new migrants who are attempting to navigate a new health system, while one participant believed that services at present are "not pro-active" in encouraging new migrants to come forward for testing, and focus remains too much on the "treatment angle" rather than a preventative approach (Participant 13, age 32, male, migrant communities).

The most cited barrier, highlighted by 19 of 20 participants, was the stigma and misconceptions that new migrant communities' hold about the key diseases. Participants identified that stigma within their own communities is the "biggest barrier to date" and the "biggest dilemma" they face when considering going for screening. Each disease has more than one different type of stigma in the different communities. According to participants, we found that TB, HIV, and hepatitis B and C can be perceived by new migrant communities as being "fatal" and/or "highly infectious", which generates fear of testing. As a result of stigma, new migrants may "run-away" from the infected individuals, not inviting infected individuals to their houses, eating with them, or wanting to be near them. Participants said this discourages people from attending screening, because they may have to face such disease-related social consequences if people know they have attended screening and an infection is found. TB specifically is perceived in the Somali and Asian community as a "disease of the poor" and in the Asian community also as "hereditary".

Participants unanimously considered HIV to still be the most stigmatised disease of the four. Issues around stigma for HIV are complex and deeply interlinked with a migrant's culture and faith. Stemming from cultural and religious beliefs, HIV is perceived as a result of a "sinful" and "immoral" lifestyle including "pre-marital sex", "drug use", "promiscuity", or "being gay". Participants said that new migrant communities see HIV as being self-inflicted, a "punishment from God" and a "well-deserved disease". This prevents people from attending screening "as nobody wants to be seen in that way" (Participant 5, age 59, male, Somali community). Two participants also indicated that in the African migrant community, HIV is strongly associated with TB. Therefore, people often misconceive patients who have TB as having HIV or vice versa. Little was known about hepatitis stigma and only three participants indicated that the stigma could be similar to the way in which HIV is perceived, "filled with things about a lifestyle, moral behaviour and stereotypical things" (Participant 2, age 44, male, Ukrainian community).

The second most important barrier reported by participants was that the screening services are not "migrant friendly". Twelve

Panel 2 I Case study on the consequences of the barriers to screening

*"I have a service user that died here [Latin American male with HIV], this was 2003 and he died because he was very ill for many months and he didn't go to any hospital - No, he didn't look for a doctor or anything because he was illegal. So the people that were living with him said that if he goes to the doctor maybe they call immigration, they call the police, they call whoever, and finally the people that bring him to the hospital are the police because he went one day to buy food and on the way from the house to the shop he collapsed in the street and so someone called the police and the police came and the police took him to the hospital. And he died in the hospital three months later.. It was too late. And many people have the same thing again, they don't go to the hospital because they think that the hospital is going to call the police. So it stops people going."* (Participant 11, age 31, male, Latin American community)

**Figure 2. Case study on the consequences of the barriers to screening.**

**Table 3.** Approaches identified to make screening more accessible.

| Approach |
|---|
| Better access features |
| Build migrants confidence to access health services |
| Engage faith-based organisations |
| Ensure confidentiality |
| Improve hospitality and cultural sensitivity, through educating front-line staff on cultural competencies and migrant health needs |
| Increase language support |
| Increase psycho-social support |
| More appropriate and accessible promotion of screening |
| Offer one package of care for migrants, a general health check incorporating infectious disease screening |
| Outreach for isolated migrants |
| Raise awareness of diseases and screening in communities |
| Stronger collaboration with community organisations |

participants expressed concerns about the cultural insensitivity experienced by new migrants within services, where sometimes assumptions are made about the patients. In addition to cultural insensitivity, eight participants indicated that new migrants were frustrated with the inhospitable and unfriendly experiences when they accessed services. Many of these participants were concerned with the inhospitality of receptionist staff in particular; one participant said that this was the case even where receptionists were from an ethnic minority or migrant background themselves. In addition, seven participants identified discrimination from health-care professionals as an important barrier. Some participants mentioned that the discrimination was against the new migrants' country of origin, for example one participant who went to ask for results was asked by a nurse, "Is this the way you guys behave in Africa?" (Participant 13, male, age 32, all migrant communities), while another participant reported patients being asked: "why don't you speak English, how long have you been here?" (Participant 20, age 36, female, all migrant communities). Language barriers may be a particular issue for new migrants on arrival; most new migrants represented in this study spoke little English (Table 1). Another participant identified that it was a combination of their migrant status, as well as their infectious disease, that lead to discrimination. Four participants, however, felt that services were culturally sensitive and had not come across any cases or complaints from within their communities.

Participants also mentioned a number of barriers that may be unique to new migrants, including the issue of a lack of entitlement to free health care and confidentiality issues (table 2). Participants commented that new migrants "have to find their own way" (Participant 5, age59, male, Somali community), that "they don't know what exists...that they have the right, that it's free" (Participant 11, age 31, male, Latin American community). New migrants "may not think they're entitled to help here and they may not think they could just go and get it" (participant 15, age 48, male, African community). New migrants may also have confidentiality issues "concerns around immigration" and whether their "disease status will be shared with immigration services" (Participant 12, age 27, male, Afro-Caribbean community). Participants report that new migrants are concerned that clinical services, especially in hospital settings, are "government bodies and attached to the government...therefore somehow linked to immigration" (Participant 10, male, age 29, Asian community). In particular, some new migrants perhaps "don't have a visa" and are scared of "exposing themselves" by attending screening as "they will be deported because of their status" (Participant 18, age 59, female, African community).

## Barriers to care have implications for health status

Participants highlighted a number of consequences that barriers can have for a new migrant patient and the wider community. Directly, the barriers stopped migrants from attending screening services as they "wait until their situation has got a little bit worse, when it's actually disabling them and they can't do any other activities" (Participant 14, age 40, male, African community) before they get tested for the diseases. "When they are screened later then the medication is not given the optimum chance to work for them...then obviously they have got a very narrow chance of recovery" (Participant 1, age 52, male, African community). Four participants mentioned that this "late diagnosis" has led to cases of death in their communities; a case study from one participant is presented in Figure 2.

Two participants mentioned that in the Eastern European community new migrants may turn to alternative forms of medication, for example, getting "herbs sent back from home" (Participant 2, age 44, male, Ukrainian community), "return back home" (Participant 7, age 31, female, Eastern European community) to do the screening or may also use services from individuals in the community "who they knew practiced medicine back in their own country" but who are not yet licensed in the UK (Participant 2, age 44, male, Ukrainian community). At the community level, participants raised concerns that by presenting late and not knowing ones status, new migrants with infections may be "putting others at risk" and increasing "the number of people being exposed to that risk" (Participant 6, age 34, female, Arabic speaking community).

## How do we improve access to screening?

Despite this lack of accessibility there was consensus among participants that screening is acceptable to new migrants, if services are promoted and offered in a tailored and sensitive manner, and uptake would be high if barriers were broken down. Participants collectively reported that between 50% and 100% of new migrants they represented would consider screening if it was more accessible to them. One participant mentioned that "in relation to their health they [the community] wouldn't hesitate to take part in the screening....because it's for their benefit." (Participant 6, age 34, female, Arabic speaking community).

Key factors to consider when making screening more accessible included ensuring better collaboration between service providers and community organisations, as well as combining the screening of diseases into one appointment (table 3). Whether with faith-based or nationality based organisations, all participants strongly conveyed the message that screening services need to be taken out into the community and that the health service must work in partnership with community organisations. Community organisations are a key "asset" because they have the link to the migrant communities and hard-to-reach individuals (Participant 13, age 32, male, migrant communities). Interventions should be "co-owned" and based on the "principles of partnership about coexistence, collaboration, and cooperation" (Participant 13, age 32, male, all migrant communities) if screening services are to be made more accessible. Statutory service providers should focus on raising awareness of diseases, promotion of screening services, language and psycho-social support, as well as designing services that are migrant friendly and culturally sensitive with input from community organisations.

Most of the participants argued that screening services need to be taken out of the hospital and into the community to make access easy, "not sticking into one building or geographical location" (Participant 13, age 32, male, all migrant communities) and "delivering the service to the people where they are" (Participant 15, age 48, male, African community). Participants identified community settings such as places of worship, football games, community centre events, and carnivals as good opportunities to run screening interventions. As one participant explained, there is a bus outside the local market where - with the assistance of community health workers - individuals can "go in there, get fully screened, come back to the market and buy your goat meat and your plantain and go home knowing your status" (Participant 15, age 48, male, African community). Another participant made the point that people would prefer screening at the site of a community organisation, compared to a hospital, as they would feel more "comfortable" having attended the organisation before, and that these organisations have "staff employed from the community itself, when people come they may have a worker on hand who can talk them through the process in a culturally sensitive manner, or in a linguistically sensitive manner" (Participant 10, male, age 29, Asian community). By bringing screening into communities screening programmes will "work better and be far more effective" (Participant 15, age 48, male, African community).

15 of 20 participants considered that the best approach is to offer new migrants a package of care to include screening for TB, HIV, and hepatitis B and C at one appointment; the majority supported the idea of this being within a community setting. Participants suggested that screening be advertised as a general "health check" which would make migrants more receptive and considerably lessen the stigma of infectious diseases. Most importantly, participants felt that offering screening for multiple diseases at one appointment would lessen the dominant barrier of stigma that can prevent migrants from attending screening. This approach could be "immensely convenient for the person as well as the service" (Participant 15, age 48, male, African community). Participants suggested that packaging screening in this integrated way will reduce stigma, or "push stigma down" (Participant 13, age 32, male, all migrant communities) and participants would say yes to screening as it "is enough for people to take a minute and think okay, I know for a fact that I might not have HIV but I might well have the others" (Participant 6, age 34, female, Arabic speaking community).

## Discussion

This research highlighted strong agreement among health-care leads that screening for infectious diseases is currently inaccessible to the new migrant community in the UK. Interestingly, a key factor in poor uptake rate among the new migrant community was stigma and misconceptions that new migrant communities' themselves hold about the key diseases, deeply interlinked with a migrants' culture and faith, as well as perceived fears around the social implications of attending screening and receiving a positive diagnosis. Participants identified numerous barriers to accessing screening services at the current time - which were considered to be non-migrant friendly and culturally insensitive. New migrants are likely to be disproportionally affected by these barriers, and delays to diagnosis and treatment may have health consequences. However, there was strong consensus that acceptability of screening of the four key diseases is high among new migrants. Participants stressed the need to bring accessible and proactive screening into the community, strengthening collaborations with community-based organisations. They supported the idea of a community-based package of health screening combining all of the diseases into a general health check-up, with the aim of lessening the associated stigma.

We are aware that the views expressed by participants will reflect their own experiences of working with the health system around West London. While this may impact on the responses they provided, as community leads, their primary role is to represent their communities. We encouraged interviewees to talk about the wider communities around them; nevertheless, it is a challenge to have one group of people speak for another, and a separate study exploring the specific views of different groups of new migrants will be of interest. In addition, we are aware that a considerable number of participants were working in HIV as oppose to other infectious diseases under discussion, which will mean there may be an inevitable focus on barriers as they relate to HIV services.

Data are limited on the issue of infectious disease screening specifically in the new migrant community; however, numerous studies exist on the use of general health services by the wider migrant community and ethnic minority groups which confirm a myriad of potential barriers to access that confer with our findings [27–29]. Studies specifically exploring HIV testing barriers in migrants, including a systematic review [30] overlap with our findings in new migrants across all four diseases – including migrants having insufficient information about diseases and their prevention, lack of knowledge about health service provision, a perceived discriminatory attitude of health-care providers (including reception staff), fear of a lack of confidentiality and deportation, and confusion over entitlement to free health care [31–33]. Furthermore, studies on tuberculosis in "vulnerable groups" report that a key barrier to screening was to do with concerns around stigma within their own communities, and a fear of death [34–36]. For hepatitis B and C, previous studies in migrants and ethnic-minority groups report barriers related to language and culture, discrimination and stigma, low confidence in health services, lack of knowledge of available services, association of hepatitis testing with sexual health, and a low perception of disease risk [12,37,38]. What is clear is that the data themes we have documented are not unique to new migrants, but common experiences of migrant and ethnic minority groups affected by these diseases. However, it is our view that new

**Table 4.** Examples of international models of community-based migrant screening collaborations for TB, HIV or hepatitis B and C.

| Study | Model |
|---|---|
| Jafferbuoy et al. Scotland, UK [46] | Mosque and Islamic centre based screening |
| | Raised awareness and promoted screening for hepatitis B and C in the mosque. After raising awareness, community offered screening in the mosque one day a week. |
| | High uptake: 177/250 attendees coming forward for testing in the mosques |
| | Only a modest investment in staff time. |
| Sadler et al. London, UK [47] | Various community settings - bars, health promotion events, community centre and social gatherings |
| | Conducted a survey of sexual attitudes in addition to HIV test. |
| | High uptake: 94/114 took test |
| Lewis et al. UK [48] | Mosque based screening promotion |
| | Distributed 5000 viral hepatitis testing cards in Mosques, following an awareness campaign, encouraging viral hepatitis testing at GP surgery. |
| | Community awareness campaigns and leaflets do not directly lead to testing for viral hepatitis |
| Gany et al. New York, USA [49] | Airport holding lot |
| | Conducted TB counselling and screening for taxi drivers in the airport holding lot - drivers drove through the lane, placed their arms out for measurement of the tuberculin skin test reaction. 123 drivers who participated, two thirds (82) were at high risk for tuberculosis. Seventy-eight (63%) of the 123 returned for test readings. |
| Brassard et al. Montreal, Canada [50] | School-based screening |
| | Newly arrived immigrant children in selected schools were screened for latent TB. Family and household associates of the TST-positive child also were screened for LTBI. 542/2524 (21%) were TST-positive. Of 342 children started on therapy, 316 (92%) demonstrated adequate adherence. 599 associates investigated from the 484 TST-positive schoolchildren seen at the TB clinic. Of 555 associates with TST results, 211 (38%) were found to be TST-positive. |
| | Programme was effective and cost-effective. |

migrants who are attempting to navigate a new health system and settle in a new community are likely to be disproportionally affected. That barriers to health care among new migrants may impact on health status has been previously reported [27,33]. That acceptability for screening of HIV, TB, and hepatitis B and C is high among migrants has also been reported elsewhere, with migrants considered to be proactive about their health and screening "valued highly" [39,40].

We found that there was a unanimous view among participants that to facilitate greater uptake of testing screening must be brought into the community, with service providers strengthening collaborations with community-based organisations. In the UK and elsewhere there are interesting examples of successful community outreach screening initiatives that target migrants for TB, HIV, or hepatitis (Table 4); however literature on community-based approaches are scarce with few high quality or controlled studies evaluating community models. We have found that data from innovative locally tested screening initiatives are often not published so the benefits of these approaches remain unclear. Conversely, international studies have reported unsuccessful community-based collaborations, in terms of uptake [41] and cost-effectiveness [42]. The Migrant-Friendly Hospitals Initiative, which resulted in The Amsterdam Declaration (Towards Migrant-Friendly Hospitals in an Ethno-culturally diverse Europe) in 2004, specifically calls for service providers to focus on developing partnerships with local community-based organisations with a view to improving service delivery to migrant groups [43]. Screening high risk groups for TB in General Practice/primary care has been formally assessed in a randomised controlled trial and found to be successful in terms of increased yield [44]. The optimum approach in high-migrant receiving countries is most likely to offer screening in a range of settings [39,45], incorporating a strong focus on community engagement and partnership with migrant organisations in both the design and implementation of screening approaches.

The idea raised by participants of combining these diseases into some kind of general health check-up, with the aim of reducing the considerable stigma associated with infectious diseases, merits further exploration. Such an approach will need to be combined with awareness raising about the benefits of screening within new migrant communities, and attempts to facilitate high uptake to services, in an attempt to tackle misconceptions and reduce stigma. The UK's Health Protection Agency previously recommended that consideration be given to the idea of an extended New Patient Health Check for certain groups of migrants in primary care [6]. To what extent such an approach can be adopted in other high-migrant receiving countries is unknown, with countries taking a wide variety of approaches to screening for infectious diseases in this patient group [22]. Further research is now urgently needed to develop evidence-based community-focussed screening models - drawing on models of best practice and lessons learned from UK and internationally – as well as exploring how healthcare professionals can work more effectively with the new migrant community to facilitate improved access to screening.

## Acknowledgments

We thank the Imperial College Healthcare Charity and the Biomedical Research Centre at Imperial College London for funding this work. We would like to thank the all the organisations that assisted us with data collection, especially: The BME Health Forum, Dalgarno Trust, Hodan Somali Community, Opportunity for All, Rain Trust, The Iranian Association, The Forum, TB Alert, and the Ukrainian Migrants Network.

## Author Contributions

Conceived and designed the experiments: SH JSF. Analyzed the data: FS SH JSF. Wrote the paper: FS SH JSF. Data collection: FS. Supported data collection: SH.

## References


1. Rechel B, Mladovsky P, Ingleby D, Mackenbach JP, McKee M (2013) Migration and health in an increasingly diverse Europe. Lancet 381(9873): 1235–45.
2. International Organization for Migration (2010) World migration report. The future of migration: building capacities for change. International Organization for Migration. Available: http://publications.iom.int/bookstore/free/WMR_2010_ENGLISH.pdf. Accessed: 2014 Sept 20
3. European Centre for Disease Prevention and Control (2009) Migrant health: Background note to the 'ECDC Report on migration and infectious diseases in the EU'. European Centre for Disease Prevention and Control. Available: http://www.ecdc.europa.eu/en/publications/publications/0907_ter_migrant_health_background_note.pdf. Accessed: 2014 Sept 20.
4. Hargreaves S, Friedland J (2012) Impact on and use of health services by new migrants in Europe. In: Thomas S, Gideon J, editors. Migration, Heath and Inequality. London: Zed Books. pp. 27–43.
5. Clark RC, Mytton J (2007) Estimating infectious disease in UK asylum seekers and refugees: a systematic review of prevalence studies. J Public Health 29: 420–428.
6. Wagner K, Jones J (2011) Migrant Health: Infectious diseases in non-UK born populations in England, Wales, and Northern Ireland. An update to the baseline report - 2011. Health Protection Agency Centre. Available: http://www.better-health.org.uk/resources/research/migrant-health-infectious-diseases-non-uk-born-populations-uk-update-baseline-rep. Accessed: 2014 Sept 20.
7. Public Health England (2013) Tuberculosis in the UK: Annual report on tuberculosis surveillance in the UK, 2013. Public Health England. Available: https://www.gov.uk/government/publications/tuberculosis-tb-in-the-uk. Accessed: 2014 Sept 20.
8. European Centre for Disease Prevention and Control (2013) Tuberculosis surveillance and monitoring in Europe. Stockholm: European Centre for Disease Prevention and Control. Available: http://www.ecdc.europa.eu/en/publications/Publications/Tuberculosis-surveillance-monitoring-2013.pdf. Accessed 2014 Sept 20.
9. Wörmann T, Krämer A (2011) Communicable disease. In Rechel B, Mladovsky P, Devillé W, Rijks B, Petrova-Benedict R, McKee M, editors. Migration and health in the European Union. Midenhead: Open University Press. pp. 121–138.
10. Doyal L, Anderson J (2005) 'My fear is to fall in love again…' How HIV-positive African women survive in London. Soc Sci Med 60: 1729–1738.
11. Deblonde J, De Koker P, Hamers FF, Fontaine J, Luchters S, et al. (2010) Barriers to HIV testing in Europe: a systematic review. Eur J Pub Health 20(4): 422–32.
12. Jones L, Atkinson A, Porcellato L, Bates G, McCoy E, et al. (2011) A systematic review of qualitative research on the views, perspectives and experiences of hepatitis B and C testing among practitioners and people at greatest risk of infection. Centre for Public Health, Research Directorate, Faculty of Health and Applied Social Sciences, Liverpool John Moores University. Available: https://www.nice.org.uk/guidance/ph43/resources/hepatitis-b-and-c-ways-to-promote-and-offer-testing-evidence-review-12. Accessed: 2014 Sept 20.
13. Stagg HR, Jones J, Bickler G, Abubakar I (2012) Poor uptake of primary healthcare registration among recent entrants to the UK: a retrospective cohort study. BMJ Open 2:e001453. doi: 10.1136/bmjopen-2012-001453.
14. Hargreaves S, Holmes AH, Saxena S, LeFeuvre P, Farah W, et al. (2008) Charging Systems for Migrants in Primary Care: The Experiences of Family Doctors in a High-Migrant Area of London. J Travel Med 15: 13–18.
15. Lewis H, Burke K, Begum S, Ushiro-Limb I, Foster G (2013) What is the best method of case finding for chronic viral Hepatitis in at-risk migrant communities? J Hepatol 56: S351.
16. Williams R, Holt AP (2013) Screening immigrants for tuberculosis? Why not for HBV infection? Lancet 381(9884): 2164–2165.
17. Hargreaves S, Carballo M, Friedland JS (2009) Screening migrants for tuberculosis - where next? Lancet Infect Dis 9: 139–140.
18. Zenner D, Zumla A, Gill P, Cosford P, Abubakar I (2013) Reversing the tide of the UK tuberculosis epidemic. Lancet 382: 1311–1312.
19. Griffiths C, Sturdy P, Brewin P, Bothamley G, Eldridge S, et al. (2007) Educational outreach to promote screening for tuberculosis in in primary care: a cluster randomised controlled trial. Lancet 369(9572): 1528–1534.
20. Pareek M, Watson JP, Ormerod LP, Kon OM, Woltmann G, et al. (2011) Screening of immigrants in the UK for imported latent tuberculosis: a multicentre cohort study and cost-effectiveness analysis. Lancet 11: 435–444.
21. Coker RJ, Bell A, Pitman R, Hayward A, Watson J (2004) Screening programmes for tuberculosis in new entrants across Europe. Int J Tuberc Lung Dis 8(8): 1022–1026.
22. Coker RJ, Bell A, Pitman R, Zellweger JP, Heldal E, et al. (2006) Tuberculosis screening in migrants in selected European countries shows wide disparities. Eur Respir J 27: 801–807.
23. Anderson J, Doyal L (2004) Women from Africa living with HIV in London: a descriptive study. AIDS Care 16: 95–105.
24. Tong A, Sainsbury P, Craig J (2007) Consolidated criteria for reporting qualitative research (COREQ): a 32-item checklist for interviews and focus groups. Int J Qual Health Care 19(6): 349–357.
25. Mays N, Pope C (2000) Assessing quality in qualitative research. BMJ 320(7226): 50–52.
26. Office for National Statistics (2011) Census: Aggregate data (England and Wales). Available: http://infuse.mimas.ac.uk. Accessed 2014 Sept 20.
27. Hargreaves S, Friedland JS, Holmes A, Saxena S (2006) The Identification and Charging of Overseas Visitors in Newham: a Consultation. London: Newham Primary Care Trust.
28. Arai L, Harding S (2002) Health and social care services for minority ethnic communities in the United Kingdom: a review of the literature on access and use. MRC Social and Public Health Sciences Unit, University of Glasgow.
29. Smaje C, Grand JL (1997) Ethnicity, equity and the use of health services in the British NHS. Soc Sci Med 45: 485–96.
30. Deblonde J, De Koker P, Hamers FF, Fontaine J, Luchters S, et al. (2010) Barriers to HIV testing in Europe: a systematic review. Eur J Pub Health 20(4): 422–32.
31. Manirankunda L, Loos J, Alou TA, Colebunders R, Nostlinger C (2009) "It's better not to know": perceived barriers to HIV voluntary counseling and testing among Sub-Saharan African migrants in Belgium. AIDS Educ Prev 21(6): 582–593.
32. Thomas F, Aggleton P, Anderson J (2010) "If I cannot access services, then there is no reason for me to test": the impacts of health service charges on HIV testing and treatment amongst migrants in England. AIDS Care 22(4): 526–531.
33. Yazdanpanah Y, Lange J, Gerstoft J, Cairns G (2010) Earlier testing for HIV - How do we prevent late presentation? Antivir Ther (Suppl 1): 17–24.
34. Johnson A (2006) Beliefs and barriers related to understanding TB amongst vulnerable groups in South East London. Health Protection Agency.
35. Gerrish K, Ismail M, Naisby A (2010) Tackling TB together: a community participatory study of the socio-cultural factors influencing an understanding of TB within the Somali community in Sheffield. Sheffield Hallam University. Available: http://shura.shu.ac.uk/7290/1/Somali_TB_report_final_14-08-10.pdf. Accessed 2014 Sept 20.
36. O'Mara A, Marrero-Guillamón I, Jamal F, Lehmann A, Cooper C, et al. (2010) Tuberculosis evidence review 1: Review of barriers and facilitators. National Institute for Health and Clinical Excellence. Available: http://www.nice.org.uk/guidance/ph37/resources/review-1-review-of-barriers-and-facilitators2. Accessed: 2014 Sept 20.
37. Guirgis M, Nusair F, Bu YM, Yan K, Zekry AT (2012) Barriers faced by migrants in accessing healthcare for viral hepatitis infection. Intern Med J 42(5): 491–496.
38. van der Veen Y, de Zwart O, Voeten H, Mackenbach J, Richardus J (2009) Hepatitis B screening in the Turkish-Dutch population in Rotterdam, the Netherlands; qualitative assessment of socio-cultural determinants. BMC Public Health 9(1): 328.
39. Brewin P, Jones A, Kelly M, McDonald E, Sturdy P, et al. (2006) Is screening for tuberculosis acceptable to immigrants? A qualitative study. J Public Health 28: 253–260.
40. Hargreaves S, Seedat F, Car J, Escombe R, Hassan S, et al. (2014) Screening for latent TB, HIV, and hepatitis B/C in new migrants in a high prevalence area of London, UK: a cross-sectional study. In press.
41. Lewis H, Burke K, Begum S, Ushiro-Limb I, Foster G (2011) What is the best method of case finding for chronic viral hepatitis in migrant communities? Gut 60: A26.
42. Adhikari N, Menzies R (1995) Community-based tuberculin screening in Montreal: a cost-outcome description. Am J Public Health 85(6): 786–90.
43. Migrant Friendly Hospitals (2004) The Amsterdam Declaration Towards Migrant Friendly Hospitals in an ethno-culturally diverse Europe. Migrant Friendly Hospitals. Available: http://www.mfh-eu.net/public/european_recommendations.htm. Accessed: 2014 Sept 20.
44. Griffiths C, Sturdy P, Brewin P, Bothamley G, Eldridge S, et al. (2007) Educational outreach to promote screening for tuberculosis in in primary care: a cluster randomised controlled trial. Lancet 369(9572): 1528–1534.
45. Van den Bosch CA, Roberts JA (2000) Tuberculosis screening of new entrants; how can it be made more effective? J Public Health 22: 220–223.
46. Jafferbhoy H, Miller MH, McIntyre P, Dillon JF (2012) The effectiveness of outreach testing for hepatitis C in an immigrant Pakistani population. Epidemiol Infect 140(6): 1048–1053.
47. Sadler KE, McGarrigle CA, Elam G, Ssanyu-Sseruma W, Othieno G, et al. (2006) Mayisha II: Pilot of a community-based survey of sexual attitudes and lifestyles and anonymous HIV testing within African communities in London. AIDS Care 18(4): 398–403.

48. Lewis H, Burke K, Begum S, Ushiro-Limb I, Foster G (2012) What is the best method of case finding for chronic viral Hepatitis in at-risk migrant communities? J Hepatol 56: S351.
49. Gany F, Trinh-Shevrin C, Changrani J (2005) Drive-by Readings: A Creative Strategy for Tuberculosis Control Among Immigrants. Am J Public Health 95(1): 117–19.
50. Brassard P, Steensma C, Cadieux L, Lands LC (2006) Evaluation of a School-Based Tuberculosis-Screening Program and Associate Investigation Targeting Recently Immigrated Children in a Low-Burden Country. Pediatrics 117(2): e148–e156.

19

# The Efficacy of Mindfulness-Based Cognitive Therapy as a Public Mental Health Intervention for Adults with Mild to Moderate Depressive Symptomatology: A Randomized Controlled Trial

**Wendy T. M. Pots[1,2]*, Peter A. M. Meulenbeek[1,3], Martine M. Veehof[1], Jorinde Klungers[3], Ernst T. Bohlmeijer[1]**

**1** University of Twente, Department of Psychology, Health & Technology, Enschede, the Netherlands, **2** Dimence, Community Mental Health Center, Almelo, the Netherlands, **3** GGNET, Community Mental Health Center, Warnsveld, the Netherlands

## Abstract

***Objective:*** Although there has been growing evidence for the efficacy of mindfulness-based cognitive therapy (MBCT) for different clinical populations, its effectiveness as a public mental health intervention has not been studied. The present study evaluates a community-based MBCT intervention for adults with mild to moderate depressive symptomatology in a large multi-site, pragmatic randomized controlled trial.

***Method:*** The participants with mild to moderate depressive symptomatology were recruited from the general population and randomized to the MBCT intervention (n = 76) or to a waiting list control group (n = 75). Participants completed measures before and after the intervention. Participants in the experimental condition also completed these measures at a 3-month follow-up.

***Results:*** In the experimental condition significant reductions in depression, anxiety, and experiential avoidance, and improvements in mindfulness and emotional- and psychological mental health were found, compared to the waiting list (effect sizes Cohen's d = 0.31–0.56). These effects were sustained at the 3-month follow-up. The likelihood of a clinically significant change in depressive symptoms was significantly higher for the MBCT group [odds ratio (OR) 3.026, $p<0.01$ at post-treatment; NNT = 5.10].

***Discussion:*** MBCT as a public mental health intervention for adults with mild to moderate depressive symptoms seems effective and applicable in a natural setting.

***Trial Registration:*** Nederlands Trial Register NTR2096

**Editor:** Gabriel S. Dichter, UNC Chapel Hill, United States of America

**Funding:** The study was funded by University of Twente (www.utwente.nl). The funder had no role in study design, data collection and analysis, decision to publish, or preparation of the manuscript.

**Competing Interests:** The authors have declared that no competing interests exist.

* Email: w.t.m.pots@utwente.nl

## Introduction

Minor depression is a highly prevalent disorder with a large negative impact on quality of life and yielding high economic costs [1]. Offering interventions for people with depressive symptomatology is a necessary public mental health strategy complementary to the treatment of depression in inpatient and outpatient settings [2]. One such effective strategy is to pro-actively offer treatments for people with mild to moderate symptoms of depression [3,4]. However, a public mental health intervention needs to be attractive for people who don't suffer from severe symptoms of depression yet [5]. Using a positive framework and promoting positive mental health as well as reducing psychological distress offers opportunities to attract more people [6–8]. Mindfulness-based cognitive therapy (MBCT) may be such an intervention, as it focuses on promoting positive mental health instead of only focusing on the reduction of psychological distress. MBCT is an 8 week group based training that combines meditation exercises with cognitive techniques. It was originally designed for prevention of relapse in people with recurrent depression [9]. In patients with three or more previous episodes of depression, MBCT significantly reduced the risk of relapse compared to the treatment as usual [10–12]. Moreover, in a recently published randomized controlled trial Williams et al. [13] found evidence that the number of episodes is a marker for those with greater vulnerability due to a history of childhood trauma and adversity. Strauss et al. [14] conducted a meta-analysis on mindfulness based interventions for people diagnosed with a current episode of an anxiety or depressive disorder and found that MBCT can also be effective for people who are currently depressed. MBCT targets processes such as avoidance of negative emotions and engaging with maladaptive thinking and rumination, that maintain depressive symptomatology in general [15,16]. Mindfulness is often referred to as intentionally paying attention to present moment experiences in a non-judgemental way [17]. Awareness and acceptance of negative experiences will reduce experiential avoidance (EA) [15]. EA has been defined as the unwillingness to remain in contact with experiences such as feelings, thoughts, and bodily sensations, as an attempted means of behavioral regulation [15]. Psychological flexibility is the counterpart of experiential avoidance. As EA could be seen as an important factor that maintains depressive symptomatology, MBCT may also be effective as a public mental health intervention for people with depressive symptomatology. This fits with a growing interest in adapting MBCT to other psychiatric disorders, such as anxiety disorders, and bipolar disorder, but also treatment-resistant major depressive disorder (for a recent review see Chiesa & Serretti [18]). Research into the potential mechanisms of action in MBCT is in its infancy. In a recent review Chiesa and Serretti [19] suggested that mindfulness-based interventions may enhance positive emotion regulation strategies, as well as self-compassion levels, and decrease rumination and experiential avoidance. They suggested that these changes are associated with several clinical benefits, including the reduction of stress and depression levels, as well as the enhancement of positive emotions. Recently, Kaviani et al. [20] found that MBCT can be effective in a non-clinical population of female students in Iran. Also, Cavanagh et al. [21] adapted MBCT as a brief online intervention and found it to be effective in a non-clinical population of students. To our knowledge, there is no research on the effectiveness of a community-based MBCT intervention for adults with depressive symptomatology. In order to modify the original MBCT as a public mental health intervention a few changes were made in time-investment. We expected a community-based MBCT with a reduced weekly time-investment to be more acceptable for the target group.

The aim of this study was to evaluate the effect of mindfulness-based cognitive therapy modified as a public mental health intervention for depressive symptomatology, in a sample of self-referred adults with mild to moderate depressive symptomatology, and offered by community mental health centers. We evaluated the effect with respect to various psychological variables, such as depression, anxiety and positive mental health. We hypothesized that changes in depressive symptoms would be mediated by psychological flexibility and mindfulness. To strengthen the trial's external validity, the intervention was studied in its natural setting.

## Method

The protocol for this trial and supporting CONSORT checklist are available as supporting information; see Checklist S1 and Protocol S1. This study was approved by the METiGG, a medical ethics committee for research in mental health settings in the Netherlands. In addition, this study has been registered in the Nederlands Trial Register, the Primary Dutch register for clinical trials (NTR2096).

### Design

A pragmatic, multi-site, randomized controlled trial was conducted comparing MBCT with a control condition. Participants were randomly assigned after receiving their written consent, either to MBCT or to the waiting list control, by means of a centrally conducted randomization process executed by an independent researcher. The randomization was carried out for the two groups with stratification on gender, using a computer generated random sequence of numbers. The control condition consisted of a waiting list, where wait-listed people were free to use other kinds of care. The wait-listed participants knew that they could start the training after the experimental condition had completed the intervention, i.e. after 3 months. The study is pragmatic as it mimics the Dutch health care system as closely as possible in terms of patient recruitment, conducting intake, offering interventions, and monitoring outcomes.

### Participants and procedure

Participants were recruited from November 2009 until October 2010, through advertisements in regional newspapers, information booklets and general practitioners. Four Dutch community mental health centers, from both urban and rural areas, participated in the study. In the advertisements, distributed within the regions of the participating community mental health services, the target group was described as adults who were hindered by depressive symptoms. Applicants were referred to a specifically developed website, where they could find detailed information about the study. When interested, they were sent an information letter and an informed consent form. For screening, the standard procedures employed by the mental health institutions were used. The community mental health centers were responsible for the procedure, and the in- and exclusion criteria were examined by experienced mental health nurses on the basis of a checklist, under supervision of a clinical psychologist. The inclusion criteria were: adults of 18 years and over, presenting depressive symptoms. Applicants were excluded if diagnosed with a current severe major depressive episode (MDE; eight or nine out of a total of nine symptoms) or when having a moderate to high suicide risk, according to the Dutch version of the Mini International Neuropsychiatric Interview (MINI) [22,23]. Other exclusion criteria were: receiving psychological or pharmacological treatment for mental complaints within the last three months, and presence of other severe mental or social problems warranting treatment or likely to interfere with participation in the group course. People meeting one of the exclusion criteria were advised to seek regular treatment.

### Power analysis

A sample of 60 participants per condition at post-intervention was needed to detect an effect size of 0.50 (Cohen's d) for the primary outcome with a statistical power of $(1-\beta)=0.80$ in a two-tailed test ($p<0.05$). Taking into account a drop-out rate of 20%, 150 eligible participants were needed.

### Measures

Measurements were taken at baseline (T0), and at post-treatment after 3 months (T1). In order to study the stability of the effect of MBCT, the patients in the experimental group received a follow-up measurement (T2) at 6 months after baseline. For the control condition, the measurement at 6 months is a post-treatment measurement. All measurements had good psychometric properties and are frequently applied in international studies.

The primary outcome measure was depressive symptomatology, measured by the Dutch version of the Center of Epidemiological Studies - Depression Scale (CES-D; 20 items, score 0–60) [24]. Higher scores mean more depressive symptoms [24,25].

Secondary outcome measures were anxiety symptoms and positive mental health. Anxiety was measured by the Hospital

Anxiety and Depression Scale - Anxiety subscale (HADS-A; 7 items, score 0–21) [26] for assessing the presence and severity of anxiety symptoms. Higher scores mean more anxiety symptoms [26,27]. Positive mental health was measured by the Mental Health Continuum - Short Form (MHC-SF) [28], that measures emotional well-being (3 items; score 0–15), social well-being (5 items; score 0–25) and psychological well-being (6 items; score 0–30). Higher scores indicate greater emotional, social, and psychological well-being [28,29].

Measures of proposed processes of change included measures of EA and mindfulness. The Acceptance and Action Questionnaire-II (AAQ-II; 10 items, score 10–70) [30] was used to measure the willingness to be in contact with aversive internal experiences, to accept these events, and to pursue values in the presence of the experiences. Higher scores indicate lower levels of EA or higher levels of psychological flexibility [30,31]. The Five Facet Mindfulness Questionnaire (FFMQ) [32] was used to measure mindfulness in five sub-dimensions: (1) observing (8 items), defined in terms of noticing or attending to internal and external experiences; (2) describing (8 items), defined in terms of labelling internal experiences with words; (3) acting with awareness (8 items), defined in terms of attending to one's activities of the moment (opposite of acting on automatic pilot); (4) non-judging of inner experience (8 items), defined in terms of taking a non-evaluative stance toward thoughts and feelings; and (5) and non-reactivity to inner experience (7 items), defined in terms of allowing thoughts and feelings to come and go, without getting caught up in or carried away by them. Facet scores range from 8 to 40 (except for the non-reactivity, which ranges from 7 to 35), with higher scores indicating more mindfulness [32,33].

To evaluate the level of satisfaction of the participants after the intervention, a self-developed evaluation questionnaire was used, including a question on how the participants evaluated the program using a scale from 1(very poor) to 10 (excellent).

## Waiting list control

Participants in the control condition participated in the MBCT training after a 3-month waiting list period. Participants were instructed to seek help from their general practitioner, family or other sources, as they normally would, should they encounter symptomatic deterioration or other difficulties during the waiting list period.

## Intervention

In this study MBCT was delivered according to the guidelines of Segal et al. [9]. The original training was adapted to suit a public mental health approach. The intervention was aimed at people with mild to moderate symptoms of depression. In order to lower the threshold for people without severe distress to participate in MBCT, the participants were asked to practice meditations for 15 minutes a day instead of the original 45 minutes a day, and the sessions were limited to 1, 5 hours instead of the original 2, 5 hours. To ensure that all of the elements of the original course were preserved, the eight-session training was extended to 11 sessions. Key themes of the sessions included awareness (sessions 1, 2, 3), acceptance (sessions 5, 7, 9, 10) and disengaging from thoughts (sessions 4, 6, 8), with the last session (session 11) focusing on evaluation and integration. The training teaches skills to become more aware of, and to relate differently to thoughts, feelings and bodily sensations. A core feature of the training is to learn to become aware of, and disengage from habitual dysfunctional (cognitive) routines, to stop reacting automatically to internal experiences, and to act more 'mindfully'. During the period of the training, the program consisted of daily homework exercises. The exercises were aimed at increasing attention to present moment experiences in a non-judgmental way, together with exercises designed to integrate application of awareness skills into daily life. To support homework assignments, participants received weekly homework registration forms, guided (taped) and unguided meditations, and information in a booklet. Group sizes varied between eight and 15 participants.

## Therapists

The MBCT instructors were all experienced psychologists and mental health nurses, with extensive former training in the original MBCT protocol by Segal [9] and Group psychotherapy. The trainers were also experienced meditators, with meditation experience ranging from 2 to 15 years.

## Statistical analyses

The statistical analyses were performed using SPSS 18. The data was analyzed on an intention-to-treat (ITT) basis. Missing values at baseline, post-intervention and follow-up were imputed with the use of SPSS Missing Value Analysis on the continuous measures with the expectation-maximization (EM) method. This method computes missing values based on maximum likelihood estimates using observed data in an iterative process [34]. The total percentage of missing data (T0-T1-T2) was 5%, due to unanswered items (0,6%) and incomplete assessments (4,4%). A comparison of results based on the imputed intention-to-treat sample versus the observed data revealed similar outcomes. Therefore, only the results from the intention-to-treat analyses are reported.

Independent sample t-tests and chi-square tests were conducted to examine differences between the two groups at baseline on sociodemographic variables and outcome measures. Analysis of covariance (ANCOVA) was conducted with depressive symptoms post-treatment as the dependent variable, treatment group as the independent variable, and five covariates consisting of pre-treatment depression score and four dummy-coded variables for each treatment site. The same analyses were conducted for the secondary measures. Analysis of variance (ANOVA) was conducted with process measures post-treatment as the dependent variable and treatment group as the independent variable. Assumptions for performing parametric analysis of (co)variance were all met. To investigate whether the effects in the intervention condition were maintained at follow-up paired-sample t-tests were carried out, comparing the scores on the follow-up (T2) with those at baseline (T0). Also, paired-sample t-tests were carried out for the control group, to measure the effect of the MBCT intervention after the waiting time period, comparing scores at post-treatment (T2 for the control group) with those at pre-treatment (T1 for the control group).

Effect sizes at post-treatment (T0-T1) were calculated with Cohen's d using the means and the pooled standard deviations of the measurements in the conditions. For the effect sizes at follow-up (T0-T2) the Cohen's d was corrected for dependence among means by using the correlation between the two means [35]. To interpret Cohen's d an effect size of less than 0.33 is considered small, while 0.33 to 0.55 is considered moderate and effect sizes of 0.56 to 1.2 are considered large [36]. Comparisons were two-tailed and interpreted with a significance value of $p<0.05$.

With the Jacobson and Truax methodology, the proportion of participants was determined who made a clinically significant change on the CES-D from baseline to post-treatment [37]. First, the reliable change was calculated with the reliable change index (RCI). Jacobson and Truax suggest that subjects can be considered to have improved when they shift from a dysfunctional distribution to a functional one, and the reliable change scores exceed measurement error (calculated by dividing the difference between the pretest and posttest scores by the standard error of the measurement). Second, the recovery criterion was defined as a post-treatment score below the cut-off value of 16 for clinically relevant depressive symptoms [38,39]. Because we studied a population with a mild to moderate symptomatology, the mean score at baseline was already at the recovery criterion (M = 16.04; range 1–43; S.D. = 8.08). A clinically significant change on the CES-D is thus defined as having a reliable change between the measurements, which required a post-treatment score below the cut-off of 16. Participants that had a clinically significant change were either coded 1 (implying a favorable treatment response, 'success') or 0 ('failure'). The binary outcome was used to calculate the odds ratio (OR) using logistic regression. Based on the clinically significant change proportions, the number needed to treat (NNT) was calculated [40]. To provide a more complete representation of the effects of the intervention, the outcomes were also analyzed for intervention completers only (somewhat arbitrarily defined as participants that attended at least 9 sessions).

The process measures were expected to be mediators between the MBCT intervention and post-treatment levels of depressive symptomatology (CES-D). Mediation was performed for all process measures that were significantly different between the intervention and control condition in the ANOVA. Then, all steps outlined by Baron and Kenny [41] were used. In the first step linear regression analysis was performed, with treatment group as independent variable and depressive symptoms post-treatment as the dependent variable. In the second step we tested the effect of the independent variable on the proposed mediators with linear regression analyses, with treatment group as independent variable and the residual change scores of the proposed mediators as the dependent variables. The third step tested the effect of the proposed mediator on the dependent variable. The indirect effect of the mediator on the outcome was assessed to examine whether an increase in psychological flexibility and mindfulness during the intervention would mediate the effects of the intervention on depressive symptomatology at post-intervention. Simple mediational analyses with bootstrapping procedures (n = 5000 bootstrap resamples) were used to assess the indirect effect of the mediator on the outcome [42]. An indirect effect was considered significant in the case zero was not contained in the 95% confidence interval.

## Results

### Enrollment, treatment adherence, satisfaction and drop-out

Figure 1 provides an overview of the flow of participants. A total of 251 persons were interested in the training. During telephone screening, 43 persons presented other psychiatric symptoms or practical restraints that precluded them from participation in the trial. The remaining 208 applicants were assessed for eligibility. Through interviewing, a further 57 were excluded. After signing the informed consent form, the included 151 participants were randomly assigned to the MBCT intervention (n = 76) and the waiting list condition (n = 75).

After randomization, two participants decided not to start with the intervention due to time constraints (n = 1) and health problems (n = 1). Four other participants in the MBCT (8%) group did not complete the intervention (attendance of at least 9 sessions). The reasons given for non-completion were that the intervention was too time consuming (n = 1), practicality reasons (n = 1), insufficient concentration (n = 1), and an unknown reason (n = 1). Two of the four community mental health centers evaluated the course resulting in anonymous evaluation forms of all participants, including those who did not participate in the study. Based on these results overall the intervention was evaluated as positive on a scale from 1 to 10 (m = 7.98, sd = 0.72, n = 130).

At T1 (post-treatment for the MBCT group and pre-treatment for the waiting list group), data was available for 143 participants (drop-out rate 5.3%) and at T2 (follow-up for the MBCT group and post-treatment for the waiting list group), data was available for 139 participants (drop-out rate 7.9%). There were no significant differences at baseline on all the measurements between participants who completed the assessments and those who did not complete all measures.

### Baseline characteristics

Table 1 shows an overview of the participants' characteristics. Participants had a mean age of 48 years (SD = 11.29, range 20–81) and were predominantly female (78.1%). The majority was of Dutch origin (96%), had a paid job (66.9%), and were living with a partner (75.5%). The level of education was high for 65.5% of the participants and intermediate for 30.5%. At the entry of the study, 2.6% met the criteria of mild MDE and 4% were diagnosed with moderate MDE. There were no significant differences at baseline between the MBCT group and the control group for any of the demographic variables or outcome measurements. Also, there were no significant changes in the waiting time period for the control group, comparing scores at baseline (T0) with pre-treatment measurement (T1), on any of the outcome measures.

## Treatment effects

### Primary outcome

The means and standard deviations for the primary outcome measure, the results of the ANCOVA and the effect sizes are presented in Table 2. Compared to the control condition, participants in the intervention condition reported significantly decreased depressive symptoms at post-treatment (Table 2). The effects of the intervention condition on depressive symptoms were maintained at follow-up compared to baseline measurement [$t(75) = -3.46$, $p<0.01$]. Moderate effect sizes were found at post-treatment ($d = 0.50$) and follow-up ($d = 0.40$). The control group also showed significant reductions in depression after they received the intervention at T2 [$t(74) = -3.03$, $p<0.01$].

### Clinically significant change

The reliable change on the CES-D appeared to be a pre-post difference of at least 7 scale points. Clinically significant change was thus defined as a recovery condition of a score ≤16 points on the CES-D (n = 138) and a RCI of 7 points. The proportion of participants with a score of ≥7 at T0 that reached a clinically significant change was 24/70 (34%) in the intervention group, versus 10/68 (15%) in the control condition [OR 3.026, 95% confidence interval (CI) 1.316–6.961, p<0.01, NNT = 5.10, under an intention-to-treat analysis]. These results compare well with completers-only findings: OR 2.916, 95% CI 1.252–6.795, p< 0.01, NNT = 5.26.

### Secondary outcome measures

The means and standard deviations for the secondary outcome measures, the results of the ANCOVA and the effect sizes are presented in Table 2. Compared to the control condition, participants in the intervention condition reported significantly decreased anxiety symptoms after the intervention. At follow-up, the effects of the intervention condition on anxiety symptoms were maintained compared to baseline measurement [$t(75) = -8.40$,

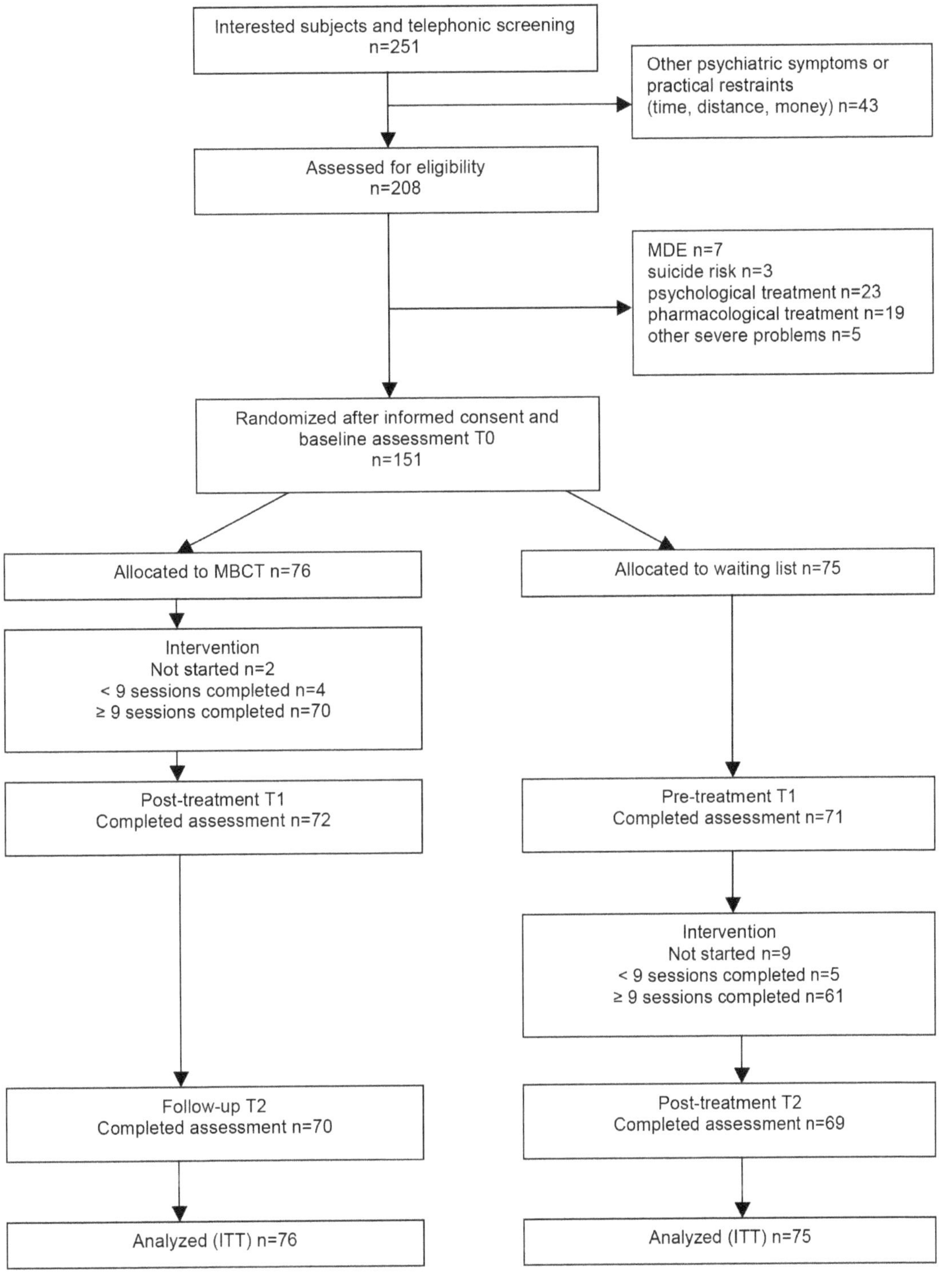


**Figure 1. Participant flow.** MDE = major depressive episode.

$p<0.001$]. The effect sizes for anxiety symptoms at post-treatment ($d = 0.56$) and at follow-up ($d = 0.97$) were large. The control group also showed significant reductions in anxiety after they received the intervention at T2 [$t(74) = -5.15$, $p<0.001$].

At post treatment, significant improvements in emotional well-being and psychological well-being were found. The effects of the intervention condition on emotional and psychological well-being were maintained at follow-up compared to baseline measurement [emotional well-being $t(75) = 4.13$, $p<0.001$; psychological well-being $t(75) = 5.20$, $p<0.001$]. Effect sizes at post-treatment were small (emotional well-being, $d = 0.31$) to moderate (psychological well-being, $d = 0.34$). The effect sizes at follow-up were moderate (emotional well-being, $d = 0.50$) to large (psychological well-being, $d = 0.56$). No significant effects were found at post-treatment for social well-being, with a small effect size ($d = 0.22$). At follow-up, there was a significant increase in social well-being compared to

**Table 1.** Baseline characteristics of the total sample, MBCT intervention and waiting list control condition.

| | | MBCT (n = 76) | | Waiting list (n = 75) | | Total (n = 151) | |
|---|---|---|---|---|---|---|---|
| | | n | % | n | % | n | % |
| *Age*[a] | Mean (SD) | 47.99 (10.59) | | 47.88 (12.02) | | 47.93 (11.29) | |
| | Range | 24–74 | | 20–81 | | 20–81 | |
| *Gender*[b] | Female | 59 | 77,6 | 59 | 78,7 | 118 | 78,1 |
| | Male | 17 | 22,4 | 16 | 21,3 | 33 | 21,9 |
| *Marital status*[b] | Single | 17 | 22,4 | 20 | 26,7 | 37 | 24,5 |
| | **Living with partner** | 59 | 77,6 | 55 | 73,3 | 114 | 75,5 |
| *Race*[b] | Dutch | 71 | 93,4 | 74 | 98,7 | 145 | 96,0 |
| | Other | 5 | 6,6 | 1 | 1,3 | 6 | 4,0 |
| *Education*[b] | Low | 2 | 2,6 | 4 | 5,3 | 6 | 4,0 |
| | Middle | 21 | 27,6 | 25 | 33,3 | 46 | 30,5 |
| | High | 53 | 69,7 | 46 | 61,3 | 99 | 65,5 |
| *Employment*[b] | Paid | 53 | 69,7 | 48 | 64,0 | 101 | 66,9 |
| | No paid | 23 | 30,3 | 27 | 36,0 | 50 | 33,1 |
| *Diagnosis*[b] | Mild MDE | 3 | 3,9 | 1 | 1,3 | 4 | 2,6 |
| | Moderate MDE | 0 | 0,0 | 6 | 8,0 | 6 | 4,0 |

*Note.* MDE, major depressive episode.
[a] No significant differences between intervention and control condition (t-test with $P<0.05$).
[b] No significant differences between intervention and control condition (chi-square-test with $P<0.05$).

**Table 2.** Means and standard deviations for outcome measures and results of ANCOVA for intervention effects, and Cohen's d.

| Measures | MBCT | | Waiting list | | | | |
|---|---|---|---|---|---|---|---|
| | (n = 76) | | (n = 75) | | | | |
| | M[a] | SD[a] | M[a] | SD[a] | F(df)[b] | P | d |
| *Primary outcome* | | | | | | | |
| CES-D baseline | 15.62 | 7.86 | 16.46 | 8.32 | | | |
| CES-D post-treatment | 11.79 | 8.76 | 16.43 | 9.94 | 10.91(1) | 0.001 | 0.50 |
| CES-D follow-up[c] | 11.77 | 8.25 | 13.60 | 8.88 | | | |
| *Secondary outcomes* | | | | | | | |
| HADS-A baseline | 7.96 | 3.40 | 8.57 | 3.58 | | | |
| HADS-A post-treatment | 6.14 | 3.52 | 8.22 | 3.89 | 12.42(1) | 0.001 | 0.56 |
| HADS-A follow-up[c] | 4.88 | 2.88 | 6.54 | 3.84 | | | |
| MHC-SF-EM baseline | 3.15 | 0.95 | 3.15 | 0.78 | | | |
| MHC-SF-EM post-treatment | 3.46 | 0.85 | 3.19 | 0.88 | 5.32(1) | 0.023 | 0.31 |
| MHC-SF-EM follow-up[c] | 3.54 | 0.95 | 3.61 | 0.78 | | | |
| MHC-SF-SOC baseline | 2.38 | 1.04 | 2.28 | 0.96 | | | |
| MHC-SF-SOC post-treatment | 2.72 | 1.08 | 2.49 | 1.05 | 1.62(1) | 0.206 | 0.22 |
| MHC-SF-SOC follow-up[c] | 2.91 | 1.12 | 2.85 | 0.86 | | | |
| MHC-SF-PSY baseline | 2.92 | 0.89 | 2.96 | 1.00 | | | |
| MHC-SF-PSY post-treatment | 3.26 | 0.98 | 2.90 | 1.11 | 8.60(1) | 0.004 | 0.34 |
| MHC-SF-PSY follow-up[c] | 3.37 | 0.93 | 3.41 | 0.89 | | | |

*Note*. ANCOVA, Analysis of covariance; CES-D, Center for Epidemiologic Studies - Depression.
Scale; HADS-A, Hospital Anxiety and Depression Scale - Anxiety subscale; MHC-SF, Mental Health Continuum - Short form; EM, emotional; SOC, social; PSY, psychological.
[a] Unadjusted condition means and standard deviations (SD).
[b] F-value, corrected for baseline values.
[c] Follow-up for intervention group and post-treatment for waiting list group.

baseline measurement [t(75) = 5.58, p<0.001], with a large effect size ($d = 0.63$).

The control group showed significant reductions on positive mental health after they received the intervention at T2 [social well-being t(74) = 4.79, p<0.001; emotional well-being t(74) = 5.47, p<0.001; psychological well-being t(74) = 6.21, p< 0.001].

### Process measures

Table 3 shows all process measurements, the results of the ANOVA, and the effect-sizes. Compared to the control condition, participants in the intervention condition showed significant improvement in psychological flexibility and all mindfulness facets (except for FFMQ-Describe). The effects of the intervention condition on all process measures were maintained at follow-up compared to baseline measurement [psychological flexibility, t(75) = 6.17, p<0.001; FFMQ observing, t(75) = 7.67, p<0.001; FFMQ describing, t(75) = 6.82, p<0.001; FFMQ acting with awareness, t(75) = 6.20, p<0.001; FFMQ non-judging of inner experience, t(75) = 6.46, p<0.001; FFMQ non-reactivity to inner experience, t(75) = 8.97, p<0.001]. The effect sizes post-treatment were small to large ($d = 0.13$–$0.84$) and large at follow-up ($d = 0.71$–$1.03$).

### Mediational analyses

Figure 2 shows the results of the first three steps of mediation. The FFMQ-Describe was excluded from the mediational analyses, having no significantly different effect in the ANOVA. The first step shows that the intervention condition had significantly decreased depressive symptoms at post-treatment, compared to the control condition. Step two shows that the intervention condition was significantly improved in psychological flexibility and mindfulness compared to the control condition. In step 3, all change scores of the process measures were significantly associated with the scores on the CES-D at post-treatment. In the last step of the mediational analysis, following Preacher & Hayes [42], results showed that the effect of the intervention on depressive symptoms was mediated by all process measures. Full mediation was found for improvement of psychological flexibility (direct effect β = .145, p = 0.057; indirect effect β = −.387, 95% CI 0.89–3.45), and mindfulness facets Observing (direct effect β = 0.132, p = 0.106; indirect effect β = −.308, 95% CI 0.98–3.60), and Non-reactivity to inner experience (direct effect β = .135, p = 0.108; indirect effect β = −.275, 95% CI 0.83−3.73). Partial mediation was found for improvement of mindfulness facets Acting with awareness (direct effect β = .176, p = 0.044; indirect effect β = −.160, 95% CI 0.18–2.84), and Non-judging of inner experience (direct effect β = .208, p = .011; indirect effect β = −.158, 95% CI 0.06–1.74).

## Discussion

### Main findings

To our best knowledge, this is the first study that evaluated MBCT as a public mental health intervention for adults with mild to moderate depressive symptomatology within a large pragmatic multi-site trial. The potential of offering MBCT to the community as a public mental health intervention is of importance, as the idea that MBCT is only effective in patients suffering from recurrent depression is superseded. In the present study the participants suffered from mild to moderate depressive symptoms but differed from severe clinical samples, as indicated by the substantially lower mean degree of severity of depressive symptoms as measured by the CES-D and the MINI. This corresponds to the nature and structure of the community-based MBCT, offered in our study.

The results from this study indicate that MBCT as a public mental health intervention is effective in reducing depressive symptoms. We found a moderate effect size for depressive symptoms at post-treatment in comparison with the control group (d = 0.50). This effect size is comparable to the effect size of 0.42 that was found for psychological treatments on subthreshold depression [43]. The only studies of MBCT in community-based samples to our knowledge are from Kaviani et al. [20] and Cavanagh et al. [21]. Both conducted a randomized controlled trial in a sample of students comparing MBCT to a waiting list control group. They showed significant reductions of depressive and anxiety symptoms over time, with effect limited by low generalizability. Our study corroborates with these findings, further showing that MBCT seems to be effective in a population of adults with mild to moderate depressive symptomatology, and that MBCT can be used as a public mental health intervention in the community. Our finding that the results are maintained at 3 months follow-up is promising, but needs to be substantiated by longer follow-up measurements under controlled conditions. Offering a public mental health intervention in a positive framework might be less stigmatizing for participants with depressive symptomatology or minor depression [5]. MBCT focuses on the enhancement of promoting positive skills and therefore has the potential to offer an alternative to stigmatization.

The likelihood of a clinically significant change in depressive symptomatology in our study was substantially higher in the intervention condition compared to the waiting-list control group. As the presence of clinically relevant depressive symptoms is known to be an important risk factor for clinical depression [44], this outcome suggests that MBCT implemented as a public mental health intervention for adults with mild to moderate depressive symptomatology may decrease the risk of developing a MDE. It is shown that the effects on clinical cases of interventions for people with sub-clinical symptomatology are most prominently found after longer periods of time [45]. However this result needs to be corroborated with longer follow-up measurement and the use of diagnostic instruments as outcome measures.

Moreover, the MBCT intervention resulted in significant reductions in anxiety symptoms with large effect sizes post-treatment and at the 3-month follow-up. The effect of MBCT on anxiety symptoms are consistent with the meta-analysis by Vøllestad et al. [46], which found a large effect size (g = 0.83) for controlled studies of mindfulness and acceptance-based interventions for patients with anxiety symptoms. Strauss et al. [14] found no effects on anxiety symptom severity in their meta-analysis, applying a more stringent definition and excluding trials with interventions based on Acceptance and Commitment Therapy. Our study supports the findings of Vøllestad et al. [46], indicating that MBCT as a public mental health intervention could be effective in not only reducing depressive symptoms, but also in significantly reducing anxiety symptoms post-treatment and, even more substantially, at the 3-month follow-up. As anxiety symptoms often coexist with depression and may precipitate depression [47], these findings could indicate that the application of MBCT has the potential to further decrease the incidence of depression. However, this needs to be substantiated by further research.

The results also show a significant effect on positive mental health. It thus seems that MBCT has the potential not only to reduce psychological distress, but also to improve emotional, psychological, and social (only at follow-up) well-being as well. This finding confirms earlier studies that show that MBCT can promote well-being in patients with anxiety or depression [20,48]. The effects of MBCT on positive mental health are of importance.

**Table 3.** Means and standard deviations for process measures, results of ANOVA and Cohen's d for intervention effects.

| Measures | MBCT | | Waiting list | | | | |
|---|---|---|---|---|---|---|---|
| | (n = 76) | | (n = 75) | | | | |
| Process outcomes | M | SD | M | SD | F(df) | P | d |
| AAQ-II baseline | 44.28 | 8.42 | 43.03 | 7.86 | | | |
| AAQ-II post-treatment | 49.59 | 8.80 | 44.36 | 10.01 | 11.62(1) | 0.001 | 0.56 |
| AAQ-II follow-up[a] | 50.93 | 9.04 | 48.91 | 8.89 | | | |
| FFMQ - Observe baseline | 24.77 | 5.58 | 25.21 | 5.77 | | | |
| FFMQ - Observe post-treatment | 27.98 | 5.15 | 25.28 | 6.29 | 8.34(1) | 0.004 | 0.47 |
| FFMQ - Observe follow-up[a] | 28.46 | 4.54 | 29.07 | 4.74 | | | |
| FFMQ - Describe baseline | 26.39 | 6.14 | 27.43 | 6.89 | | | |
| FFMQ - Describe post-treatment | 28.60 | 5.56 | 27.80 | 6.35 | 0.68(1) | 0.410 | 0.13 |
| FFMQ - Describe follow-up[a] | 29.24 | 6.03 | 29.77 | 6.76 | | | |
| FFMQ - ActAware baseline | 20.92 | 5.45 | 22.61 | 5.48 | | | |
| FFMQ - ActAware post-treatment | 25.31 | 5.53 | 22.67 | 6.05 | 7.86(1) | 0.006 | 0.46 |
| FFMQ - ActAware follow-up[a] | 25.08 | 5.51 | 26.31 | 5.30 | | | |
| FFMQ - NonJudge baseline | 23.64 | 6.04 | 22.87 | 5.48 | | | |
| FFMQ - NonJudge post-treatment | 27.68 | 5.16 | 24.72 | 5.66 | 11.28(1) | 0.001 | 0.55 |
| FFMQ - NonJudge follow-up[a] | 28.16 | 5.57 | 28.05 | 5.52 | | | |
| FFMQ - NonReact baseline | 19.73 | 4.29 | 19.31 | 4.29 | | | |
| FFMQ - NonReact post-treatment | 23.86 | 4.27 | 20.24 | 4.32 | 26.82(1) | 0.000 | 0.84 |
| FFMQ - NonReact follow-up[a] | 24.24 | 4.04 | 23.54 | 4.22 | | | |

*Note.* AAQ-II, Acceptance and Action Questionnaire-II; ANOVA, Analysis of variance; FFMQ, Five Facet Mindfulness Questionnaire; Observe, observing; Describe, describing; ActAware, acting with awareness; NonJudge, non-judging of inner experience; NonReact, non-reactivity to inner experience.

[a] Follow-up for intervention group and post-treatment for waiting list group.

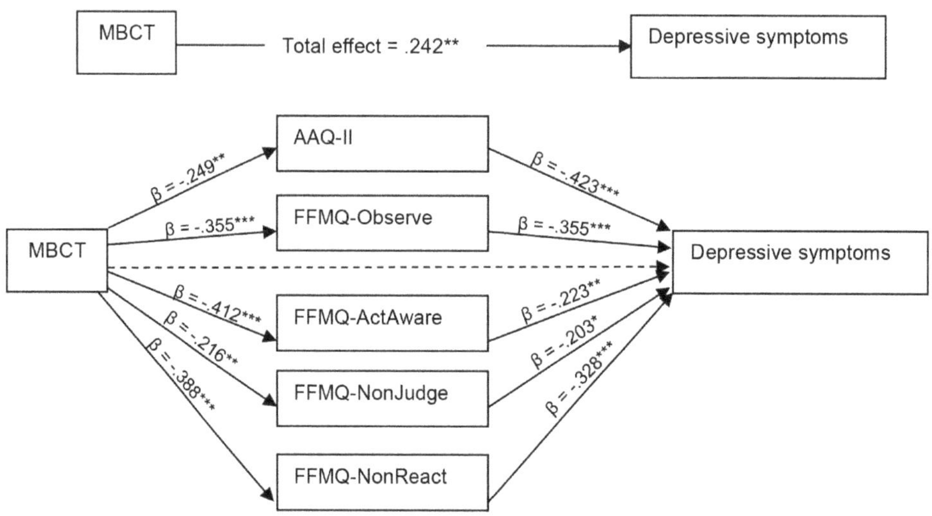


**Figure 2. Mediation model of psychological flexibility and mindfulness as mediators.** *Note.* AAQ-II, Acceptance and Action Questionnaire-II; FFMQ, Five Facet Mindfulness Questionnaire; Observe, observing; ActAware, acting with awareness; NonJudge, non-judging of inner experience; NonReact, non-reactivity to inner experience. $^{*}P<0.05$; $^{**}P<0.01$; $^{***}P<0.001$.

There is growing evidence that positive mental health and psychopathology are related but different dimensions of mental health [49], and that positive mental health is a protective factor against mental illnesses [6,7]. Several researchers suggest that aspects of psychological well-being (e.g. meaning, mastery, autonomy, goals) increase personal resilience [50–52]. The findings of this study suggest that adults with mild to moderate depressive symptomatology that participated in this public mental health intervention will be able to better cope with life adversity in the future. Moreover, offering a public mental health intervention in a positive framework might be less stigmatizing for participants with depressive symptomatology [5].

Mediational analyses show that the efficacy of MBCT compared to the control group on reducing post-treatment depressive symptoms is mediated by an increase in psychological flexibility and all mindfulness skills, except for the subscale 'describe'. Our results are in line with Kuyken et al. [53], which showed that 15-month follow-up level of depression were mediated by mindfulness skills and self-compassion. Developing a compassionate attitude toward one's own negative thoughts and feelings mediated the effect of MBCT on depressive symptoms and relapse. These findings are also in line with earlier studies that demonstrated the association between low psychological flexibility (i.e. experiential avoidance) and mindfulness and psychopathology [15,54,55]. The increase of psychological flexibility and mindfulness that mediated the effects of MBCT on depressive symptomatology suggests that participants have gained additional adaptive emotion regulation skills in response to negative affect-producing stressors [19,54].

The original MBCT training was designed for people with a history of depression and requires participants to commit to a 2.5-hour group session and to 45 to 60 minutes of mindfulness practice each day for 8 weeks [9]. The current study suggests that mindfulness exercises of a total of 15 minutes a day may be effective for adults with mild to moderate depressive symptomatology. Much of the research on the effects of MBCT is conducted based on a clinical population. For the non-clinical population, mostly still working and active socially, the required time commitment on a weekly and daily basis may be a barrier to effectively integrate exercises into daily life. Carmody and Baer [56] concluded in their review that the correlation between mean effect size and number of in-class hours was non-significant for both clinical and non-clinical samples. They suggested that adaptations that include less class time may be worthwhile for populations for whom reduction of psychological distress is an important goal and for whom longer time commitment may be a barrier to their ability or willingness to participate. Our findings are in line with a number of studies which have shown that short-term meditation can lead to more tolerance, and a lower distress of pain and perceived stress (e.g. [57,58]). For example, Klatt et al. [57] showed that a 60-minute training together with 20 minutes of daily practice of meditation can have a significant positive effect on levels of perceived stress in healthy working adults ($p = .0025$). Also, Cavanagh et al. [21] effectively adapted their online MBCT to a brief intervention with daily mindfulness meditation practices of 10 minutes. Our finding that an 11-week MBCT training with 15 minutes of daily mindfulness meditation practice can sufficiently and significantly reduce depressive symptomatology seems promising from a public mental health perspective and is in line with Carmody and Baer [56]. The finding that the community-based MBCT intervention was very positively evaluated by the participants (scoring 7.98 out of 10), and that very few people dropped out of the intervention or dropped out of the study, underscores the feasibility and the attractiveness of the intervention.

## Limitations

Some limitations must also be acknowledged. First, for the design of the study as a waiting-list compared RCT, controlling for the influence of possible non-specific factors, such as attention and social interaction, was unlikely. Future research should use an active control intervention or an attention placebo controlled design to overcome this limitation. Secondly, the study used a short follow-up period of 3 months for which the follow-up was limited to a within group analysis. For ethical reasons, the time until the control group could receive the intervention was limited to 3 months. For future research, a longer follow-up (e.g. 1-year follow-up) is recommended to study the impact of MBCT on the incidence of depression. Third, the design was a pragmatic randomized controlled trial with self-referred participants, so the results of the study may have been influenced by a selection bias. All measures were self-report: no psychiatric diagnoses were available because participants were recruited from the general public. Generalizability of the findings to patients seeking treatment cannot be assumed. On the other hand, no restrictions were made to the level of depressive symptoms, as is customary to the procedures applied in community mental health centers. In this regard, the study was representative for standard general practice.

## Conclusion

This study shows that MBCT as a public mental health intervention for adults with mild to moderate depressive symptomatology is effective by not only reducing depressive symptoms and anxiety symptoms, but also enhancing positive mental health and psychological flexibility. Furthermore, this study shows that the intervention is applicable and effective in a natural setting.

## Acknowledgments

The authors wish to thank the therapists and participants that took part in this study.

## Author Contributions

Conceived and designed the experiments: WTP PAM MMV JJK ETB. Performed the experiments: JJK. Analyzed the data: WTP PAM MMV. Contributed reagents/materials/analysis tools: WTP PAM MMV JJK ETB. Wrote the paper: WTP PAM MMV JJK ETB.

## References


1. Cuijpers P, Smit F, Oostenbrink J, De Graaf R, Ten Have M, et al. (2007) Economic costs of minor depression: A population-based study. Acta Psychiatr Scand 115: 229–236.
2. Muñoz RF, Cuijpers P, Smit F, Barrera AZ, Leykin Y (2010) Prevention of major depression. Annu Rev Clin Psychol 6: 181–212.
3. Jané-Llopis E, Barry M, Hosman C, Patel V (2005) Mental health promotion works: a review. Promot Educ Suppl 2: 9–25, 61, 67.
4. Cuijpers P, Beekman ATF, Reynolds CF (2012) Preventing depression: A global priority. JAMA 307: 1033–1034.
5. Cuijpers P, Van Straten A, Warmerdam L, Van Rooy MJ (2010) Recruiting participants for interventions to prevent the onset of depressive disorders: Possibile ways to increase participation rates. BMC Health Serv Res 10: 181.
6. Keyes CLM, Dhingra SS, Simoes EJ (2010) Change in level of positive mental health as a predictor of future risk of mental Illness. Am J Public Health 100: 2366–2371.
7. Wood AM, Joseph S (2010) The absence of positive psychological (eudemonic) well-being as a risk factor for depression: A ten year cohort study. J Affect Disord 122: 213–217.
8. Fledderus M, Bohlmeijer ET, Smit F, Westerhof GJ (2010) Mental health promotion as a new goal in public mental health care: A randomized controlled trial of an intervention enhancing psychological flexibility. Am J Public Health 100: 2372–2378.
9. Segal ZV, Williams JMG, Teasdale JD (2002) Mindfulness-based Cognitive Therapy for Depression: A New Approach to Preventing Relapse. New York: The Guilford Press.
10. Ma SH, Teasdale JD (2004) Mindfulness-Based Cognitive Therapy for Depression: Replication and Exploration of Differential Relapse Prevention Effects. J Consult Clin Psychol 72: 31–40.
11. Teasdale JD, Segal ZV, Williams JMG, Ridgewaya VA, Soulsby JM, et al. (2000) Prevention of relapse/recurrence in major depression by mindfulness-based cognitive therapy. J Consult Clin Psychol 68: 615–623.
12. Piet J & Hougaard E (2011) The effect of mindfulness-based cognitive therapy for prevention of relapse in recurrent major depressive disorder: A systematic review and meta-analysis. Clin Psychol Rev, 31: 1032–1040.
13. Williams JMG, Crane C, Barnhofer T, Brennan K, Duggan DS, et al. (2014) Mindfulness-based cognitive therapy for preventing relapse in recurrent depression: A randomized dismantling trial. J Consult Clin Psychol 82: 275–286.
14. Strauss C, Cavanagh K, Oliver A, Pettman D (2014) Mindfulness-based interventions for people diagnosed with a current episode of an anxiety or depressive disorder: A meta-analysis of randomised controlled trails. PLOS ONE 9:e96110. doi: 10.1371/journal.pone.0096110
15. Hayes SC, Luoma JB, Bond FW, Masuda A, Lillis J (2006) Acceptance and Commitment Therapy: Model, processes and outcomes. Behav Res Ther 44: 1–25.
16. Aldao A, Nolen-Hoeksema S (2010) Specificity of cognitive emotion regulation strategies: A transdiagnostic examination. Behav Res Ther 48: 974–983.
17. Kabat-Zinn J (1990) Full catastrophe living: Using the wisdom of your body and mind to face stress, pain and illness. New York: Delacorte.
18. Chiesa A, Serretti A (2011) Mindfulness based cognitive therapy for psychiatric disorders: A systematic review and meta-analysis. Psychiatry Res 187: 441–453.
19. Chiesa A, Anselmi R, Serretti A (2014) Psychological mechanisms of mindfulness-based interventions: What do we know? Holist Nurs Pract 28: 124–148.
20. Kaviani H, Hatami N, Javaheri F (2012) The impact of Mindfulness-based Cognitive Therapy (MBCT) on mental health and quality of life in a sub-clinically depressed population. Arch Gen Psychiatry 14: 21–28.
21. Cavanagh K, Strauss C, Cicconi F, Griffiths N, Wyper A, et al. (2012) A randomised controlled trial of a brief online mindfulness-based intervention. Behav Res Ther 51: 573–578.
22. Sheehan DV, Lecrubier Y, Sheehan KH, Amorim P, Janavs J, et al. (1998) The Mini-International Neuropsychiatric Interview (M.I.N.I.): the development and validation of a structured diagnostic psychiatric interview for DSM-IV and ICD-10. J Clin Psychiatry 59: 22–33.
23. Van Vliet IM, De Beurs E (2007) The MINI-International Neuropsychiatric Interview (M.I.N.I.). A brief structured diagnostic psychiatric interview for DSM-IV and ICD-10 psychiatric disorders [in Dutch]. Tijdschr Psychiatr 49: 393–397.
24. Radloff LS (1977) The CES-D scale, a self report depression scale for research in the general population. Appl Psychol Meas 1: 385–401.
25. Haringsma R, Engels GI, Beekman ATF, Spinhoven P (2004) The criterion validity of the Center for Epidemiological Studies Depression Scale (CES-D) in a sample of self-referred elders with depressive symptomatology. Int J Geriatr Psychiatry 19: 558–563.
26. Zigmond AS, Snaith RP (1983) The hospital anxiety and depression scale. Acta Psychiatr Scand 67: 361–370.
27. Spinhoven P, Ormel J, Sloekers PPA, Kempen GIJM, Speckens AEM, et al. (1997) A validation study of the hospital anxiety and depression scale (HADS) in different groups of Dutch subjects. Psychol Med 27: 363–370.
28. Keyes CLM, Wissing M, Potgieter JP, Temane M, Kruger A, et al. (2008) Evaluation of the mental health continuum-short form (MHC-SF) in Setswana-speaking South Africans. Clin Psychol Psychother 15: 181–192.
29. Lamers SMA, Westerhof GJ, Bohlmeijer ET, Ten Klooster PM, Keyes CLM (2011) Evaluating the psychometric properties of the mental health Continuum-Short Form (MHC-SF). J Clin Psychol 67: 99–110.
30. Bond FW, Hayes SC, Baer RA, Carpenter KM, Guenole N, et al. (2011) Preliminary Psychometric Properties of the Acceptance and Action Questionnaire-II: A Revised Measure of Psychological Inflexibility and Experiential Avoidance. Behav Ther 42: 676–688.
31. Fledderus M, Oude Voshaar MAH, ten Klooster PM, Bohlmeijer ET (2012) Further evaluation of the psychometric properties of the acceptance and action questionnaire-II. Psychol Assess 24: 925–936.
32. Baer RA, Smith GT, Hopkins J, Krietemeyer J, Toney L (2006) Using self-report assessment methods to explore facets of mindfulness. Assessment 13: 27–45.
33. Bohlmeijer E, Klooster PM, Fledderus M, Veehof M, Baer R (2011) Psychometric properties of the five facet mindfulness questionnaire in depressed adults and development of a short form. Assessment 18: 308–320.
34. Dempster AP, Laird NM, Rubin DB (1977) Maximum likelihood from incomplete data via the EM algorithm. J R Stat Soc Series B Stat Methodol 39: 1–38.

35. Morris SB, DeShon RP (2002) Combining effect size estimates in meta-analysis with repeated measures and independent-groups designs. Psychol Methods 7: 105–125.
36. Lipsey MW, Wilson DB (1993) The efficacy of psychological, educational, and behavioral treatment: Confirmation from meta-analysis. Am Psychol 48: 1181–1209.
37. Jacobson NS, Truax P (1991) Clinical significance: A statistical approach to defining meaningful change in psychotherapy research. J Consult Clin Psychol 59: 12–19.
38. Beekman ATF, Deeg DJH, Van Limbeek J, Braam AW, De Vries MZ, et al. (1997) Criterion validity of the Center for Epidemiologic Studies Depression scale (CES-D): Results from a community-based sample of older subjects in the Netherlands. Psychol Med 27: 231–235.
39. Smit F, Ederveen A, Cuijpers P, Deeg D, Beekman A (2006) Opportunities for cost-effective prevention of late-life depression: An epidemiological approach. Arch Gen Psychiatry 63: 290–296.
40. Cook RJ, Sackett DL (1995) The number needed to treat: A clinically useful measure of treatment effect. Br Med J 310: 452–454.
41. Baron RM, Kenny DA (1986) The moderator-mediator variable distinction in social psychological research: conceptual, strategic, and statistical considerations. J Pers Soc Psychol 51: 1173–1182.
42. Preacher KJ, Hayes AF (2008) Asymptotic and resampling strategies for assessing and comparing indirect effects in multiple mediator models. Behav Res Methods 40: 879–891.
43. Cuijpers P, Smit F, Van Straten A (2007) Psychological treatments of subthreshold depression: A meta-analytic review. Acta Psychiatr Scand 115: 434–441.
44. Cuijpers P, Smit F (2004) Subthreshold depression as a risk indicator for major depressive disorder: A systematic review of prospective studies. Acta Psychiatr Scand 109: 325–331.
45. Cuijpers P, Van Straten A, Smit F, Mihalopoulos C, Beekman A (2008) Preventing the onset of depressive disorders: A meta-analytic review of psychological interventions. Am J Psychiatry 165: 1272–1280.
46. Vøllestad J, Nielsen MB, Nielsen GH (2012) Mindfulness- and acceptance-based interventions for anxiety disorders: A systematic review and meta-analysis. Br J Clin Psychol 51: 239–260.
47. Horn PJ, Wuyek LA (2010) Anxiety disorders as a risk factor for subsequent depression. Int J Psychiatry Clin Pract 14: 244–247.
48. Kuyken W, Byford S, Taylor RS, Watkins E, Holden E, et al. (2008) Mindfulness-Based Cognitive Therapy to Prevent Relapse in Recurrent Depression. J Consult Clin Psychol 76: 966–978.
49. Lamers SMA, Westerhof GJ, Kovács V, Bohlmeijer ET (2012) Differential relationships in the association of the Big Five personality traits with positive mental health and psychopathology. J Res Pers 46: 517–524.
50. Fava GA, Tomba E (2009) Increasing psychological well-being and resilience by psychotherapeutic methods. J Pers 77: 1903–1934.
51. Ruini C, Fava GA (2012) Role of Well-Being Therapy in Achieving a Balanced and Individualized Path to Optimal Functioning. Clin Psychol Psychother 19: 291–304.
52. Ryff CD, Friedman EM, Morozink JA, Tsenkova V (2012) Psychological resilience in adulthood and later life: Implications for health. Annu Rev Gerontol Geriatr 32: 73–92.
53. Kuyken W, Watkins E, Holden E, White K, Taylor RS, et al. (2010) How does mindfulness-based cognitive therapy work? Behav Res Ther 48: 1105–1112.
54. Kashdan TB, Rottenberg J (2010) Psychological flexibility as a fundamental aspect of health. Clin Psychol Rev 30: 865–878.
55. McCarney RW, Schulz J, Grey AR (2012) Effectiveness of mindfulness-based therapies in reducing symptoms of depression: A meta-analysis. European Journal of Psychotherapy and Counselling 14: 279–299.
56. Carmody J, Baer RA (2009) How long does a mindfulness-based stress reduction program need to be? A review of class contact hours and effect sizes for psychological distress. J Clin Psychol 65: 627–638.
57. Klatt MD, Buckworth J, Malarkey WB (2009) Effects of low-dose mindfulness-based stress reduction (MBSR-ld) on working adults. Health Educ Behav 36: 601–614.
58. Liu X, Wang S, Chang S, Chen W, Si M (2012) Effect of Brief Mindfulness Intervention on Tolerance and Distress of Pain Induced by Cold-Pressor Task. Stress Health 29: 199–204.

# 20

# Maternity Care Services and Culture: A Systematic Global Mapping of Interventions

**Ernestina Coast[1]*, Eleri Jones[1], Anayda Portela[2], Samantha R. Lattof[1]**

1 Department of Social Policy, London School of Economics and Political Science, London, United Kingdom, 2 Department of Maternal, Newborn, Child and Adolescent Health, World Health Organization, Geneva, Switzerland

## Abstract

***Background:*** A vast body of global research shows that cultural factors affect the use of skilled maternity care services in diverse contexts. While interventions have sought to address this issue, the literature on these efforts has not been synthesised. This paper presents a systematic mapping of interventions that have been implemented to address cultural factors that affect women's use of skilled maternity care. It identifies and develops a map of the literature; describes the range of interventions, types of literature and study designs; and identifies knowledge gaps.

***Methods and Findings:*** Searches conducted systematically in ten electronic databases and two websites for literature published between 01/01/1990 and 28/02/2013 were combined with expert-recommended references. Potentially eligible literature included journal articles and grey literature published in English, French or Spanish. Items were screened against inclusion and exclusion criteria, yielding 96 items in the final map. Data extracted from the full text documents are presented in tables and a narrative synthesis. The results show that a diverse range of interventions has been implemented in 35 countries to address cultural factors that affect the use of skilled maternity care. Items are classified as follows: (1) service delivery models; (2) service provider interventions; (3) health education interventions; (4) participatory approaches; and (5) mental health interventions.

***Conclusions:*** The map provides a rich source of information on interventions attempted in diverse settings that might have relevance elsewhere. A range of literature was identified, from narrative descriptions of interventions to studies using randomised controlled trials to evaluate impact. Only 23 items describe studies that aim to measure intervention impact through the use of experimental or observational-analytic designs. Based on the findings, we identify avenues for further research in order to better document and measure the impact of interventions to address cultural factors that affect use of skilled maternity care.

**Editor:** Irene Petersen, UCL, United Kingdom

**Funding:** The study was funded by the WHO Department of Maternal, Newborn, Child, and Adolescent Health, the UN Population Fund and The Norwegian Agency for Development. The funders had no role in study design, data collection and analysis, decision to publish, or preparation of the manuscript.

**Competing Interests:** The authors have declared that no competing interests exist.

* Email: e.coast@lse.ac.uk

## Introduction

Global strategies to reduce maternal and newborn mortality and health have emphasised the need for scaling up the use of skilled maternity care [1]. Yet, experience has shown that provision of skilled care and availability of maternity care facilities does not necessarily lead to increased utilisation. A large body of literature describes how cultural factors affect women's use of services [2–4], including those resulting from differing 'cultures' of maternity care between service providers and populations served [5].

### What is culture?

There is no one agreed definition of culture, but a focus on culture means emphases placed on aspects such as shared norms, beliefs and expectations, spoken language and behavioural customs [6]. In reality, it is difficult to separate out culture from social, economic and geographical context [7]. For example, members of a cultural group might not use a particular health service because they are too poor or because they know they will be discriminated against – highlighting the danger of conflating poverty with culture. Culture includes components that are both explicit and implicit. Hall [8] describes different levels of culture: a level that is explicit or manifest to outsiders (e.g., language, rituals, dress), a level of rules and norms that are known to group members but rarely shared with outsiders, and a level that is known and followed but not stated. Most societies have more than one culture within them. These cultural sub-divisions might take the form of social groups or strata (e.g., ethnic groups, religious groups, social classes, castes, ranks) marked by distinctive cultural attributes (e.g., beliefs, behaviour, perceptions, attitudes to illness and health, religion, language, manners, dress, housing, diet) alongside social and economic attributes (e.g., wealth, power, gender, education).

### Culture and maternity care services

Childbirth, and the time around birth, is a social and cultural event that is often governed by norms. However, in most societies, the dominant culture, expressed through social institutions such as the health care system, regulates how health issues are both perceived and addressed. Differences between the cultures of health care services and service users have been recognised as a major issue in service delivery. Perceived or actual cultural insensitivity or incompetence of professionals can lead to perceptions of poor quality care by users or discrimination of certain users by providers, resulting in a lack of trust in services and service providers [9–11].

Many authors have recommended that cultural factors should be taken into account in the planning and delivery of services in order to effectively encourage service uptake as an important step in reducing maternal and newborn mortality [5,12–16]. Intercultural approaches to the design and delivery of national policies are well-established in some countries, particularly in Latin America [17]. The need for 'culturally-appropriate' health facilities is core to the World Health Organization's (WHO) mandate on 'health for all' [18] and its strategy for improving maternal and newborn health [5]. However, research reveals the complexity of such endeavours. [19]. It is known that some interventions have been implemented in different world regions to address cultural factors that affect the use of maternity care services. However, the literature has not been synthesised.

### Aims and objectives

This systematic mapping of the literature aims to understand the range of interventions that have been implemented to address cultural factors affecting women's use of skilled maternity care services. The study's objectives were to methodically identify and develop a map of the literature; categorise the range of interventions, the type of literature and the study designs included; and identify knowledge gaps.

## Methods

### Methods

The methodology for systematic mapping used in this study was developed from work at the Evidence for Policy and Practice Information and Co-ordinating Centre and is increasingly used in a range of social sciences [20–24]. The scope and types of literature included in a systematic mapping are normally broader than in a systematic review. The aim in this mapping is to describe as widely as possible all of the literature relating to the topic without limiting to studies that assess the strength or direction of the relationship, or even to empirical studies. We developed a protocol that was reviewed by an advisory group composed of content and method experts.

### Inclusion/exclusion criteria

Potentially eligible studies included journal articles, and published and unpublished information from governments and other agencies, whether available in print or online, published in English, French and/or Spanish. Since the aim is to describe the nature and coverage of the literature, quality was not assessed and was not a criterion for inclusion. Multiple references based on the same sample were also not excluded (as would be the case in a systematic review in order to avoid bias).

Table 1 provides the specification of the items to be mapped. Whilst intervention aims and outcomes relate only to women's use of services during pregnancy, childbirth and after birth, intervention recipients may include, for example, household or family members, community leaders or maternity care providers. Skilled care is defined in this mapping as those services provided by a skilled attendant: an "accredited health professional – such as a midwife, doctor or nurse – who has been educated and trained to proficiency in the skills needed to manage normal (uncomplicated) pregnancies, childbirth and the immediate postnatal period, and in the identification, management and referral of complications in women and newborns. Traditional birth attendants, trained or not, are excluded" [25]. Where the distinction between skilled and unskilled care is not clear, an inclusive approach is adopted. However, interventions that focused primarily on traditional birth attendants' (TBAs) roles in the direct provision of childbirth services were excluded, as the focus of the paper is on skilled maternity care services. Interventions concerned with improving satisfaction, but not also the use of services, are excluded.

Items must describe an *implemented* intervention in which a primary, focused aim or strategy is to address cultural factors as a vehicle to change use of maternity care services. This criterion excludes the following:

- Interventions that exclusively address economic or geographical access barriers for a defined cultural group, although overlaps between cultural factors on the one hand and economic and geographical factors on the other are acknowledged [7];
- Generic quality improvement interventions that consider and/or accommodate cultural factors explicitly or implicitly, but not as a primary, focused aim or strategy. Whilst it is acknowledged that an "important question may be what combination of interventions and ways of incorporating culture into generic quality improvement are most likely to improve quality of care and outcomes" [6], this question is beyond the scope of this mapping; and
- Items in which 'cultural appropriateness' is evaluated, but not incorporated in intervention design or implementation.

### Search strategy

Electronic databases, registers and websites were assessed for their availability, relevance and likely coverage of the eligible literature. Ten electronic databases and two targeted websites were included and searched for items published from 1 January 1990 to 28 February 2013. Combinations of relevant search terms were developed and tested in a sample of databases for sensitivity to a list of references that were known to the research team and judged to be potentially relevant. Table 2 presents the final combinations of search terms used. Electronic searches were adapted to each database using appropriate truncations/wildcards. Titles and abstracts were normally searched, and Medical Subject Headings (MeSH) terms were included where possible. A call for papers was sent by the WHO to various organisations and topic experts. The references received were combined with the electronic search results.

### Screening process

All items identified through the search were screened initially on the basis of title and abstract. Where inclusion or exclusion could not be determined on the basis of title and abstract, the full text was screened. Figure 1 illustrates the screening process. EC, EJ, EH and SK contributed to screening the items individually. The following measures were taken for quality assurance: 1/all team members involved in screening independently screened the first 100 items. The whole team subsequently met to compare results, and discuss and resolve any differences in understanding of the

**Table 1.** Specification of systematic mapping.

| | |
|---|---|
| **Population** | The outcomes apply to women during pregnancy, childbirth and after birth in any world region. The intervention population may be broader, including other community members or health providers. |
| **Intervention** | An implemented intervention that is primarily and explicitly designed to accommodate or address a cultural group's shared norms, values and/or beliefs; behavioural customs; and/or spoken language/s. Cultural group is defined broadly to include any form of group or social stratum that is (considered to be) marked by its own distinctive cultural characteristics [7,128], such as ethnic groups, groups defined by religion, language groups, indigenous groups, tribal communities, caste-based groups/strata or geographically defined populations. |
| **Aim/outcome** | Items must state an aim to increase, or measure as an outcome, women's use of skilled care during pregnancy, childbirth and after birth. |
| **Study design** | Reviews are not included. No other criteria are specified for study design. |

inclusion/exclusion criteria. The criteria were further elaborated where necessary; 2/at the full text screening stage, any items that a team member considered borderline or problematic were noted. At the end of the process, EJ and EH independently screened all of the problematic items. Again, the whole team met to compare results, debate and resolve any differences. Decisions were made in favour of an inclusive approach where questions remained.

## Analysis

Data were extracted for analysis from all items in the map, including background information; a description of the intervention; details of the type of literature (and study if relevant); and details of relevant outcomes measured. Based on the map, we inductively developed and defined intervention categories. It was unfeasible to create perfectly discrete categories since many interventions are complex. Where an intervention could have

**Table 2.** Search terms and their combinations.

| 1. Intervention/study type terms | 2. Access/use terms | 3. Care terms | 4. Population terms | 5. Culture terms |
|---|---|---|---|---|
| Arrangement* | Accept* | Advice | ***Antepartum terms*** | Attitud* |
| Evaluat* | Access | ANC | Ante*natal | Behaviour* |
| Initiative* | Appointment* | "Birth attendan*" | Ante*partum | Behavior* |
| Intervention* | Attend* | Care | Expect*[a] | Belief* |
| Model* | Availab* | Doctor* | Pregnan* | Believ* |
| Package* | Obtain | Centre | Prenatal | Caste* |
| Pilot* | Outreach | Center | Trimester | Communit* |
| Program* | Recei* | Clinic* | ***Intrapartum terms*** | Culture* |
| Project* | Seek* | Counsel* | Birth* | Cultural |
| Provision* | Uptake | Department* | Child*birth | Custom* |
| Regime* | Use | Facilit* | Intra*partum | Ethnic* |
| Scheme* | Utilisation | Healthcare | Maternity | Indigen* |
| Strateg* | Utilization | Health care | Obstetric* | Language* |
| Trial* | Visit* | "Health system" | Parturition | Minorit* |
| | | Hospital* | Partus | Norm* |
| | | Institution* | Peri*natal | Race* |
| | | Midwif* | Deliver*[a] | Racial* |
| | | Nurs* | Labour[a] | Religio* |
| | | Physician* | Labor[a] | Ritual* |
| | | PNC | ***Postpartum terms*** | Sub*cultur* |
| | | Service* | Maternal | Sub*population* |
| | | Treatment* | "New mother" | Tradition* |
| | | Unit* | Post*natal | Tribal* |
| | | | Post*partum | Tribe* |
| | | | PPC | Value* |
| | | | Puerper* | Participatory |

[a]These terms have multiple meanings. Due to their presence in a column that narrowed a search that was otherwise very broad, they were included only in searches where their inclusion did not yield an unfeasible number of references.

Table 2 provides the basic template that was adapted to the particulars (e.g., wildcards using the asterisk symbol (*) and truncations, capacity for complex searches, MeSH facility) of each electronic database. The full protocol is available from the corresponding author or from WHO Department of Maternal, Newborn, Child and Adolescent Health at portelaa@who.int.

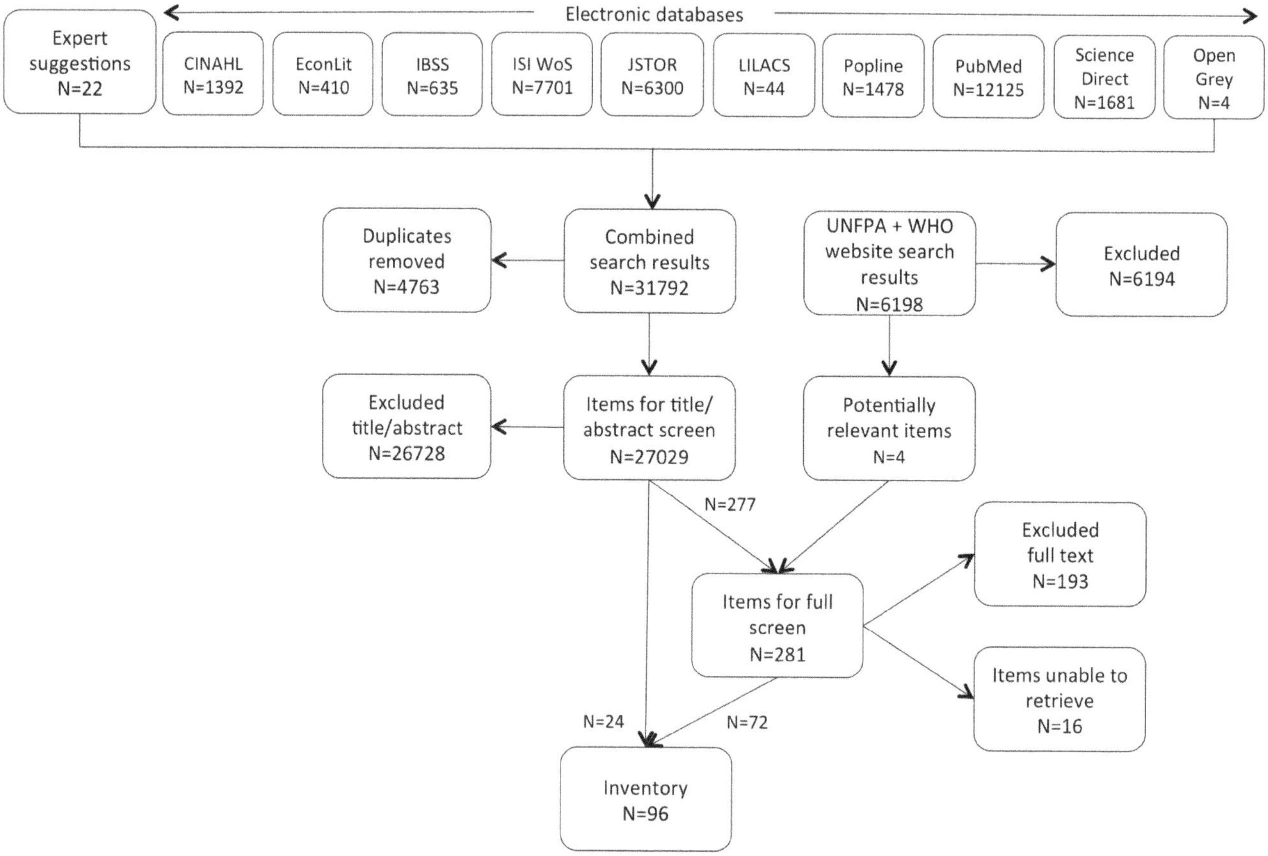


**Figure 1. Mapping results.**

fitted into more than one category, did not fit neatly into any category, or was not described in sufficient detail to understand its content, the item was placed in the category in which it was deemed to fit best. Data are presented in tables along with a narrative synthesis.

## Results

After removing duplicates, the electronic database searches and website searches, combined with references suggested by experts, generated a total of 33,227 items for screening. The majority of items were not relevant. Following the screening, a total of 96 items were included in the map. The research team was unable to retrieve or screen a further 16 items.

Interventions addressing cultural factors affecting the use of skilled maternity care are not confined to a specific type of country. The map includes items from 35 countries across all world regions and the whole range of country income levels. Thirty-nine of the items were based in high-income countries, of which the majority were from the United States of America (USA), followed by Australia, Canada and the United Kingdom (UK). Items from the USA and UK predominantly included interventions targeting specific immigrant or ethnic minority groups, whilst items from Australia and Canada predominantly targeted indigenous communities. Only one item was based in continental Europe, although this may partly reflect the systematic mapping's restricted language coverage.

Of the remaining items, 25 were from low-income countries and 29 from middle-income countries, with three items located in multiple countries that cut across these categories. Sixteen items described interventions across nine countries in Eastern and Western Africa, and 14 items described interventions in Latin America. Twenty-seven items from Asia were dominated by literature from southern Asia.

### Description of interventions

The five intervention categories we developed were: (1) service delivery models, (2) service provider interventions, (3) health education interventions, (4) participatory approaches, and (5) mental health interventions. We define the categories and describe the range of interventions within each below.

**1. Service delivery models.** This category includes 24 items describing models of service delivery specifically designed (or adapted from existing models of service delivery) to provide culturally-appropriate services for targeted groups (Table 3). These models are largely complex interventions taking a broad range of measures, often including elements of the 'service provider interventions' and 'participatory approaches' described below as well as adaptations to the service setting, practices, materials and/or language. The category is dominated by interventions from Australia and Latin America.

Several items from Australia describe comprehensive service delivery models for Aboriginal communities, implemented through a targeted health service [26–30]. For example, Nel and Pashen describe an indigenous medical centre managed by a community board and staffed by indigenous service providers [28]. Service users are seen in familiar surroundings, and Aboriginal health workers visit them to ensure attendance. Moreover,

**Table 3.** Included items: Service delivery models.

| Author and year | Country (ies) | Intervention | Literature/study type | Maternal care outcomes measured |
|---|---|---|---|---|
| Affonso et al. 1993 [37] | USA (Hawaii) | Culturally-sensitive nursing care and community outreach interventions (prenatal) congruent with the lifestyles of ethnic groups in Hawaii | Narrative description of intervention | |
| Ahmed and Jakaria 2009 [42] | Bangladesh | Cadre of skilled birth attendants developed for home births (with a culture-based rationale). | Descriptive study (qualitative + performance monitoring surveys) | Number and proportion of women covered |
| Bender et al. 2005 [36] | Bolivia | Community-based intervention. Emphasis on quality care to provide culturally-acceptable services appropriate to women's needs. Used popular education in the community's meeting centre as a first point of entry. | Descriptive study (monitoring data) | Utilization of antenatal care (ANC) (number of first visits in 1st trimester; total of at least 4 visits) |
| Blum et al. 2006 [43] | Bangladesh | A national level initiative to post skilled birth attendants at community level (with a culture-based rationale). | Qualitative study | |
| Dickerson et al. 2010 [129] | China (Tibet) | A programme to train rural healthcare workers and laypersons to provide outreach to pregnant women and families (with a partly culture-based rationale), emphasizing a continuum of community-level care. | Descriptive study (survey) | Number of antepartum care visits; birth place |
| Eckermann and Deodato 2008 [31] | Lao PDR | Introduction of maternity waiting homes, incorporating research findings on traditional practices, and social and cultural (among other) factors | Descriptive study (formative study + monitoring data) | Number of women using facility |
| Gabrysch et al. 2009 [35] | Peru | Culturally-appropriate delivery care model developed in cooperation with Quechua indigenous communities and health professionals. Involves features such as a rope and bench for vertical delivery position, inclusion of family and TBAs and use of the Quechua language. | Descriptive study (formative study + survey) | Proportion of births delivered in health facility |
| Greenberg et al. 1996 [130] | USA | Various strategies by Washington State Department of Health to ensure access to health care for ethnic minority groups, including culturally-competent staff; targeted outreach; development of partnerships with community organizations and other agencies. | Narrative description of intervention | |
| Homer et al. 2012 [26] | Australia | Community outreach service developed into a comprehensive model of care known as the Malabar Community Midwifery Link Service. Prioritises Aboriginal and Torres Strait Islander communities and aims to provide culturally-appropriate services. Aboriginal Health Education Officers work alongside midwives and nurses, ensuring community engagement and cultural safety, and providing a link between the community and the service. Aboriginal midwives are mentored. | Descriptive study (clinical data + qualitative component) | Number of women accessing the service; starting ANC before 20 weeks |
| Jan et al. 2004 [27] | Australia | Daruk Aboriginal Medical Service is a community-controlled health service initiated by local Aboriginal communities and aiming to deliver holistic and culturally appropriate health care. Includes a full-time Aboriginal health worker and cultural awareness sessions for local hospital staff. | Observational analytic study (retrospective cohort study) + qualitative component | Gestational age at first visit; number of antenatal visits |
| Kenney et al. 2005 [41] | Kazakhstan | Holistic, family-centred and culturally-appropriate approach to de-medicalise care. Elements include involving women in decision-making on care; evaluating new interventions in a national context for their impact on cultural attitudes and facilitating their acceptance through information and discussion; and introduced change through understanding and agreement with local people (rather than orders). | Descriptive study (analysis of trends using clinical data, pre-post surveys and official statistics + qualitative component) | Place of ANC; provider of ANC; number of ANC visits; initiating ANC in 1st trimester; referral to specialists; prenatal hospitalisation; type of birth (normal vs complicated) |
| Kim 2003 [40] | Korea | Sanhujori centres to provide more systematic professionalised care for postpartum women as an alternative to traditional sanhujori postpartum care provided by family members. Centres accommodate traditional beliefs while providing quality postpartum care and support (not exclusively concerned with health). | Descriptive study (cross-sectional survey) | Number of women admitted to a care centre |
| Larson et al. 1992 [131] | USA | A bilingual Migrant Health Project Team assisted staff at migrant health centres in designing culturally-appropriate strategies for delivering care to migrant groups. A migrant-specific maternal care coordination programme was developed that used bilingual staff, outreach services and migrant lay health advisers. | Descriptive study (clinical data + trends in outcomes) | First trimester entry into prenatal care; receiving 9+ prenatal visits |

**Table 3.** Cont.

| Author and year | Country (ies) | Intervention | Literature/study type | Maternal care outcomes measured |
|---|---|---|---|---|
| Mayberry et al. 1999 [38] | USA (Hawaii) | The Caring for Pregnant Women health care programme (Malama Na Wahine Hapai) is purposefully built on values and customs of Native Hawaiian, Filipino, and Japanese women - ethnic groups with late or no entry into prenatal care. Complementary to standard obstetric care. Informed by focus groups, it aims to provide culturally competent care through attention to training and monitoring by local cultural and ethnic healers and neighbourhood leaders. | Narrative description of intervention | |
| McAree et al. 2010 [132] | UK | Midwifery group practice compared to standard maternity care in an ethnically-diverse area (with a partly culture-based rationale). | Qualitative study | |
| Moreno and Lopez 2013 [34] | Ecuador | National Plan adapted to Kichwa indigenous communities. It involves intercultural health strategies to overcome barriers that were mainly cultural in nature; respect for and use of indigenous knowledge and implementation of culturally-appropriate birth houses; and training of traditional Kichwa birth attendants. | Descriptive study (project output statistics) | Number of births in institutions |
| Nel and Pashen 2003 [28] | Australia | Service changes in local and regional ANC services. Consultation with health providers and Aboriginal communities to address cultural and family needs. The programme includes a separate indigenous medical centre managed by a community board and staffed by indigenous people. Pregnant women are seen in familiar surroundings, initially by indigenous staff. Aboriginal health workers make home visits to ensure service use. Pregnant women are allowed to bring children and family members. | Descriptive study (pre-post comparison of outcome counts) | Number of women presenting for birth without any ANC; attendance at the medical centre |
| Nurena 2009 [133] | Peru | Integration of an intercultural focus into health policies, in this case specifically reorienting services and including approaches to respond to and address the needs and cultural preferences of indigenous populations, focusing on respect for a vertical birth position. | Narrative description of intervention | |
| Panaretto et al. 2005 [29] | Australia | Collaboration with indigenous community to improve antenatal services, producing an integrated model of antenatal shared care delivered from the community-controlled Townsville Aboriginal and Islander Health Service. | Observational analytic study (Prospective cohort study) | Total visits per pregnancy; Total TAIHS ANC visits per pregnancy; weeks of gestation at first visit; pregnancies with inadequate care; pregnancies with late first visit |
| Panaretto et al. 2007 [30] | Australia | Sustained, community-based collaborative approach to ANC services for indigenous women. | Observational analytic study (Prospective cohort study) | ANC visits per pregnancy; gestation at first visit; pregnancies with inadequate care; pregnancies with late first visit |
| Reavy et al. 2012 [39] | USA | Culturally Appropriate Resources and Education (CARE) clinic is a nurse-led clinical programme providing healthcare services and education. | Descriptive study (qualitative study + clinical data) | Missed clinical appointments derived from chart reviews (all other data qualitative, although aim was to address barriers in accessing healthcare services) |
| Schooley et al. 2009 [32] | Guatemala | The Casa Materna maternity waiting home and community outreach strategy seeks to bridge traditional and western approaches to health care services. Built on principles of respect, caring and culturally-appropriate care, the strategy uses TBAs and volunteer health advocates, and involves men as advocates. | Qualitative study | |
| Tucker et al. 2013 [33] | Mexico | Intercultural birthing house established as a place where women can give birth with their TBAs with access to skilled birth attendants to reduce maternal mortality among indigenous women. | Qualitative study | |
| Zangari 2009 [134] | Bolivia | A strategy to culturally adapt maternal health services, through training health workers to improve intercultural care, strengthening institutional management, and developing recommendations for a model of maternal care with an intercultural focus, with local participation. | Descriptive study | |

pregnant women are allowed to bring children and family members, in recognition of the cultural importance of extended family links. Several items in this category, particularly from Latin America, describe the introduction of culturally-appropriate 'maternity waiting homes' or 'birthing houses' [31–33]. Moreno and Lopez [34] describe this model of service delivery as part of a broad strategy to adapt a national plan in Ecuador for indigenous communities.

Different types of culturally-appropriate models of service delivery have been designed for indigenous communities [35,36], ethnic groups [37,38], refugees [39] and the general population [40]. For example, Gabrysch et al. [35] describe a delivery care model that was developed in Peru in cooperation with Quechua indigenous communities and health professionals, featuring a rope and bench for vertical childbirth, inclusion of family and TBAs in the service delivery process and during childbirth, and use of the Quechua language. One item in this category [41] is an outlier; in the item from Kazakhstan, the aim of a new culturally-appropriate service delivery approach is to introduce less medicalised care.

Some interventions refer to the provision of skilled home-based childbirth services explicitly in order to accommodate cultural norms [42,43]. Several further interventions in which a culture-based rationale was cited for training TBAs were excluded since the TBA was solely responsible for the direct provision of childbirth services [44–49]. However, these interventions also aimed to harness the TBAs' cultural role to facilitate linkages with the formal health system and improve referral for obstetric complications.

**2. Service provider interventions.** This category encompasses a range of interventions characterised by their focus on service providers. Analysis within this category revealed several sub-categories. One sub-category refers to three interventions in which the service provider is selected to match service users in terms of cultural characteristics [50–52] (Table 4). For example, Bilenko et al. [50] described an intervention in Israel in which a clinic for Bedouin families was staffed by an Arabic speaking Bedouin public health nurse. Few items describe this type of intervention as the sole focus. However, several items placed in other categories, particularly in the 'service delivery model' category, include this as one element of a broader intervention [26,27].

A large sub-category comprises 14 interventions in which people who share cultural characteristics with a target service user group are employed to bridge the cultural gap between this group and service providers (Table 4) [53–66]. They may fulfil various roles including encouraging and helping women to access care [57,59]; assisting women in communicating with healthcare providers [55,56]; and advocating on their behalf [62]. They are sometimes referred to as 'linkworkers,' 'peer health workers' or 'cultural brokers'. The category is dominated by items from the USA and the UK, where interventions have been implemented with specific immigrant or ethnic minority groups. This type of intervention has a long history, with many interventions implemented as early as the 1980s and 1990s. Again, several items placed in other categories, particularly in the 'service delivery model' category, include this position as one element of a broader intervention [26,32].

The final sub-category refers to eight interventions with existing staff to enhance their cultural awareness or sensitivity. These interventions have been implemented across diverse contexts and include various teaching and/or learning approaches [67–74] (Table 4). For example, Smith and Davies [74] describe a knowledge exchange intervention in Canada that brings "communities together to enable them to understand each other's goals and cultures."

**3. Health education interventions.** Within this category, 22 items from diverse settings describe a wide range of strategies employed with the aim of designing culturally-appropriate health education activities (Table 5). Interventions may use one or more strategies. Several interventions use preliminary studies investigating cultural factors to inform health education activities, although they differ in the extent to which they describe how these cultural factors were addressed in the actual intervention [75–80]. This finding may reflect different levels of emphasis on these factors in intervention design, but may also simply be a reporting issue. For example, Opoku et al. [79] and Olaniran et al. [80] both refer to the same intervention in Nigeria. However, whilst Opoku et al. [79] make a brief mention of using research on cultural factors to inform design, Olaniran et al. [80] describe in more detail the measures taken to address cultural factors. Culturally-appropriate health education messages were developed, trainers were selected who were fluent in the local language, and campaigns were carried out in churches.

Related to a sub-category within 'service provider interventions,' one strategy within the category of health education interventions is to employ facilitators or trainers who share cultural characteristics with the relevant population [80–84]. For example, both Gennaro et al. [82] and Yeshi et al. [84] describe interventions employing village leaders as trainers.

Several items describe developing culturally-appropriate health education materials and practices, in terms of messages, language, modalities and/or images [80,85–90]. For example, Omer et al. [89] describe using an education tool in Pakistan that reflects local materials and skills in embroidery, and DeStephano et al. [86] describe a culturally-tailored health education video series for Somali women in the USA. Finally, health education interventions have used participatory approaches [75,84,91–94]. These are distinguished from the 'participatory approaches' category on the basis that their primary focus is the delivery of education interventions.

**4. Participatory approaches.** An inclusive approach was adopted for participatory interventions in this systematic mapping because a population's participation in intervention design and implementation may be considered inherently to address or accommodate cultural factors. Thus, all items in which the population's participation in intervention design and implementation was a primary and explicit strategy were included. Analysis of items in this category indicates different levels of explicit emphasis on 'cultural' factors, a distinction that is highlighted with sub-categories (Table 6).

The first sub-category comprises four items that describe the participatory approach adopted as an explicit strategy to address or accommodate cultural factors affecting the use of skilled maternity care [95–98]. For example, Hounton et al. [96] describe their intervention in Burkina Faso as one that involved "investment in communities through an understanding of their social structure and health seeking behaviours, through identification and partnership with credible community leaders, and through identification of culturally-sensitive and locally-acceptable approaches to address transport and referrals." Jewell and Russell [97] describe another approach implemented in the USA of forming a state-wide network of grassroots county minority health coalitions to develop projects to eliminate cultural barriers to prenatal care for minority women.

The second sub-category includes four items [99–102] that explicitly refer to cultural factors affecting use of skilled maternity

**Table 4.** Included items: Service provider interventions.

| Author and year | Country (ies) | Intervention | Literature/study type | Maternal care outcomes measured |
|---|---|---|---|---|
| **Service provider matched on cultural characteristics** | | | | |
| Bilenko et al. 2007 [50] | Israel | A new MCH clinic in desert areas for Bedouin extended families living in tribal units, staffed by an Arabic speaking Bedouin public health nurse. | Descriptive study (review of clinical data for successive pregnancies before and after the intervention) | ANC utilisation; physician examination; at least 3 nursing visits |
| Dundek 2006 [51] | USA | Provision of labour support by Somali women (doulas) educated and certified in methods of labour support. The programme is based on identified barriers to culturally-competent care. | Descriptive study (clinical data and surveys) | |
| Nauman 1995 [52] | Mexico | The Mexican Social Security Institute (IMSS) began a rural midwife programme in a region where transport is limited and people speak indigenous languages. TBAs, IMSS-trained midwives and apprentices have a cultural role. Midwives are encouraged to use their knowledge of native herbal remedies and swap modern for traditional healthcare information. | Descriptive study (project output counts) | Number of pregnancies assisted; number of births assisted |
| **Bridging the gap between service providers and specific service user groups** | | | | |
| Chowdhury 1998 [53] | Bangladesh | A programme to involve TBAs in a safe delivery system (with a culture-based rationale), in which the TBA becomes a catalyst for the creation of a relationship between a pregnant woman and the formal health system. | Narrative description of intervention | |
| Friedsam et al. 2003 [54] | USA | Addresses cultural discrimination through 'outstationing' Medicaid eligibility workers to community locations. Counsellors advocate on behalf of the targeted population to improve health insurance uptake. | Descriptive study (enrolment indicators) | |
| Hazard et al. 2009 [55] | USA | Bilingual Hispanic community women ('Hispanic Labour Friends') are assigned to pregnant Hispanic immigrant women to assist communication with healthcare providers and provide social support. | Qualitative study | |
| Hicks and Hayes 1991 [56] | UK | The Asian Mother and Baby Campaign aims to improve communication between mothers and health professionals by employing linkworkers from the same social class and background as the client. | Descriptive study (Survey of health districts) | |
| Julnes et al. 1994 [57] | USA | Norfolk Resource Mothers Program is a community outreach programme using 'resource mothers' to assist with non-medical dimensions of pregnancy and childcare, including getting prenatal care. 'Resource mothers' are lay people often from the culture of the adolescents. | Observational Analytic (retrospective cohort study) | Month of pregnancy when prenatal care begins; number of prenatal visits completed; place of delivery (hospital or no hospital) |
| Ley et al. 2011 [58] | USA | "Women of color" often forego health services perceived as intimidating and/or culturally insensitive. The Healthy Start Initiative is a major community-based programme that encourages participation. Qualified community residents are employed as outreach workers and home visitors to facilitate the delivery of culturally-competent services. | Descriptive study (survey + qualitative component) | Use of services |
| Marsiglia et al. 2010 [59] | USA | The Familias Sanas intervention was designed to bridge the cultural gap between Latinas and the health care system. Prenatal Partners (Compañeras) are used as cultural brokers to reinforce among pregnant Latinas the importance of the postpartum visit and of caring for one's health. | Experimental study (RCT) | Compliance with the 6–8 week postpartum visit |
| Mattson and Lew 1992 [60] | USA | The South East Asian Health Project (SEAHP) provides culturally-sensitive maternal and child care to south-east Asian refugees. Bilingual, bicultural outreach workers provide education about the importance of care and act as interpreters. Information is printed in three languages. Providers are educated on health care practices and beliefs of south-east Asians. | Descriptive study (survey + clinical data) | Number using the clinic; current active caseload; class attendance |
| Meister et al. 1992 [61] | USA | A prenatal outreach and education intervention for low-income, Hispanic women in migrant and seasonal farmworker communities. Includes a Spanish language prenatal curriculum; indigenous health promoters; and a support network of local health professionals. | Narrative description of intervention | |

**Table 4.** Cont.

| Author and year | Country (ies) | Intervention | Literature/study type | Maternal care outcomes measured |
|---|---|---|---|---|
| Parsons and Day 1992 [62] | UK | A health advocacy programme to improve obstetric outcomes in non-English speaking women. Advocates both interpret and mediate between the service users and professionals. | Observational analytic (retrospective cohort study) | Gestation at booking; non-attendance of ANC appointments; uptake of antenatal investigations |
| Stamp et al. 2008 [63] | Australia | Anangu Bibi Family Birthing Program provides culturally-focused perinatal care for aboriginal mothers and families, with cultural guidance from an Aboriginal Women's advocacy group. Aboriginal maternal and infant care workers take a leadership role. | Qualitative study | |
| Thompson et al. 1998 [64] | USA | Rural Oregon Minority Prenatal Program seeks to provide culturally-appropriate care through using a bilingual and bicultural outreach worker as a cultural broker. | Observational analytic (retrospective cohort study) | Adequacy of prenatal care utilization index, including adequacy of prenatal care initiation; adequacy of total number of visits; distribution of prenatal visits |
| Warrick et al. 1992 [65] | USA | Peer health workers with similar cultural and community characteristics as the target population are employed in a community-based prenatal education programme to bridge the socio-cultural gap between providers and families. | Descriptive study (survey + qualitative components) | Number of prenatal visits; trimester prenatal care began; Birth attendant |
| Woodard and Edouard 1992 [66] | Canada | An advisory committee is created, made up of influential native women. The programme initially employs native women as counsellors, and includes native liaison workers with language abilities and cultural knowledge. | Descriptive study (service records) | Programme coverage |
| **Staff training** | | | | |
| Adams et al. 2005 [67] | China (Tibet) | A culturally-appropriate village birth attendant training programme. A committee ensures the curriculum used in training health workers is appropriate for the Tibetan context. Ethnographic research informed intervention design. | Qualitative study | |
| Andrus et al. 1997 [68] | USA | A prenatal outreach programme (Opening Doors) for a culturally-diverse population. Focusing on 'cultural competence,' peer health consultants work with providers to address barriers to care, and staff development and training programmes focus on cultural awareness. | Narrative description of intervention | |
| Bardack and Thompson 1993 [69] | USA | A prenatal programme in which medical students are taught to be humane, culturally sensitive and competent, with a focus on indigent women. | Narrative description of intervention | |
| Clapham et al. 2008 [70] | Nepal | An intervention to address the negative attitudes of some providers due to a combination of cultural influences and health system factors. | Descriptive study (project reviews + monitoring data) | |
| Fahey et al. 2013 [71] | Guatemala | PRONTO is an inter-professional obstetric and neonatal simulation training programme including components that deal with culturally-appropriate care. This intervention deals with cultural humility, informed by preliminary qualitative studies. | Formative qualitative study + narrative description of intervention | |
| Kreiner 2009 [72] | Canada | Initiatives to address the issue of accessible, quality maternity services to First Nation, rural and immigrant communities. Includes the development of an Aboriginal midwifery degree programme, and efforts to increase ethnic diversity and cultural competence in midwifery. | Descriptive study (qualitative + documentary sources) | |
| Sathar et al. 2005 [73] | Pakistan | A programme to make the individual client a focus of services and address some of the gender-related and familial constraints to health care service use. | Experimental (cluster non-RCT) | |
| Smith and Davies 2006 [74] | Canada | A programme to initiate the transfer and exchange of knowledge to improve prenatal care by bringing communities together to understand each other's goals and cultures. | Descriptive study (participant feedback) | |

**Table 5.** Included items: Health education interventions.

| Author and year | Country (ies) | Intervention | Literature/study type | Maternal care outcomes measured |
|---|---|---|---|---|
| Belizan et al. 1995 [76] | Argentina, Brazil, Cuba & Mexico | Prenatal care home visits where trained staff use a manual based on specially conducted ethnographic studies in each site on needs, fear, expectations and social support. | Experimental (RCT) | Utilisation of antenatal services; postpartum attendance at 40 days |
| Bhagat et al. 2002 [75] | Canada | Focus groups to tailor prenatal sessions to the needs and beliefs of the Punjabi community. The Punjabi language is used for materials and the event is launched during a cultural festival. | Narrative description of intervention | |
| Clemmons and Coulibaly 1995 [135] | Mali | The strategy used indigenous knowledge and cultural resources, including three traditional communication channels, for behaviour change (see [81]). | Descriptive study | |
| Clemmons and Coulibaly 1999 [81] | Mali | The strategy used indigenous knowledge and cultural resources, including three traditional communication channels, for behaviour change. | Descriptive study (survey) | Skilled birth assistance; prenatal consultations |
| Clemmons and Coulibaly 1999 [136] | Mali | The strategy used indigenous knowledge and cultural resources, including three traditional communication channels, for behaviour change (see [81]). | Descriptive study | |
| Coley 2012 [85] | USA | The Moms Matter support group employs cultural competence techniques, including the use of interpreters, hand-outs in other languages, respect for various cultures and inclusion of mothers' support people. | Qualitative study | Mother's care after childbirth |
| DeStephano et al. 2010 [86] | USA | A culturally-tailored health education video series for Somali women emphasising the importance of prenatal care. | Descriptive study (participant feedback + obstetric provider surveys) | |
| Doctor et al. 2012 [77] | Nigeria | Community education designed on the basis of a study of cultural beliefs and practices relevant to demand for antenatal care and facility-based childbirth. | Descriptive study (Baseline survey and qualitative data + preliminary evaluation with service utilisation data) | 1 antenatal visit; facility-based delivery |
| Dynes et al. 2011 [91] | Bangladesh | A skill-based programme disseminated through a training cascade, with emphasis on respectful consideration of local knowledge and agreement on actions to be taken during an obstetric or neonatal emergency. | Descriptive study (clinical data, performance testing + qualitative component) | |
| Gennaro et al. 2001 [82] | Malawi | A train the trainer intervention in which village leaders teach other villagers how to improve health (with a partly culture-based rationale). | Descriptive study (cross-sectional surveys pre and post intervention) | Prenatal care; postnatal care; birth site (home, TBA, clinic, or hospital) |
| Gies et al. 2008 [78] | Burkina Faso | Female community leaders are trained to promote specifically-designed health messages. Messages are based on a previous socio-anthropological survey investigating local perceptions and beliefs. | Experimental study cluster (part-RCT)) | 3+ ANC visits; 1st ANC visit in 3rd trimester; 2+ doses IPT-SP |
| Gummi et al. 1997 [92] | Nigeria | Community education with key messages developed by a team of leaders and women from the community. Cultural factors to seeking care are identified and addressed, such as men's role as decision-makers. | Descriptive study (preliminary studies + clinical data + qualitative component + repeat survey) | Utilisation of obstetric services |
| Karl-Trummer et al. 2006 [87] | Austria, Italy | The European 'Migrant-Friendly Hospitals' project conducted workshops on how to design services for migrant/ethnic minority pregnant women and their families. Tailored ethno-culturally sensitive information material and prenatal training courses were developed, informed by a needs assessment. | Qualitative study | |
| Midhet and Becker 2010 [88] | Pakistan | An information and education programme with cultural elements incorporated in design, such as the testing of materials for suitability to the local culture and consideration of the local dynamics of decision-making power. | Experimental study (cluster-RCT) | Visiting a qualified healthcare provider during 1st/2nd trimester for routine prenatal check-up; tetanus immunisation; type of birth attendant; in case of obstetric complication, referral to district hospital |

**Table 5.** Cont.

| Author and year | Country (ies) | Intervention | Literature/study type | Maternal care outcomes measured |
|---|---|---|---|---|
| Olaniran et al. 1997 [80] | Nigeria | Community health education and mobilisation informed by preliminary studies exploring knowledge, attitudes and practices. The intervention is discussed with community leaders and incorporates people fluent in the local dialect. Culturally-appropriate health education messages are developed in the local language or dialect, communicated through posters, drama and songs, and distributed in churches, markets and to clan heads. | Descriptive study (surveys, hospital statistics, financial records + qualitative component) | From polyclinic registers: total obstetric admissions; total deliveries; admissions for major obstetric complications |
| Omer et al. 2008 [89] | Pakistan | A health education intervention with participation at every stage from framing issues to planning and implementation. Communication tools are user-friendly and indigenous. | Experimental study (cluster-RCT) + qualitative component | Prenatal check-ups |
| Opoku et al. 1997 [79] | Ghana | Community health mobilisation, informed by preliminary studies exploring cultural and other factors. The project is discussed with the community and messages are communicated through role play and drama. | Descriptive study (health facility records, financial records, community data + qualitative component) | From hospital records: obstetric admissions |
| Perreira et al. 2002 [90] | Guatemala | Three health education interventions, including a clinic-based intervention using images of indigenous women with staff using buttons to identify the language they speak. | Observational analytic study (repeat cross-sectional studies) | Prenatal care utilisation |
| Ratnaike and Chinner 1992 [83] | Cambodia, Vietnam, Laos | A community health education system that seeks to address the unique cultural beliefs concerning medicine and health in Indochina. Cultural sensitivity and community participation are sought through minimal involvement of non-national health professionals. | Narrative description of intervention | |
| Sibley et al. 2001 [93] | India and Ethiopia | A community and competency-based program taking into consideration the social context of childbirth. A community self-assessment is conducted for community mobilisation and to provide information about local norms. | Narrative description of intervention | |
| Turan et al. 2011 [94] | Eritrea | Volunteers are trained to lead participatory educational sessions on safe motherhood. | Experimental study (non-RCT) + qualitative component + descriptive component | Birth at a health facility; % having recommended 4+ ANC visits |
| Yeshi et al. 2009 [84] | China (Tibet) | The programme involves village leadership in training and change promotion. | Descriptive study (project output data + survey) | Antenatal and delivery care |

care but do not explicitly describe whether or how the intervention addressed these cultural factors.

While the final sub-category comprises 14 items [103–116] that neither discuss cultural factors affecting the use of care nor explicitly frame the intervention as a strategy to address cultural factors, they are mentioned because participatory interventions are considered within the inclusive approach of this mapping as ones that inherently accommodate cultural factors.

Manandhar et al. [110] and Osrin et al. [116] describe a participatory, community-based women's group intervention with a marginalised population with low access to services in Nepal, facilitated through a community action cycle. They do not frame the intervention as one designed to address cultural factors. Yet, Morrison et al. [98], referring to the same intervention in Nepal, was placed in the subcategory of 'participatory approaches that focus explicitly on cultural factors,' because the item describes formative research that was used to design the intervention to be acceptable and sensitive to the local culture. The implication is that the distinction between the three sub-categories may not always be a reflection of differences in intervention content; it may in some cases simply be a result of the emphasis in authors' reporting. This attests to the elusiveness of how culture is incorporated and addressed in many health interventions.

**5. Mental health interventions.** This small category includes three fairly recent interventions focusing on perinatal depression, all aiming to overcome treatment barriers for Latina women in the USA [117–119] (Table 7). All three items describe adaptations to existing interventions and models. They use strategies for addressing cultural factors that are similar to those used in other categories, such as service providers sharing cultural characteristics of the target group, a more appropriate service setting, and/or more appropriate materials or therapy in terms of language or content.

## Description of types of literature and study designs

The map includes a wide range of literature, from narrative descriptions of interventions to studies using randomised controlled trials (RCTs) to evaluate impact. Eleven items provide only narrative descriptions of the intervention, including details of the design process, the content or its implementation. Some items

**Table 6.** Included items: Participatory approaches.

| Author and year | Country (ies) | Intervention | Literature/study type | Maternal care outcomes measured |
|---|---|---|---|---|
| **Approaches that explicitly focus on cultural factors** | | | | |
| Bhattacharyya and Murray 2000 [95] | Ethiopia | A community assessment for health staff and communities to jointly identify and prioritise health problems and develop plans to solve them. | Descriptive study (pre/post intervention surveys + qualitative component) | At least 2 ANC visits for last pregnancy |
| Hounton et al. 2009 [96] | Burkina Faso | Community mobilisation strategies include building awareness through engaging local traditional healers, administrative and religious leaders. Capacity is strengthened through facilitating community problem-solving, and culturally sensitive and locally acceptable approaches are identified to address barriers to care. | Experimental study (cluster non-RCT) | Institutional births |
| Jewell and Russell 2000 [97] | USA | Minority communities form a state-wide network of grassroots county minority health coalitions and a state coalition. Coalitions develop projects to increase access to early prenatal care for minority women with the intent of eliminating cultural barriers to care. Strategies include use of minority professional and paraprofessional staff, and monitoring of projects by minority health coalition boards. | Observational Analytic study (retrospective cohort study) | Kessner Adequacy of Prenatal Care Index (including timing of 1st prenatal visit; number of prenatal visits); Adequacy of Prenatal Care Utilization (including month prenatal care begins; ratio of actual number of visits to expected number) |
| Morrison et al. 2008 [98] | Nepal | A participatory, community-based women's group intervention informed by formative research. Aiming for sensitivity to local needs and beliefs, it addresses negotiation within families, and tailors information to the needs of local groups and stakeholders such as mothers-in-law and traditional healers. It aims to be a forum in which to discuss cultural ideas. | Descriptive study (survey, health service audit + qualitative component) | |
| **Approaches that refer to cultural factors affecting use only** | | | | |
| Orozco-Nuñez et al. [102] | | A key action was the coordination of a network to strengthen the links between communities, local authorities and health services. | Qualitative study | |
| Kaur 1994 [99] | Malaysia | The intervention is informed by an in-depth survey of the community's culture, beliefs and health status. Participatory planning meetings are held with relevant agencies. | Narrative description of intervention | |
| Mushi et al. 2010 [100] | Tanzania | In collaboration with villagers, representatives and health service providers, a community-based intervention package for Safe Motherhood is developed, relying heavily on community volunteers. | Descriptive study (surveillance data + qualitative component) | Deliveries with a skilled birth attendant; ANC attendance |
| O'Rourke et al. 1998 [101] | Bolivia | The Warmi project involves participatory women's groups, which identify problems and implement an action plan to address them. | Observational analytic study (case control study pre/post intervention) | Received prenatal care; utilisation of trained birth attendants (including TBAs, health promoters, physicians and nurses) |
| **Approaches that inherently address cultural factors** | | | | |
| Afsana 2012 [103] | Bangladesh | BRAC develops partnerships with communities to develop capacity and to build human resources for health at the community level. | Descriptive study (district indicators) | Receiving 4+ antenatal visits; referral to hospital for problems; place of delivery; 3+ postnatal visits |
| Ahluwalia et al. 2003 [104] | Tanzania | The Community Capacity Building and Empowerment Project is designed to promote problem solving in part through increasing participation by community members in planning and decision making. | Descriptive study (formative research + monitoring data, survey) | Timely referral to appropriate health facilities |
| Azad et al. 2010 [105] | Bangladesh | Participatory women's learning and action cycle groups. | Experimental study (cluster-RCT) | Uptake of antenatal and delivery services; health-care seeking behaviour (for any maternal illness or complication) |
| Kaseje et al. 2010 [106] | Kenya | A model engaging both the service delivery system and communities in an iterative process of dialogue for assessment, planning and action. | Experimental study (cluster non-RCT) + qualitative component + descriptive component | 4+ ANC attendance; health facility childbirth |

**Table 6.** Cont.

| Author and year | Country (ies) | Intervention | Literature/study type | Maternal care outcomes measured |
|---|---|---|---|---|
| Keyser and Pincus 2010 [107] | USA | A learning collaborative made up of various stakeholders, families and researchers is convened with the goal of building a model system of care. | Descriptive study (performance measures + qualitative component) | Programme enrolment; screening; referral; completed referral |
| Kwast 1995 [108] | Bolivia, Indonesia, Uganda, Nigeria, Guatemala | The MotherCare Project strengthened maternal health and family planning programmes through policy reform, behaviour change, and improved service delivery. | Descriptive study (case report) | ANC; trained birth attendant use |
| Lewycka et al. 2010 [109] | Malawi | Community mobilisation through women's groups. | Experimental study (cluster-RCT) | ANC (use of malaria prophylaxis in pregnancy + tetanus toxoid); facility based skilled attendant; uptake of prevention of mother-to-child transmission; postpartum check-ups; referral patterns. |
| Manandhar et al. 2004 [110] | Nepal | Participatory intervention with women's groups. | Experimental (cluster-RCT) | Any ANC; visited health facility in event of illness; institutional delivery |
| More et al. 2012 [111] | India | Participatory intervention with women's groups. | Experimental (cluster-RCT) | 1st antenatal visit before 3rd trimester; 3 or more ANC visits; institutional delivery; postnatal check |
| Morrison et al. 2011 [112] | Nepal | Community mobilisation through women's groups. | Protocol for cluster-RCT | None presented (but will measure Primary- 1. Deliveries conducted by trained health workers. 2. Institutional deliveries; Secondary- 1. ANC uptake. 2. Postnatal care uptake.) |
| Osrin et al. 2003 [116] | Nepal | A community-level participatory intervention with mothers and other key members of the community. | Reporting on implementation, but not results, of a cluster-RCT | NA (evaluation results not reported. Will include ANC service use, health-care seeking behaviour) |
| Rath et al. 2010 [113] | India | Participatory intervention with women's groups. | Descriptive study (qualitative component + monitoring data) | No |
| Skinner and Rathavy 2009 [114] | Cambodia | A community-development approach to birth preparedness. | Descriptive study (qualitative component + provider statistics + financial data) | Number receiving ANC, Number who gave birth with health centre midwife, Number who gave birth with a TBA, Number of referrals to hospital |
| Tripathy et al. 2010 [115] | India | A participatory intervention with women's groups. | Experimental study (cluster-RCT) | Any ANC; 3+ ANC visits; visited health facility in case of illness during pregnancy; institutional; birth attended by formal provider |

report on studies used to inform the design of an intervention now being implemented.

All other items present some type of evaluation data, whether for monitoring, outcome evaluation or impact evaluation. The majority of items present various forms of quantitative or qualitative data used for monitoring the intervention and/or to evaluate outcomes. Only 23 items describe studies that aim to measure intervention impact through the use of experimental or observational analytic designs. Of these, 14 use experimental designs including nine RCTs and five non-RCTs, and nine use observational-analytic designs including seven cohort studies.

Differences in study designs are evident across intervention categories. A large proportion of the studies with designs that aim to measure impact, particularly those with experimental designs, are in the 'participatory approaches' category. This is followed by a smaller proportion in the 'health education interventions' and 'service provider interventions' categories, and very few in the other categories combined.

## Discussion

Global recognition of the need to address cultural factors affecting the use of skilled maternity care has led to a wide range of interventions being implemented across diverse settings in all world regions and across all country income levels. Overall, the map provides a rich source of information on the types of intervention options that have been attempted to address or accommodate cultural factors that affect the use of skilled maternity care. The articles included in the systematic mapping and others indicate a growing awareness of the need to incorporate culture into the design of appropriate care to improve maternal and newborn outcomes [120,121] and to deliver more responsive, effective maternity care services.

The mapping reveals examples of good practice and success stories. However, some of the literature identified, whilst stating a clear aim of addressing cultural factors, provides insufficient detail to understand exactly how they were addressed. It is clear that the complexities of formulating and implementing culturally-responsive

**Table 7.** Included items: Mental health interventions.

| Author and year | Country (ies) | Intervention | Literature/study type | Maternal care outcomes measured |
|---|---|---|---|---|
| Baker-Ericzen et al. 2012 [117] | USA | A culturally-sensitive, short-term telemedicine, collaborative care intervention for addressing maternal depression among Mexican-American mothers during the perinatal period. Elements include bilingual, bicultural Mexican-American staff; training on Latina mental health issues; practices adapted to the Latino community; and intervention modules on sociocultural influences. | Descriptive study (qualitative component + monitoring data) | Treatment engagement; treatment adherence |
| Grote et al. 2004 [118] | USA | A culturally-relevant version of brief interpersonal psychotherapy (IPT-B) for perinatal depression. Additions include a pre-treatment engagement strategy consisting of an ethnographic interview accompanied by psycho-education to engage women in treatment; convenient service delivery location; flexible scheduling of treatment sessions at the clinic or on the phone; and facilitation of access to social services. | Qualitative study | |
| Le et al. 2010 [119] | USA | Cultural adaptation of an evidence-based cognitive–behavioural therapy intervention to prevent perinatal depression. Culturally-specific topics are addressed, such as immigration status, acculturation, and discrimination, and the discussion is tailored to Latinas' personal realities. Manuals are developed in Spanish and English. | Narrative description of intervention | |

programmes remain [16,122–126]. In some of the literature found, culture is positioned as a barrier to maternal health service use, rather than an attribute of the population that services seek to serve. The type of cultural groups in a setting and the nature of cultural factors that affect use of skilled maternity care are context-specific, and give rise to a need for different kinds of intervention approaches that both anticipate and respect a community's culture, values and beliefs. This finding is reflected in the map by the clustering of items from specific contexts in specific categories of intervention.

Cultural beliefs and behaviour are impossible to isolate from the social and economic context in which they occur [7]. Interventions research around culture and maternal health service use is heavily weighted in favour of evidence focusing on sub-populations in high-income countries. We know that 99% of maternal deaths occur in low income settings and that scaling up the use of skilled maternity care will reduce global maternal morbidity and mortality [18]. We know that focusing only on the supply side of maternity care does not necessarily lead to increased use, and that culture is often invoked as an explanation for this supply-demand gap. Our systematic mapping shows that there is a critical need for better documentation of interventions, with an emphasis on lower-income countries, and better study methods to evaluate the ways in which cultural factors can be systematically mainstreamed into programmes to increase maternity care service use. Literature on interventions addressing cultural factors as evaluated models of practice remains limited. This finding may be to some extent related to the small-scale, context-specific nature of many interventions of this type.

We exclude several interventions with TBAs providing childbirth services because our focus is on use of skilled maternal health care (see category 1). However, within these items, there are several examples where the TBAs cultural role is also harnessed to facilitate linkages with formal health services. Although WHO guidance has moved away from promoting approaches that involve TBAs in the direct provision of care at birth, it also emphasises the importance of building links with TBAs and finding new roles so that this valuable resource can continue to support women during pregnancy, childbirth and after birth, and serve as an important link between services and communities [127]. Future interventions incorporating WHO guidance on the need for women to be attended by health care workers with the appropriate skills and training may consider employing traditional health workers in alternative roles. Going beyond public health programmes, there is also a need to incorporate cultural knowledge and responsiveness into health education, the development of health policies, and the delivery of culturally-competent health care.

## Limitations

Limitations arising from the inevitable conceptual challenges of any attempt to map or categorise items focusing on 'culture' are acknowledged. Culture is a complex, elusive concept that is challenging to define, leading to diverse definitions and operationalisations in the literature. Usages of the term are not always helpful, and the concept is susceptible to assumptions and overgeneralisation. Making distinctions between interventions that address cultural factors and those that address other factors that affect use of skilled care was not a straightforward task. Distinguishing between interventions that address cultural factors as the primary and explicit aim on the one hand, and those in which cultural sensitivity is incorporated as part of generic quality improvement on the other, inevitably involves subjective judgement.

One particular challenge was the research question's focus not on what was actually 'done' in the intervention, but rather on what the intervention sought to address, which was reflected in the search terms. However, what the intervention seeks to address is not always carefully described by authors.

The above conceptual challenges all had implications for what was eventually identified and included. Identifying relevant items depended in part on the research team's judgement of where the line should be drawn around those to be included (outlined in Table 1). This effort was the first attempt of its kind to map such interventions; however, the range of interventions was unknown at the design stage, making it necessary for the research team to confer frequently and to continue drawing lines throughout the screening process. Moreover, at both the searching and screening stages, identifying relevant items depended in part on how authors of potentially relevant items framed their reporting, and also on the research team's ability to overcome challenges to identifying (from the text available) those that meet the criteria. The research team was aware of the challenges at the outset and continuously sought to address them from the design stage through to the final synthesis. Nevertheless, any shortcomings remain a limitation of this systematic mapping.

Relevant items may have been missed through method limitations. More specifically, any relevant literature in languages other than English, French or Spanish would have been missed. Because searches were not designed to focus on participatory approaches, some literature on these interventions may have been missed. Also, since it would have been unfeasible to search all of the infinite potential sources of grey literature, the possibility that some items of this type were missed is high. The possibility that some in-service reports on small-scale interventions that were not intended or prepared for wider circulation were missed is particularly high. Finally, we were unable to retrieve 16 items for screening that may have been eligible for inclusion. These 16 items largely represented interventions implemented in low- and middle-income countries.

## Conclusion

The map provides a rich source of information on interventions attempted in diverse settings that might have relevance elsewhere. However, many sources lack sufficient description or robust designs that allow us to draw firm conclusions. This may be to some extent related to the small-scale, context-specific nature of interventions of this type. Addressing the impacts of interventions to address cultural factors affecting the use of maternity care services is an issue of importance for researchers, programmers, and policy makers. It requires an inter-disciplinary approach and active dialogue with communities in order to understand their cultural systems, health beliefs, health practices and preferences. In order to better serve the varied needs of communities with culturally-diverse populations, the following recommendations are made for future research and reviews:

- The interventions in this map are inherently context-specific. Nevertheless, further intervention studies with harmonised outcomes, appropriate research methods and robust designs are warranted, which may provide valuable evidence on the impact (including benefits or potential harms) of a type of intervention model.
- Where an intervention is designed explicitly to address cultural factors, sufficient detail should be provided in reporting for the audience to understand how they were addressed (i.e., by specifying the links between the cultural factors identified and the content of the intervention).
- A full systematic review may be warranted of the more cohesive set of interventions designed to provide culturally-appropriate skilled maternity care for defined ethno-linguistic or religious groups. This would allow both the quality and outcomes of intervention studies to be examined.

## Acknowledgments

Brian Gaschler (LSE) and Stephanie Kumpunen (LSE) (SK) provided research assistance during the design of the search strategy. Dr Eleanor Hukin (LSE) (EH) and Stephanie Kumpunen (SK) provided research assistance during the search, screening and coding phases. The authors wish to thank the members of the advisory group for their support throughout the process including: Jessica Davis, Sebanti Ghosh, Azza Karam, Cicely Marston, and Tina Miller. Disclaimer: Anayda Portela (AP) is a staff member of the WHO. The author alone is responsible for the views expressed in this publication, and they do not necessarily represent the decisions or policies of the WHO.

## Author Contributions

Conceived and designed the experiments: EC EJ AP. Performed the experiments: EC EJ SL. Analyzed the data: EC EJ AP SL. Contributed reagents/materials/analysis tools: EC EJ AP SL. Wrote the paper: EC EJ AP SL.

## References


1. WHO (2005) The World Health Report 2005: Make every mother and child count. Geneva: World Health Organization.
2. Acsadi GT, Johnson-Acsadi G (1991) Social and cultural factors influencing maternal and child mortality in Sub-Saharan Africa with special reference to eastern African countries. New York, New York, Defense for Children International-USA, 1991. pp. 73–96.
3. Evans EC (2012) A review of cultural influence on maternal mortality in the developing world. Midwifery.
4. Thaddeus S, Maine D (1994) Too far to walk: maternal mortality in context. Soc Sci Med 38: 1091–1110.
5. WHO (2003) Working with individuals, families and communities to improve MNH. Geneva: World Health Organization.
6. Fisher TL, Burnet DL, Huang ES, Chin MH, Cagney KA (2007) Cultural leverage: interventions using culture to narrow racial disparities in health care. Med Care Res Rev 64: 243S–282S.
7. Helman C (2000) Culture, health, and illness. Oxford; Boston: Butterworth-Heinemann. 328p p.
8. Hall ET (1984) The Dance of Life: The Other Dimension of Time. Garden City, New York: Anchor.
9. Gabrysch S, Campbell OM (2009) Still too far to walk: literature review of the determinants of delivery service use. BMC Pregnancy Childbirth 9: 34.
10. Gabrysch S, Lema C, Bedrinana E, Bautista MA, Malca R, et al. (2009) Cultural adaptation of birthing services in rural Ayacucho, Peru. Bull World Health Organ 87: 724–729.
11. Glei DA, Goldman N, Rodriguez G (2003) Utilization of care during pregnancy in rural Guatemala:does obstetrical need matter? Social Science and Medicine 57: 2447–2463.
12. Camacho AV, Castro MD, Kaufman R (2006) Cultural aspects related to the health of Andean women in Latin America: A key issue for progress toward the attainment of the Millennium Development Goals. International Journal of Gynaecology and Obstetrics 94: 357–363.
13. Mackian S, Bedri N, Lovel H (2004) Up the garden path and over the edge: where might health-seeking behaviour take us? Health Policy and Planning 19: 137–146.
14. Miller T (1995) Shifting boundaries: Exploring the influence of cultural traditions and religious beliefs of Bangladeshi women on prenatal interactions. Women's Studies International Forum 18: 299–309.
15. Simwaka BN, Theobald S, Amekudzi YP, Tolhurst R (2005) Meeting millennium development goals 3 and 5. British Medical Journal 331: 708–709.
16. UNFPA (2005) Cultural Programming: Reproductive health challenges and strategies in East and South-East Asia. Bankgkok, Thailand: UNFPA.
17. Castro MD (2012) SISTEMATIZACIÓN DE BUENAS PRÁCTICAS EN EL DESARROLLO DE MODELOS DE ATENCIÓN A LA SALUD MATERNA CON PERTINENCIA INTERCULTURAL: Informe basado en el análisis de experiencias de Bolivia, Ecuador, Guatemala y Perú UNFPA-FCI. 51 p.
18. WHO (2007) Maternal mortality in 2005: estimates developed by WHO UNICEF, UNFPA, and the World Bank. Geneva: WHO.
19. WHO (2007) Engaging men and boys in changing gender based inequity in health: evidence from programme interventions. Geneva: WHO.
20. Greenhalgh T, Robert G, Macfarlane F, Bate P, Kyriakidou O, et al. (2005) Storylines of research in diffusion and innovation: a meta-narrative approach to systematic review. Social Science and Medicine 61: 417–430.
21. Oakley A, Gough D, Oliver S, James T (2005) The politics of evidence and methodology: lessons from the EPPI-Centre. Evidence and Policy 1: 5–31.
22. Abrami PC, Bernard RM, Wade CA (2006) Affecting policy and practice: issues involved in developing an Argument Catalogue. Evidence and Policy 2: 417–437.
23. Coast E, Leone T, Jones E, Hirose A (2012) Poverty and postnatal depression in low and middle income countries: a systematic mapping. Health and Place.
24. Leone T, Coast E, Narayanan S, Graft Aikins A (2012) Diabetes and depression comorbidity and socio-economic status in low and middle income countries (LMICs): a mapping of the evidence" Globalisation and Health 8.
25. WHO (2004) The critical role of the skilled attendant. Geneva: World Health Organization.
26. Homer CSE, Foureur MJ, Allende T, Pekin F, Caplice S, et al. (2012) 'It's more than just having a baby' women's experiences of a maternity service for

Australian Aboriginal and Torres Strait Islander families. Midwifery 28: E449–455.

27. Jan S, Conaty S, Hecker R, Bartlett M, Delaney S, et al. (2004) An holistic economic evaluation of an Aboriginal community-controlled midwifery programme in Western Sydney. J Health Serv Res Policy 9: 14–21.
28. Nel P, Pashen D (2003) Shared antenatal care for indigenous patients in a rural and remote community. Aust Fam Physician 32: 127–131.
29. Panaretto KS, Lee HM, Mitchell MR, Larkins SL, Manessis V, et al. (2005) Impact of a collaborative shared antenatal care program for urban Indigenous women: a prospective cohort study. Med J Aust 182: 514–519.
30. Panaretto KS, Mitchell MR, Anderson L, Larkins SL, Manessis V, et al. (2007) Sustainable antenatal care services in an urban Indigenous community: the Townsville experience. Med J Aust 187: 18–22.
31. Eckermann E, Deodato G (2008) Maternity waiting homes in southern Lao PDR: The unique 'silk home'. Journal of Obstetrics and Gynaecology Research 34: 767–775.
32. Schooley J, Mundt C, Wagner P, Fullerton J, O'Donnell M (2009) Factors influencing health care-seeking behaviours among Mayan women in Guatemala. Midwifery 25: 411–421.
33. Tucker K, Ochoa H, Garcia R, Sievwright K, Chambliss A, et al. (2013) The acceptability and feasibility of an intercultural birth center in the highlands of Chiapas, Mexico. BMC Pregnancy Childbirth 13: 94.
34. Moreno E, Lopez N (2013) Mother and child health in Ecudaor: Working together to build the Sumak Kawsay. Bulletin von Medicus Mundi Schweiz 127.
35. Gabrysch S, Lema C, Bedrinana E, Bautista MA, Malca R, et al. (2009) Cultural adaptation of birthing services in rural Ayacucho, Peru. Bulletin of the World Health Organization 87: 724–729.
36. Bender D, Santander A, Balderrama A, Arce A, Medina R (1995) Transforming the Process of Service Delivery to Reduce Maternal Mortality in Cochabamba, Bolivia. Reproductive health matters 3: 52–59.
37. Affonso DD, Mayberry LJ, Graham K, Shibuya J, Kunimoto J (1993) Prenatal and postpartum care in Hawaii: a community-based approach. Journal of Obstetric and Gynecological Neonatal Nursing 22: 320–325.
38. Mayberry LJ, Affonso DD, Shibuya J, Clemmens D (1999) Integrating cultural values, beliefs, and customs into pregnancy and postpartum care: Lessons learned from a Hawaiian public health nursing project. Journal of Perinatal & Neonatal Nursing 13: 15–26.
39. Reavy K, Hobbs J, Hereford M, Crosby K (2012) A new clinic model for refugee health care: adaptation of cultural safety. Rural & Remote Health 12: 1–12.
40. Kim J (2003) Survey on the programs of Sanhujori centers in Korea as the traditional postpartum care facilities. Women & Health 38: 107–117.
41. Kenney AM, Siupsinskas G, Sharman D, Adilbekova R, Zues O (2005) Technical report: Introducing international approaches to safe motherhood in Zhezkazgan: results of a pilot project in Kazakhstan. Almaty, Kazakhstan, Abt Associates, ZdravPlus, 2005 Apr. [55] p. p.
42. Ahmed T, Jakaria S (2009) Community-based skilled birth attendants in Bangladesh: attending deliveries at home. Reproductive health matters 17: 45–50.
43. Blum LS, Sharmin T, Ronsmans C (2006) Attending Home vs. Clinic-Based Deliveries: Perspectives of Skilled Birth Attendants in Matlab, Bangladesh. Reproductive Health Matters 14: 51–60.
44. Alto WA, Albu RE, Irabo G (1991) An alternative to unattended delivery–a training programme for village midwives in Papua New Guinea. Soc Sci Med 32: 613–618.
45. Bailey PE, Szaszdi JA, Glover L (2002) Obstetric complications: does training traditional birth attendants make a difference? Revista Panamerica de Salud Publica Pan American Journal of Public Health 11: 15–23.
46. Dehne KL, Wacker J, Cowley J (1995) Training birth attendants in the Sahel. World Health Forum 16: 415–419.
47. Hoff W (1997) Traditional health practitioners as primary health care workers. TROPICAL DOCTOR 27 Suppl 1: 52–55.
48. Rowen T, Prata N, Passano P (2011) Evaluation of a traditional birth attendant training programme in Bangladesh. Midwifery 27: 229–236.
49. Smit JJ (1994) Traditional birth attendants in Malawi. Curationis 17: 25–28.
50. Bilenko N, Hammel R, Belmaker I (2007) Utilization of antenatal care services by a semi-nomadic Bedouin Arab population: evaluation of the impact of a local Maternal and Child Health Clinic. Matern Child Health J 11: 425–430.
51. Dundek LH (2006) Establishment of a Somali doula program at a large metropolitan hospital. Journal of Perinatal & Neonatal Nursing 20: 128–137.
52. Nauman T (1995) Mexico: birth revolution. POPULI 22: 8.
53. Chowdhury M (1998) The role of traditional birth attendants in a safe delivery programme in Bangladesh. TROPICAL DOCTOR 28: 104–106.
54. Friedsam D, Haug G, Rust M, Lake A (2003) Tribal benefits counseling program: Expanding health care opportunities for tribal members. American Journal of Public Health 93: 1634–1636.
55. Hazard CJ, Callister LC, Birkhead A, Nichols L (2009) Hispanic Labor Friends Initiative Supporting Vulnerable Women. Mcn-the American Journal of Maternal-Child Nursing 34: 115–121.
56. Hicks C, Hayes L (1991) Linkworkers in antenatal care: facilitators of equal opportunities in health provision or salves for the management conscience? Health Services Management Research 4: 89–93.
57. Julnes G, Konefal M, Pindur W, Kim P (1994) Community-based perinatal care for disadvantaged adolescents: evaluation of The Resource Mothers Program. J Community Health 19: 41–53.
58. Ley CE, Copeland VC, Flint CS (2011) Healthy Start Program Participation: The Consumers' Perspective. Social Work in Public Health 26: 17–34.
59. Marsiglia FF, Bermudez-Parsai M, Coonrod D (2010) Familias Sanas: an intervention designed to increase rates of postpartum visits among Latinas. Jouranl of Health Care for the Poor & Underserved 21: 119–131.
60. Mattson S, Lew L (1992) Culturally sensitive prenatal care for Southeast Asians. Journal of Obstetric & Gynecological Neonatal Nursing 21: 48–54.
61. Meister JS, Warrick LH, de Zapien JG, Wood AH (1992) Using lay health workers: case study of a community-based prenatal intervention. J Community Health 17: 37–51.
62. Parsons L, Day S (1992) Improving Obstetric Outcomes in Ethnic-Minorities - An Evaluation of Health Advocacy in Hackney. Journal of Public Health Medicine 14: 183–191.
63. Stamp GE, Champion S, Anderson G, Warren B, Stuart-Butler D, et al. (2008) Aboriginal maternal and infant care workers: partners in caring for Aboriginal mothers and babies. Rural and Remote Health 8.
64. Thompson M, Curry MA, Burton D (1998) The effects of nursing case management on the utilization of prenatal care by Mexican-Americans in rural Oregon. Public Health Nursing 15: 82–90.
65. Warrick LH, Wood AH, Meister JS, de Zapien JG (1992) Evaluation of a peer health worker prenatal outreach and education program for Hispanic farmworker families. J Community Health 17: 13–26.
66. Woodard GRB, Edouard L (1992) Reaching Out - A Community Initiative for Disadvantaged Pregnant Women. Canadian Journal of Public Health-Revue Canadienne De Sante Publique 83: 188–190.
67. Adams V, Miller S, Chertow J, Craig S, Samen A (2005) Having a "safe delivery": conflicting views from Tibet. Health Care for Women International 26: 821–851.
68. Andrus NC, Partner SF, Leppert PC (1997) Analyzing strategies for developing a prenatal health care outreach program to reduce social and cultural barriers. J Health Hum Serv Adm 20: 230-241.
69. Bardack MA, Thompson SH (1993) Model prenatal program of Rush Medical College at St. Basil's Free Peoples Clinic, Chicago. Public Health Rep 108: 161–165.
70. Clapham S, Pokharel D, Bird C, Basnett I (2008) Addressing the attitudes of service providers: increasing access to professional midwifery care in Nepal. TROPICAL DOCTOR 38: 197–201.
71. Fahey JO, Cohen SR, Holme F, Buttrick ES, Dettinger JC, et al. (2013) Promoting Cultural Humility During Labor and Birth. Journal of Perinatal & Neonatal Nursing 27: 36–42.
72. Kreiner M (2009) Delivering diversity: newly regulated midwifery returns to Manitoba, Canada, one community at a time. Journal of Midwifery & Womens Health 54: e1–e10.
73. Sathar Z, Jain A, RamaRao S, ul Haque M, Kim J (2005) Introducing Client-Centered Reproductive Health Services in a Pakistani Setting. Studies in Family Planning 36: 221–234.
74. Smith D, Davies B (2006) Creating a new dynamic in Aboriginal health. Can Nurse 102: 36–39.
75. Bhagat R, Johnson J, Grewal S, Pandher P, Quong E, et al. (2002) Mobilizing the community to address the prenatal health needs of immigrant Punjabi women. Public Health Nursing 19: 209–214.
76. Belizan JM, Barros F, Langer A, Farnot U, Victora C, et al. (1995) Impact of health education during pregnancy on behavior and utilization of health resources. Latin American Network for Perinatal and Reproductive Research. American journal of obstetrics and gynecology 173: 894–899.
77. Doctor HV, Findley SE, Ager A, Cometto G, Afenyadu GY, et al. (2012) Using community-based research to shape the design and delivery of maternal health services in Northern Nigeria. Reproductive health matters 20: 104–112.
78. Gies S, Coulibaly SO, Ouattara FT, Ky C, Brabin BJ, et al. (2008) A community effectiveness trial of strategies promoting intermittent preventive treatment with sulphadoxine-pyrimethamine in pregnant women in rural Burkina Faso. Malar J 7: 180.
79. Opoku SA, KyeiFaried S, Twum S, Djan JO, Browne ENL, et al. (1997) Community education to improve utilization of emergency obstetric services in Ghana. International Journal of Gynecology & Obstetrics 59: S201–S207.
80. Olaniran N, Offiong S, Ottong J, Asuquo E, Duke F (1997) Mobilizing the community to utilize obstetric services, Cross River State, Nigeria. The Calabar PMM Team. International Journal of Gynaecology & Obstetrics 59 Suppl 2: S181–189.
81. Clemmons L, Coulibaly Y (1999) Cultural resources and maternal health in Mali. Washington, D.C., World Bank, Africa Region, Knowledge and Learning Center, 1999 Sep. 4 p. p.
82. Gennaro S, Thyangathyanga D, Kershbaumer R, Thompson J (2001) Health promotion and risk reduction in Malawi, Africa, village women. Journal of Obstetric and Gynecological Neonatal Nursing 30: 224–230.
83. Ratnaike RN, Chinner TL (1992) A community health education system to meet the health needs of Indo-Chinese women. J Community Health 17: 87–96.
84. Yeshi C, Wangdui P, Holcombe S (2009) Health and Hygiene Behaviour Change: Bottom-Up Meets Top-Down in Tibet. Development in Practice 19: 396–402.

85. Coley SL (2012) New Baby in a New Country: Supporting Local Immigrant Pregnant Mothers through "Moms Matter". International Journal of Childbirth Education 27: 57–62.
86. DeStephano CC, Flynn PM, Brost BC (2010) Somali prenatal education video use in a United States obstetric clinic: A formative evaluation of acceptability. Patient Education and Counseling 81: 137–141.
87. Karl-Trummer U, Krajic K, Novak-Zezula S, Pelikan JM (2006) Prenatal courses as health promotion intervention for migrant/ethnic minority women: high efforts and good results, but low attendance. Diversity in Health & Social Care 3: 55–58.
88. Midhet F, Becker S (2010) Impact of community-based interventions on maternal and neonatal health indicators: Results from a community randomized trial in rural Balochistan, Pakistan. Reproductive Health.
89. Omer K, Mhatre S, Ansari N, Laucirica J, Andersson N (2008) Evidence-based training of frontline health workers for door-to-door health promotion: A pilot randomized controlled cluster trial with lady health workers in Sindh Province, Pakistan. Patient Education and Counseling 72: 178–185.
90. Perreira KM, Bailey PE, de Bocaletti E, Hurtado E, Recinos de Villagran S, et al. (2002) Increasing awareness of danger signs in pregnancy through community- and clinic-based education in Guatemala. Maternal & Child Health Journal 6: 19–28.
91. Dynes M, Rahman A, Beck D, Moran A, Rahman A, et al. (2011) Home-based life saving skills in Matlab, Bangladesh: a process evaluation of a community-based maternal child health programme. Midwifery 27: 15–22.
92. Gummi FB, Hassan M, Shehu D, Audu L (1997) Community education to encourage use of emergency obstetric services, Kebbi State, Nigeria. International Journal of Gynecology & Obstetrics 59: S191–S200.
93. Sibley L, Buffington ST, Beck D, Armbruster D (2001) Home based life saving skills: Promoting safe motherhood through innovative community-based interventions. Journal of Midwifery & Womens Health 46: 258–266.
94. Turan JM, Tesfagiorghis M, Polan ML (2011) Evaluation of a Community Intervention for Promotion of Safe Motherhood in Eritrea. Journal of Midwifery & Womens Health 56: 8–17.
95. Bhattacharyya K, Murray J (2000) Community assessment and planning for maternal and child health programs: A participatory approach in Ethiopia. Human Organization 59: 255–266.
96. Hounton S, Byass P, Brahima B (2009) Towards reduction of maternal and perinatal mortality in rural Burkina Faso: communities are not empty vessels. Global health action 2.
97. Jewell NA, Russell KM (2000) Increasing access to prenatal care: an evaluation of minority health coalitions' early pregnancy project. J Community Health Nurs 17: 93–105.
98. Morrison J, Osrin D, Shrestha B, Tumbahangphe KM, Tamang S, et al. (2008) How did formative research inform the development of a women's group intervention in rural Nepal? Journal of Perinatology 28: S14–S22.
99. Kaur P (1994) Providing choices for a marginalized community. A community-based project with Malaysian aborigines. PLANNED PARENTHOOD CHALLENGES: 23–25.
100. Mushi D, Mpembeni R, Jahn A (2010) Effectiveness of community based Safe Motherhood promoters in improving the utilization of obstetric care. The case of Mtwara Rural District in Tanzania. BMC Pregnancy Childbirth 10: 14.
101. O'Rourke K, Howard-Grabman L, Seoane G (1998) Impact of community organization of women on perinatal outcomes in rural Bolivia. Revista Panamerica de Salud Publica Pan American Journal of Public Health 3: 9–14.
102. Orozco-Nunez E, Gonzalez-Block M, Kageyama-Escobar L, Hernandez-Prado B (2009) The experience of the Mexican maternal health care program Arranque Parejo en la Vida. Salud Publica De Mexico 51: 104–113.
103. Afsana K (2012) Empowering the Community: BRAC's Approach in Bangladesh; Hussein J, McCawBinns A, Webber R, editors. Cambridge, MA: CABI Publishing. 170–180 p.
104. Ahluwalia IB, Schmid T, Kouletio M, Kanenda O (2003) An evaluation of a community-based approach to safe motherhood in northwestern Tanzania. International Journal of Gynecology & Obstetrics 82: 231–240.
105. Azad K, Barnett S, Banerjee B, Shaha S, Khan K, et al. (2010) Effect of scaling up women's groups on birth outcomes in three rural districts in Bangladesh: a cluster-randomised controlled trial. Lancet 375: 1193–1202.
106. Kaseje D, Olayo R, Musita C, Oindo CO, Wafula C, et al. (2010) Evidence-based dialogue with communities for district health systems' performance improvement. Global public health 5: 595–610.
107. Keyser DJ, Pincus HA (2010) From community-based pilot testing to region-wide systems change: lessons from a local quality improvement collaborative. Programme in Community Health Partnerships 4: 105–114.
108. Kwast BE (1995) Building a Community Based Maternity Program. International Journal of Gynecology & Obstetrics 48: S67–S82.
109. Lewycka S, Mwansambo C, Kazembe P, Phiri T, Mganga A, et al. (2010) A cluster randomised controlled trial of the community effectiveness of two interventions in rural Malawi to improve health care and to reduce maternal, newborn and infant mortality. Trials 11: 88.
110. Manandhar DS, Osrin D, Shrestha BP, Mesko N, Morrison J, et al. (2004) Effect of a participatory intervention with women's groups on birth outcomes in Nepal: cluster-randomised controlled trial. Lancet 364: 970–979.
111. More NS, Bapat U, Das S, Alcock G, Patil S, et al. (2012) Community mobilization in Mumbai slums to improve perinatal care and outcomes: a cluster randomized controlled trial. PLoS Med 9: e1001257.
112. Morrison J, Tumbahangphe KM, Budhathoki B, Neupane R, Sen A, et al. (2011) Community mobilisation and health management committee strengthening to increase birth attendance by trained health workers in rural Makwanpur, Nepal: study protocol for a cluster randomised controlled trial. Trials 12: 128.
113. Rath S, Nair N, Tripathy PK, Barnett S, Rath S, et al. (2010) Explaining the impact of a women's group led community mobilisation intervention on maternal and newborn health outcomes: the Ekjut trial process evaluation. Bmc International Health and Human Rights 10.
114. Skinner J, Rathavy T (2009) Design and evaluation of a community participatory, birth preparedness project in Cambodia. Midwifery 25: 738–743.
115. Tripathy P, Nair N, Barnett S, Mahapatra R, Borghi J, et al. (2010) Effect of a participatory intervention with women's groups on birth outcomes and maternal depression in Jharkhand and Orissa, India: a cluster-randomised controlled trial. Lancet 375: 1182–1192.
116. Osrin D, Mesko N, Shrestha BP, Shrestha D, Tamang S, et al. (2003) Reducing childhood mortality in poor countries - Implementing a community-based participatory intervention to improve essential newborn care in rural Nepal. Transactions of the Royal Society of Tropical Medicine and Hygiene 97: 18–21.
117. Baker-Ericzen MJ, Connelly CD, Hazen AL, Duenas C, Landsverk JA, et al. (2012) A Collaborative Care Telemedicine Intervention to Overcome Treatment Barriers for Latina Women With Depression During the Perinatal Period. Families Systems & Health 30: 224–240.
118. Grote NK, Bledsoe SE, Swartz HA, Frank E (2004) Culturally relevant psychotherapy for perinatal depression in low-income ob/gyn patients. Clinical Social Work Journal 32: 327–347.
119. Le HN, Zmuda J, Perry DF, Munoz RF (2010) Transforming an evidence-based intervention to prevent perinatal depression for low-income Latina immigrants. Americal Journal of Orthopsychiatry 80: 34–45.
120. Pell C, Meñaca A, Were F, Afrah NA, Chatio S, et al. (2013) Factors Affecting Antenatal Care Attendance: Results from Qualitative Studies in Ghana, Kenya and Malawi. PLoS ONE 8: e53747.
121. Finlayson K, Downe S (2013) Why Do Women Not Use Antenatal Services in Low- and Middle-Income Countries? A Meta-Synthesis of Qualitative Studies. PLoS Med 10: e1001373.
122. Goodburn E, Campbell O (2001) Reducing maternal mortality in the developing world: Sector-wide approaches may be key. Social Science and Medicine 35: 967–977.
123. UNFPA (2005) Culture Matters - Working with Communities and Faith-based Organizations: Case Studies from Country Programmes. United Nations Population Fund (UNFPA). 1–103 p.
124. UNFPA (2008) Culture Matters - Lessons From a Legacy of Engaging Faith-Based Organizations as Cultural Agents of Change. United Nations Population Fund (UNFPA). 1–113 p.
125. UNFPA (2010) Promoting Equality, Recognizing Diversity - Intercultural Sexual and Reproductive Health among Indigenous Peoples in Latin America. United Nations Population Fund (UNFPA). 1–27 p.
126. UNFPA (2011) Social and Cultural Determinants on Sexual and Reproductive Health - Studies From Asia and Latin America. United Nations Population Fund (UNFPA). [Online]. Available from: http://www.unfpa.org/public/home/publications/pid/8825.
127. WHO (2010) Working with individuals, families and communities to improve maternal and newborn health. Geneva: World Health Organization.
128. Kreuter MW, Lukwago SN, Bucholtz RD, Clark EM, Sanders-Thompson V (2003) Achieving cultural appropriateness in health promotion programs: targeted and tailored approaches. Health Educ Behav 30: 133–146.
129. Dickerson T, Crookston B, Simonsen SE, Sheng XM, Samen A, et al. (2010) Pregnancy and Village Outreach Tibet A Descriptive Report of a Community- and Home-Based Maternal-Newborn Outreach Program in Rural Tibet. Journal of Perinatal & Neonatal Nursing 24: 113–125.
130. Greenberg EL, Perz M, Sockalingam S, Hayes M (1996) Multicultural maternal and child health outreach: Washington State strategies to assure access for Asian and Pacific Islander women and children. Journal of Public Health Management and Practice 2: 66–71.
131. Larson K, McGuire J, Watkins E, Mountain K (1992) Maternal care coordination for migrant farmworker women: program structure and evaluation of effects on use of prenatal care and birth outcome. Journal of Rural Health 8: 128–133.
132. McAree T, McCourt C, Beake S (2010) Perceptions of group practice midwifery from women living in an ethnically diverse setting. Evidence Based Midwifery 8: 91–97.
133. Nurena CR (2009) Incorporation of an intercultural approach in the Peruvian health care system: the vertical birth method. Revista Panamerica de Salud Publica Pan American Journal of Public Health 26: 368–376.
134. Zangari A (2009) El enfoque intercultural en la atención de la salud materna: una estrategia de aplicación -The intercultural approach in maternal health care: an implementation strategy. In: Menardi LC, Zangari A, Navarro RC, editors. Yachay Tinkuy: Salud E Interculturalidad en Bolivia Y America Latina. Bolivia: PROHISABA, Cooperacion Italiana, Editorial Gente Comun. pp. 454–478.
135. Clemmons L, Coulibaly Y (1995) Africare/Mali: creative communication for maternal health. PVO CHILD SURVIVAL TECHNICAL REPORT 4: 5–6.
136. Clemmons L, Coulibaly Y (1999) Turning the ordinary into the extraordinary: The Green Pendelu and maternal health in Mali. Arlington, Virginia, Partnership for Child Health Care, Basic Support for Institutionalizing Child Survival [BASICS], 1999 Oct. pp. [15]p.

# 21

# Challenges and Opportunities: What Can We Learn from Patients Living with Chronic Musculoskeletal Conditions, Health Professionals and Carers about the Concept of Health Literacy Using Qualitative Methods of Inquiry?

**Charlotte Salter*, Julii Brainard, Lisa McDaid, Yoon Loke**

Norwich Medical School, Faculty of Medicine & Health Sciences, University of East Anglia, Norwich, NR4 7TJ, United Kingdom

**Abstract**

The field of health literacy continues to evolve and concern public health researchers and yet remains a largely overlooked concept elsewhere in the healthcare system. We conducted focus group discussions in England UK, about the concept of health literacy with older patients with chronic musculoskeletal conditions (mean age =73.4 years), carers and health professionals. Our research posed methodological, intellectual and practical challenges. Gaps in conceptualisation and expectations were revealed, reiterating deficiencies in predominant models for understanding health literacy and methodological shortcomings of using focus groups in qualitative research for this topic. Building on this unique insight into what the concept of health literacy meant to participants, we present analysis of our findings on factors perceived to foster and inhibit health literacy and on the issue of *responsibility* in health literacy. Patients saw health literacy as a result of an inconsistent interactive process and the implications as wide ranging; healthcare professionals had more heterogeneous views. All focus group discussants agreed that health literacy most benefited from good inter-personal communication and partnership. By proposing a *needs-based* approach to health literacy we offer an alternative way of conceptualising health literacy to help improve the health of older people with chronic conditions.

**Editor:** Karen Spilsbury, The University of York, United Kingdom

**Funding:** This research was funded by the National Institute for Health Research under its Research for Patient Benefit Programme (RfPB). The funders had no role in study design, data collection and analysis, decision to publish, or preparation of the manuscript.

**Competing Interests:** The authors have declared that no competing interests exist.

* Email: c.salter@uea.ac.uk

## Background

Health literacy (HL) is an evolving concept [1]. Definitions and practical intervention models vary widely [2–5]. The most common perspective is that HL is a personal asset, a package of competencies relevant to personal healthcare, and a skill-set typically ascribed mostly or solely to individual patients rather than to context or healthcare delivery systems. Estimates are that 15–26% of adults in developed nations have poor HL, while a further 20–29% have HL skills that are at best 'problematic' or 'marginal' [6–8]. HL is measured as poorest in the oldest age cohorts. This may be due to fewer years of formal education amongst this age group, increased complexity of healthcare and medical needs and/or decline in cognitive function [9].

This paper discusses methodological challenges in using focus groups to undertake qualitative research into HL in older adults. We explore how the HL concept is interpreted by patients, their carers and health professionals, and how these interpretations may differ from predominant research directions and academic models. We propose that HL might be more accurately described as a 'whole-system' construction rather than as either an individual asset (something that can be promoted) or an individual risk (something that is missing and needs correcting). This perspective seems to ally more with the minority model of HL as a risk, arising from a set of attributes belonging to patient, setting, modes of delivery and other provider features [3], [4]. However, much focus in the field of HL at the risk level concentrates on the notion of individual time and place specific clinical risk and only measured cross-sectionally. The emergence of a broader conceptualisation of a risk model of HL in patients' understanding allows us to revisit shortcomings in both the traditional asset and risk models. We explore some of the limitations in previous interpretations of the risk view of HL, and how it might be redeveloped and perhaps even integrated with the asset model. The contrast between an asset model and a whole-system attributes approach is significant and has many implications for healthcare delivery. However, the observations are framed by the characteristics of the study participants and to some extent by the data collection techniques. The research was also undertaken within the context of how health care is usually obtained in the UK, which is through the National Health Service (NHS), a taxpayer funded service which provides the vast majority of medical care in the UK. We therefore present our suggestions in the context of methodological challenges in undertaking such qualitative research.

## Introduction

Early (1990s) definitions and conceptual models of health literacy (HL) were concerned with identifying patients with significant shortcomings in literacy and numeracy skills. These basic deficits were observed to comprise >40% of US adults unable to read complex text [10] and one in five UK adults with less literacy than expected of an 11 year old child and up to 40% of adults with significant numeracy problems [11]. It was anxiety raised by these statistics that fuelled an interest in health literacy where in the context of the US and UK healthcare systems both rely extensively on complex written and verbal information to guide patients. Nutbeam (2000) [12] categorised HL into 3-levels: functional, interactive and critical. Functional HL is concerned with basic skills (reading and numeracy). Interactive HL further involves communicative and social skills necessary to understand and apply new information in changing situations. Critical HL is a 'higher level' set of cognitive and social skills used to critically examine health information. Chinn [13] described critical HL as a social asset (whereas functional HL may be seen as a health knowledge deficit). Numerous assessment instruments have been developed to measure functional and sometimes interactive HL in individuals [14], [15]. Most such instruments are relatively easy to administer but are quite simplistic in what they assess, focusing primarily on word or short sentence comprehension. Much research exists that establishes a consistent deleterious association between low HL levels as indicated by those instruments and health outcomes [16], [17] although the full causal pathways remain uncertain [16–18].

The view of HL as an individual attribute (or asset) has dominated and indeed is the basis of many intervention and health promotion efforts. However, variations on the perspective have emerged. Baker [19] described HL as an individual's ability to function in a healthcare environment, while Volandes and Paasche-Orlow [20] argued that HL can only be addressed and understood in the context of other health-related inequalities. Nutbeam (2008) [4] described Baker's work as a 'risk' model of HL and critiqued it as too limited in scope for development of interventions but welcomed perspectives which might better integrate the risk and assets models. Most practical guidance to address poor HL (e.g. Nielsen-Bohlman et al. [10]) has stated that while HL levels are individual patient assets, health professionals have joint responsibility with patients for tackling problems of low HL. Other recent definitions and models [2], [21] describe HL as an individual or population asset, while simultaneously portraying it as a product of both context (including external mediators) and patient capacities. Common to all such research is an untested underlying assumption that if people are given the conditions (skills, awareness, information etc) to make individual informed decisions, then they will 'do the right thing': i.e. adopt public health and (bio)medical strategies deemed necessary and important to promote and maintain good health. As a result, poor health literacy has become almost synonymous with undesirable health choices. We will return later to the tangled problems of low HL and non-adherence.

## Methods

This research was part of a National Institute for Health Research study to evaluate the impact of low HL on older people with chronic conditions and identify areas for improvement in patient care and future research. Musculoskeletal conditions were chosen because we had conducted a systematic review and collected published data on these conditions. The specific aim of the focus group discussions (FGD) was to explore with older people, carers and healthcare professionals the concept of HL and issues they believed might impact on the HL of older people with musculoskeletal conditions. All FGD took place in 2012 in the East of England. Ethical approval was granted by East of England National Research Ethics Committee – 09/H0310/30.

We conducted six interactive focus groups with older patients living with musculoskeletal conditions, carers and their health professionals (HP) recruited from secondary care, primary care and community settings run by the National Health Service (NHS). See Table 1. We employed a three-prong approach to recruitment as we envisaged it might be challenging. In the event three focus groups were conducted (n = 15) with older patients (mean age = 73.4 years) recruited through the local hospital rheumatology department; a community support group for people with rheumatoid conditions, and via a specialist rheumatology nurse at a large primary care medical centre. Prominent posters advertised the research and staff were asked to give information packs to suitable patients. Although we aimed for a purposive sample to represent a broad a range of characteristics including social class, gender and education, recruitment was challenging and we became reliant on HP to give information packs to potentially eligible consecutive patients with at least one long-term musculoskeletal condition. The researcher (LM) then followed up potential participants with a phone call to explain the study in full and ask if they were willing to take part. Everyone approached agreed to take part although at least one person dropped out on the day of each of the patient focus groups (n = 5). Rheumatoid arthritis was the main chronic illness reported by patients (n = 10), with four other musculoskeletal conditions and type II diabetes also represented. All bar one patient considered their health to be fair to good at the time of the FGDs. Two thirds of participants were female. We achieved a range of socio-economic backgrounds. Nearly two thirds left school by age 15 and three went on to higher education. All but one gave their current employment status as retired. Focus group discussions were held at the university research park and the primary care medical centre respectively.

Two focus groups were conducted with HPs (n = 16); one in secondary care and one in primary care. See Table 1. Details of individual participants are not included in order to maintain confidentiality. The primary care focus group included 6 general practitioners, two of whom were male, plus five nurse practitioners. The hospital based focus group was an all-female group that consisted of five members of the specialist practitioner multidisciplinary rheumatology team including nurses, a healthcare assistant and occupational therapists but no physicians. Unfortunately, recruitment of carers proved difficult, despite over a thousand leaflets being distributed within a local charity newsletter (Norwich Age UK). The leaflet asked 'can you help improve services for older people living with chronic illnesses' and carers were specifically invited to attend a group discussion about accessing, using and understand health care services. Travel and replacement carer costs plus refreshments were offered to all. We eventually recruited 2 carers (only) via an existing carers support group at the same primary care medical centre and had another carer in attendance at a patient FGD to support her husband's personal care needs and speak for him when he got exhausted during the discussion. A fourth potential carer sadly declined to participate after he found the consent forms too stressful to fill in. Recently bereaved, he had 'had enough of red tape and paper work to last a lifetime'. This highlighted to us the excess burden

**Table 1.** Focus Group Participants by Recruitment Site.

| Group Number | Type of participant | No of participants |
|---|---|---|
| FG1 | Patients recruited in primary care setting | 5 |
| FG2 | Patients recruited in community Group | 6 |
| FG3 | Patients recruited in hospital setting | 5 |
| FG4 | Carers recruited in primary care setting | 2 |
| FG5 | Health professionals in primary care | 11 |
| FG6 | Health professionals in hospital setting | 5 |

that constant form filling and applications for support services can place on vulnerable people.

## Data collection

A topic guide was used to ensure the same domains were covered in each focus group and open-ended questions and prompts used to encourage participants to talk about their own experiences and views as well as those of their peers. Domains included: i) understanding of the concept of HL and how it might impact on the experience of older people living with long term chronic health conditions; ii) experiences of accessing, navigating and engaging with the healthcare system; and, iii) factors that might enhance or impede HL. We aimed not to impose any existing theoretical framework on the discussions. The focus group discussions lasted average 81 minutes (range 72–91) and were interactive as after approximately one hour 'trigger material' was presented to participants to stimulate further discussion. This took the form of a short 2 minute video clip about health literacy with Professor Rima Rudd talking about how words can get in the way of understanding and access to health (https://www.youtube.com/watch?v=_d-dtYTpdCw) and a brief summary of our findings from the literature about the issues facing older people with low HL and chronic conditions [22], [23]. FGD were audio recorded, transcribed verbatim and all identifiers removed.

Two experienced moderators (CS and LM) were present at each FGD and reassurance given that the views of all participants would be respected equally and all identifiers removed from transcripts and subsequent documentation. All groups aimed to maintain a friendly and approachable (casual and non-intimidating) atmosphere and moderators invited contributions from all participants. The HP were known to one another and talked informally and openly. Some of the patients and carers knew one another by sight through support groups. Travel expenses and replacement carer expenses were offered and refreshments were provided. All participants gave written consent and completed a simple baseline questionnaire including information on age, gender, educational attainment, subjective well-being and chronic conditions experienced. Although females predominated in all 5 focus groups the male patients were equal contributors. However, the two male GPs were more reticent than their female clinical and nursing colleagues. Respondents were offered a copy of their transcript for the purpose of checking they were still happy for us to use their contribution. Findings were fed back to a multidisciplinary group of health professionals (HP) at an education meeting at the regional hospital.

## Data analysis

A thematic analysis was applied to the fully transcribed focus group transcripts. Familiarisation, data management, coding and categorisation were carried out by the three members of the interdisciplinary research team. Iteration within and between patient, carer and HP data sets and the research literature helped inform the analysis at the explanatory level. Participant attributes such as occupation and gender were mapped and considered during the analysis stage. The principles of framework analysis [24] were used to order, chart and search the data both manually and supported by relevant software (NVivo 9 Software, MSWord and Framework). In particular, attempts were made in the beginning to map findings across existing models of HL but this was found to be difficult and ultimately inappropriate.

# Findings

Building from our starting point of exploring what the concept of HL meant to participants, we present the analysis of our findings under two broad themes: i) the meaning of health literacy for patients and carers, and health professionals; and, ii) health literacy, governance and responsibility. Study findings are presented as both extracts of participants' social interactions [25] and illustrative individual quotes. Extracts are labelled using participant pseudonym (first names for patients and carers, and surnames for HP) and focus group attended. All identifiers have been removed.

## i) The meaning of health literacy

**Patients and carers.** Discussion of the term 'health literacy' was problematic with only one participant across all six focus groups (Nurse Ford in FG6) having any prior knowledge of the concept. Patients and carers had some strong views about the term 'health literacy' with several feeling it was an unhelpful term, too much linked to formal learning and literacy. On several occasions in the non-HP groups participants tried to help each other out as in this exchange between two carers in FG4:

Diane: *I mean you earlier mentioned this word health literacy and I've actually tried to avoid using it because I think it's a very academic term which actually when you say to someone like yourself (Linda) or myself what does it actually mean? I suppose they're now trying to refer to this area about how patients and carers use and understand health information and services and does it make sense to them*

Linda: *Well then understanding about your health like any other literacy uh 'computer literate' means you know how to use a computer so presumably (it's the same)*

When asked to state initial impressions of the term 'health literacy', typical responses from carers and patients concerned comprehension and understanding. These could be at both a very personal and intrinsic level where ill health hindered comprehension, and at a more extrinsic or practical level. This exchange between patients and a carer in FG3 illustrates both levels:

James: *I would like to understand more I must admit and uh that's the difficult bit I have various illnesses um I just can't, sometimes it's completely gobbledygook*

Vivien: *I'm Vivien James's wife and um health literacy to me first of all means understanding how you can get appointments quickly, understanding the forms that come through, also understanding when doctors talk to you and consultants speak. Sometimes they speak very fast because they know what they're speaking about, they use words that you're not always used to and you'd like to very much be able to stop them in full flow and say 'what is this' 'what do you mean?' can you explain'?*

Jill: *I agree with Vivien largely but I think it means understanding my problems and being able to ask questions which over the years I've had my condition now for 18 years I do feel more confident to ask questions*

Being able to follow and adhere to doctor's instructions was another common way patients and carers interpreted the notion of health literacy for others. However for themselves, patients and carers cited the importance of knowing many 'tricks' of the system to more efficiently get their needs met. These tricks ranged from being able to get suitable appointments and ask questions through to the ability to interrogate information and do their own research. Joan and Barbara's in FG2 exchange examples of their expertise in note making:

Joan: *The other thing, after that consultation on Monday, as soon as I got out I wrote down everything she said so that when I go to see the GP in two weeks' time I will remember it*

Barbara: *Well I always write everything down as well because as you say you tend to get in there and you think oh what am I going to ask? So if I write it down I find that very helpful*

Many of our patients had become expert patients over years of living with their chronic conditions (mean = 19 years; range 4–35) and routinely engaged with their health needs. These 'tricks' and skills that had developed over time illustrate increasingly sophisticated competencies (see Nutbeam 2008) and include the ability to interpret and critique healthcare information. Furthermore participants saw themselves as well informed about their own conditions and even able to support friends and family as Barbara again highlights here:

> *I don't know. Because if I I've got anyone close to me that's got something wrong with them I sort of do investigate. But I don't feel your GP tell you exactly what you've got, and how you can cope with it. Is there any preventive cures etc?* (Barbara:FG2)

Patients and carers portrayed the attainment and maintenance of health literacy as an ongoing process. Many described their learning journeys including mistakes made by themselves or HP. Patients often voiced frustration that they were expected to rise to the expectations of the healthcare system and manage inadequate communication rather than the system adapting itself to meet their needs. They implied that for them personally, any lack of HL was a defect in the system, a system that did not give them, or help them, discover and develop the information or skills they need. Also, patients did not suggest that good HL was a one-sided attribute. They often described HL as the result of good two-way communication, particularly between patient and professional, with both sides needing to bring equal interest and skills to the relationship. However, patients were not surprised to be informed that measured HL is lowest among older adults. Many had anecdotes about older friends, family or neighbours who struggled with health management. They cited social isolation as a causal factor, and lack of awareness about choices or rights to access services. There was talk of how chronic illness undermines self-confidence and the risks of dementia were mentioned:

> *I used to go to a bungalow where an old couple lived. She could hardly see at all. They were in their 80's. The chemist would deliver to them a box full of medication and there he was trying to sort his wife's out and his own out getting utterly mixed up and in fact he went by colour. So I used to go in and help him sort out what was what and how many times a day and so on [they were] totally incapable of sorting it.* (Jean:FG1)

**Health Professionals.** Health professionals were quick to grapple with the idea of HL and what it meant in their work. They also saw significant barriers in identifying HL levels including embarrassment and stigma, and described 'gauging' (but not directly asking about) patients understanding and need for information. Most HP had anecdotes about patients whose social needs or literacy shortcomings they had failed to recognise. HP were keen to provide healthcare information at the appropriate level of complexity, but noted it was difficult when patients might not be open if asked 'can you read that okay' as the following extract exemplifies:

> *I had a little lady who nearly starved once. Her elderly brother used to look after her and it wasn't [until] he died, that I realised that she couldn't read. And she couldn't shop, do you know what I mean? You forget you've made assumptions about people's literacy levels all the time.* (Dr Shelley:FG5)

Professionals (and patients) agreed that the best way to identify patient HL needs was by spending enough time talking to patients. HP could see deficits in their own approach to information giving as the following exchange in the primary care professional FG5 reveals. Here the doctors are aware that by comparison much of their own communication and institutional literature is poorly worded and targeted, especially when compared to the way in which the media was able to construct and target an idea:

Dr Gregory: *The literacy level of the information given doesn't match the understanding level of the patient so you can blame the professional instead of the patient.*

Dr Jones: *[Newspapers] always pitch their literacy levels better. I mean that was always something you were aware of and I think they still do, which is why we get so many people coming forward with things that they have understood from their newspaper article but haven't accessed other things that we probably provided.*

Dr Patel: *The moral of that is get them [journalists] to write the health information leaflets.*

Health professionals also identified difficulties in communicating information that went beyond their ability to present information in a clear and accessible manner. In particular they discussed the difficulties posed when patients struggled to understand or accept a diagnosis, or had personal views and preferences about their health management that would preclude acceptance of a diagnosis or treatment. Thus another integral part of health literacy communication was ensuring information is relevant as these exchanges in FG5 illustrate (including when a doctor becomes a patient himself):

Nurse Rowan: *The amount of people that are coming in post op and they don't seem to know how much exercise they can do or when the dressing needs to be changed or … you think they must have been told and they must have had some written information.*

Nurse Castle: *Exactly*

Dr Jones: *But it's whether you think it's applicable to you as well. Cos from uh looking at it from my experience of being a patient, if you're given a leaflet of a certain condition with a grey haired lady on the front, you don't relate to them very well. See what I'm saying? So it's whether you're buying into what you've been given. Even if you can, as you say, even if you can read it and understand the words. If you don't think it's actually applicable because you decide that it's, you know?*

Moderator: *Can you see how someone could not know they're got a heart problem but they are on a heart drug?*

Dr Jones: *Yes yes!*

Dr Gregory: *Very common.*

Dr Gregory: *'Well I've had a heart attack and I've got better hence I haven't got heart disease'.*

Nurse Rowan: *Or, 'It was a bit irregular once but that's sorted out'.*

On the thorny issue of measuring HL and although only given brief attention by HP in these focus group discussions, there was a general (if not fully elaborated) dismissal of using an instruments to measure HL. In the context of the average ten minute appointment in UK primary care such measures were considered impractical due to lack of time and a perceived likely patient reluctance to reveal any literacy problems. Yet incomplete understanding or explanation of instructions was a common problem frustrating to patients and professionals. This is revealed in the following comment about lengthy appointment letters highlighting that communication can break down even before HP and patient meet leading to potential no-shows, underprepared and already confused patients:

> *The appointment letter is two page and they never read the second page. They look at the second page when they get here when we point it out to say they should have bought a clean specimen of urine with them. And they say: 'No, I never got asked to bring that'* (Mrs Robinson: FG6)

Patients, carers and professionals conceptualised and discussed health literacy at both the individual and system level. This key findings will be explored in further detail below. Analysis across the six focus groups found that participant understanding of health literacy could be fostered and facilitated as well as inhibited or challenged at both the system (or structural) and the individual (or agentic) level. The next section addresses participants' views on governance and responsibility for health literacy. Sub-themes are: interpersonal communication; intra-organisational communication and continuity of care; information management; and responsibility for health literacy.

## ii) Health literacy, governance and responsibility

**Interpersonal communication.** A problematic part of healthcare delivery and accessing information was poor interpersonal relationships. Patients identified the importance of communication, continuity and a sense of partnership or personal alliance that could be disrupted by both poor individual practice or by larger organisational obstacle. At the individual level approachable doctors who gave the appearance of having time and invited patients and carers to share in the consultation made a huge difference to how patients described that they felt about getting and comprehending the information they wanted. Something as simple as extra time for their routine appointments was very helpful:

> *One doctor we have always used, when my husband went, always used to book a double appointment. And I invariably went in with him and he would look at me and say 'Have you got any questions today'?* (Rosemary:FG2)
>
> *Dr Chandler was fantastic. He made you feel you were the only patient in the world and discussed everything.* (Michael:FG2)
>
> *There's many occasion [when] they've left the young doctors with us who has explained things and that's helped tremendously.* (Diane:FG3)

Continuity *within* a care sector facilitated good communication and as far as these patients were concerned, the key factor in good HL was effective communication and a relationship with their HP. In other words care could facilitate HL:

> *I believe it starts with the GP. I've experienced both extremes and I had one GP who would say: 'Oh yes, you've got this, take them'. [It] just was 'get rid of you'. The GP I've got now is just the opposite: 'Hello Christina, how are you, sit down, what's the problem'? And then he will tell me all about it and provide me literature on the problem. And you feel then that you want to know more. It's definitely beneficial having a good GP who explains things and makes you feel welcome.* (Christina:FG2)
>
> *Well, if you have a good GP that is the answer. That can answer a whole lot of questions; you don't need to go any further. [A good GP has] communication, interest, knowledge. Dr Sinclair and Dr Russell were both splendid … nothing was too much trouble for them. You know you felt they'd got all the time in world. You knew they hadn't so you weren't foolish enough to think you'd got them for half an hour, but they gave you that feeling that you were of great interest and they wanted to help you.* (Jennifer:FG1)

Stable organisational structures allowing patients to see familiar members of their health team facilitated these 'caring' relationships. However, what is also revealed is how evidently patient health literacy needs might vary, especially if explanations and information are poor or rushed. The issues of continuity and partnership in health, especially around comprehension and adherence to recommended advice could be both difficult to transmit or receive depending on a patient's emotional and physical state as these participants affirm:

*When you're anxious you don't remember things you may be told very clearly* (Jean:FG1)

*They're also at the point of least being able to understand the information that they're presented with because they're most poorly* (Dr Gregory:FG5)

*People are so shocked it's like a mini bereavement when you're diagnosed with rheumatoid arthritis* (Rosemary:FG2)

**Intra-organisational communication and continuity of care.** Continuity *between* care sectors was also regarded as essential to the promotion of health literacy and the experience of lack of continuity and fragmentation exemplified in both community and hospital settings was seen as deleterious to patient understanding, feeling cared for and ultimately use of health services. This concept emerged in the HP discussion too, whether this was because patients never saw the same doctor twice or (as a result of their complex and multi-faceted condition) on referral they saw several consultants from different specialities who did not seem to communicate with each other, or due to terse hospital letters. Lack of a holistic approach and continuity often led to negative clinical outcomes and patient dissatisfaction, typically arising from poor interpersonal and intra-organisational communication. Furthermore, both HP and patients had stories of professionals making erroneous assumptions about what information had previously been given to a patient particularly when these encounters has occurred in another care setting. Patients strongly believed that HP often could not appreciate properly the full range of challenges patients faced because of the wide-ranging impacts of their chronic conditions, or the long term impacts on them as individuals:

*I think it would help more if we saw the same person every time, if possible. Because you go in there and you think, 'Well, do they know all about me?' They haven't had time to read all the information, and I think it would be good if people could see the same person each time.* (Michael:FG2)

This experience of fragmentation both between and within services and concomitant burden placed on individual HP, patients and carers was discussed in all focus groups. Everyone had experience or evidence of 'departments not working together' (Vivien:FG3). Primary care doctors were conscious of the communication void between the two sectors:

*[Patients] often come to ask us what happened and then we've got a [discharge summary] letter with three lines and we try to work out from that what actually happened in hospital* (Dr Gregory:FG5)

For carers this could create a double burden leaving them feeling very isolated:

*I just think everything has become so impersonal so far removed as to make you feel unimportant I suppose. Lost, that's probably another word you feel that you're abandoned ...you're on your own that's how you feel you're on your own."* Diane FG4

However, an example of good practice in secondary care was mentioned in three different groups. It highlights how the practice of patient focused care could enhance patient understanding and sense of wellbeing. Here it is discussed in FG3:

*Vivien: Dr Evans dictates the letter that's going [to the GP] because if you hear anything you say, 'Oh excuse me a moment' and he stops dictating, doesn't he? And he explains and then he sends you a copy of the letter that he's dictated which is fantastic. You've heard it once but, um, the words they use are not always lay words that we would use. He is brilliant like that*

*Flo: That must be very handy I've never had that happen*

*Keith: There's not many people do that, he does it to me too*

**Information management.** Most patients expected to supplement consultations with health professionals with their own endeavours such as searching out written material, media reports, anecdotal research and Internet searches. As the following extracts highlight, they recognised that the deluge of available information often is not helpful or relevant, they wanted to truly understand their condition not read unreliable opinions about it.

*[There are] some very good leaflets ... they're nice and simple and then you've got the internet which is the other extreme where you've got reams and reams and reams of it so somewhere in-between, you know. First of all you know you start off with the general knowledge and you move onto something a bit more (in-depth). You want to be able to find out how it actually affects you personally because we're all different.* (Richard:FG1)

*I also see the other side, of the drivel printed every week [in the tabloid newspaper] which for most parts is very unhelpful at times shall we say.* (Keith, retired HP:FG3)

Similarly, GPs believed that it was their job to act as a conduit or filter to the 'reams of information' available to patients:

*We here get quite a lot of people who actually come with their reams [of information]. I think there are problems with information filtering as well as problems of informing people.* (Dr Shelley:FG5)

However, impersonal information sources alone were not adequate and patients were adamant that the relationship with HP was fundamental to understanding, specifically the caring relationship. Much effort in the HL field has to date gone into simplifying information and instructions. However, our data suggests patients and carers perceived the need for 'layering' of types information but with the key being not the information *per se* but it's delivery mode and context. David in FG1 sums it up as follows:

*Personally I think [a leaflet] should add to what you've been told it shouldn't be instead of; it should be in addition to. So that if something is talked about in the consultation you can take away something and look at it which would then give you more information rather than expecting that information to take the place of the human interaction cos the piece of paper can't look at you and see whether you're stressed, whether it's worrying you.*

These (well engaged) patients tried hard to get expert advice and perspectives, and were mostly willing to accept the limitations of imperfect medical opinion as long as it did not become a barrier. The following exchange in FG2 exemplifies this and highlights a structural determinant governing access to healthcare in the UK where primary care doctors tend to be generalists, while specialists reside in the secondary care hospital setting and are accessed only after referral from primary care:

Rosemary: *So something you said that when you were talking to your GP and talking about your joints. And he basically told you to take pain killers. The GP might not know the difference between rheumatoid or osteo or whatever kind of arthritis*

Barbara: *Which I don't know*

Rosemary: *He's not paid to know. He's paid to see there's a problem and refer you to someone who does know. I think sometimes the GP can be a brick wall, as well*

**Shifting responsibilities in health literacy.** This final sub-theme illustrates a significant debate that permeated these focus group discussions about whose responsibility it was to ensure patients understand and use healthcare services and treatment appropriately. Participants deliberated how roles and responsibilities had shifting from 'doctor knows best' to a situation today where patients were encouraged to be more autonomous. Despite the current political rhetoric in the UK to encourage responsibility and empowerment, older people in particular and for deeply ingrained cultural reasons were deemed to be far less likely to question the doctor or contribute to discussion about their health. Here are just two examples of this common debate:

*I think a lot of old people, especially in their 80's, those sort of age groups, the doctor was the saint and you don't question him.* (Joan:FG2)

*They're afraid you know afraid to ask the doctor because he's more important than they are, more educated than they are. Some don't want to know any further than what's wrong and what tablets they've got give them, but I suppose I'm a bit inquisitive I like to know what things are all about.* (Deborah:FG1)

In terms of health literacy specifically, HP appeared to see the responsibility as theirs and spoke of patients at all levels of HL and their engagement (or lack thereof) with their own health management. The following extract between HP illustrates the complexity of the perceived struggle for patients (and professionals) with too much information, and a resistance to the expectation that they become medical experts:

Dr Shelley: *Maybe you've got to think about, when you take your car into the garage and they start gabbling on, you think: 'I don't care - just sort it'. Well, you're not stupid, but you've got no idea what theymyre talking about.*

Nurse Rowe: *I've had quite a few people who [come back from hospital saying]: 'They said I was to decide'. So then I tend to say to them, 'Well, if they genuinely believed this then that is the emphasis they put and if it was genuinely a choice then that's why they're saying it'. But people are feeling that healthcare professionals are a bit passing the buck.*

Dr Hunter: *Yes, telling them, 'You decide', and then not empowering them or giving them enough information.*

Patients did not advocate a paternalistic style of healthcare delivery, and were critical of peers with little interest in managing their own health. Nor did they advocate a delivery model which gave too much apparent choice or empowerment. Patients perceived that HL was just as much the responsibility of the patient as the professional but the HP had a responsibility to answer questions and impart information in such a way that enhanced health literacy:

*I had one doctor say 'I wonder whether dispensing it prophylactically would help' and I said 'just remind me what prophylactically means'? And she said 'oh I'm worrying you about something that might never happen'. And I said 'never worry about telling patients what you're thinking and what the options are'. We want to know, that helps us to work with you to get the best possible outcome. So I think we've got to play our part.* (Rosemary:FG2)

Furthermore, many patients saw it as a privilege of their role as consumers to choose if or when to be noncompliant. Enhanced health literacy gave them greater moral legitimacy to disagree with diagnosis or disregard recommended treatment:

*How things have changed in the last 20 well even in 5 years. There is so much that we can understand about what we've got and because we understand what we've got to a certain extent we can take responsibility for our own problems. And, well, not decide what drugs we'll take but bend the rules may I say it a little bit.* (Jennifer:FG1)

Our patients and carers saw themselves as their own advocates and described querying details as part of their role especially with medication, including spotting mistakes, but said that this was a challenge for a lot of older people due to persisting cultural perceptions about the doctor:

*[What] patients ought to do is to question whether they still need to take a particular medicine or if you are on 3 or 4 things.* (Richard:FG1)

*Because they believe the doctors are right they believe the doctors are god more or less they think the doctors know everything and so they abide by them but I've had two or three occasions where mistakes have been made on my part and I've lost the centre of my eye because of failure and also given the wrong antibiotics by a doctor.* (Florence:FG3)

However, there was a sense that by taking responsibility and getting involved in decision making patients could potentially threaten their relationship with HP. In contrast, primary care professionals spoke about a recent shift from 'offering choices' or 'option sharing' with patients, to engaging patients in the management of their own care and 'sharing the management'. Even so, there was a concern in both primary and secondary care from HP not knowing how much information it was appropriate to give. Concerns included frightening and/or confusing patients. Primary care HP spoke of their biases or preferences inevitably 'creeping in'. Both patients and professionals described inhibitions relating to asking about understanding: both parties said that older patients could be reticent to ask questions – this was described as a 'generational thing'; HP were anxious about asking if a person understood or could read. Asking about 'illiteracy' and even about understanding was compared to being as challenging as asking about sex.

## Discussion

Initially patients and professionals tended to interpret health literacy fairly narrowly, as compliance to medical treatment or self-directed research. They quickly expanded the concept, linking it to notions of empowerment through knowledge of their own conditions. Our patients, carers and professionals mostly saw HL not as an individual attribute or skill but rather as a result of interaction between patients and the healthcare system. Discussants agreed there was much scope for improved communication between patients and professionals. Patients expressed frustration at the perceived certainty that professionals knew more than they were saying; professionals voiced frustration that patients did not seem to have absorbed what professionals believed had been said or written down. Although patients praised support groups and certain practices, good face-to-face consultation experiences were the most valuable means of improving and maintaining HL. Despite limitations to our findings, patient perspectives were in some ways revelatory. Rather than dwelling on individual assets and skills patients saw HL as a *whole-system outcome*, highly dependent upon good communication, particularly in one-to-one consultations.

Health literacy research has placed emphasis on the individualised assets model while tending to overlook how to improve delivery. However, the need for a switch in emphasis has been advocated by others [26]–[28], and fits well with recent research on HL and shared decision making [29], [30]. That healthcare systems can form barriers to adequate health literacy – particularly in communication, and that professionals need to provide high quality care regardless of low HL has been recognised in practical guidance [10], [31]. A drawback of the traditional risk model is to see HL as prone to inevitable decline over time, especially as increasingly complex conditions develop in the adult lifespan. An alternative within the risk model perspective that allows for a dynamic understanding of HL is to focus on mitigating risk by improving both patient and professional assets (e.g. [32]). We suggest at the simplest level a *needs*-based understanding of HL is required. Just as patients have medical needs, they have needs in terms of skills, self-efficacy and for information to best manage their health related behaviour. These needs vary depending on social, cultural, temporal and medical context. A focus on HL needs can provide the foundations of many other proposed HL models. Rather than describe HL as a set of fixed patient assets across settings, perhaps it is a mismatch between variable assets and fluctuating needs that contributes highly to poor outcomes. A needs approach allows for change over time and for variations depending on patient, context, professional, disease and types of treatment – aspects particularly pertinent to ageing. Diverse approaches to health literacy needs and understanding patient roles have been suggested previously [33]. In practice many HL initiatives are run with more of a need than an asset based understanding. The simplistic functional-interactive-critical divisions for understanding HL [4] are inadequate for capturing the emotional needs and quite variable negotiation and communication skills of patients and professionals, particularly in a shared decision making environment. For instance, Smith et al found that some patients with nominally tested low functional literacy skills exhibited quite well-developed critical literacy skills, whereas some patients with tested high functional HL skills displayed relatively poor interactive or critical HL skills [34]. Other research highlights that patients often fail to fully engage in medical encounters because of perceived power imbalance or expectations that arise from previous social and cultural experiences [35], [36].

The needs-understanding of HL also promotes the value of personal relationships in medical care to make assessments, exchange information and teach skills. This might better be described as care rather than education and could fit better with the needs of an ageing population. These suggestions are sympathetic with Mol [37]. She argues that the apparent empowering model of *choice* is a poor focus in the delivery of healthcare and advice for individuals with chronic conditions. A *logic of choice* places an over-emphasis on empowerment of the patient, dismissing the emotional complexities of managing chronic illness, and the reality that even when individuals are highly informed and perfectly adherent, the nature and progress of their disease may still mean a poor outcome. Instead she advocates an emphasis on care rather than choice for patients with chronic conditions. Others have criticised excessive promotion of healthcare choices and the notion of personal independency or autonomy, arguing that what most patients would like and what would benefit them most, is not to decide for themselves the best treatment option, or to be compelled to go along with the choice determined by the health expert, but rather to know that the default and routine choice will mean excellent care without any need for them to personally apply critical analysis to various options [38], [39]. Although much data on health care quality and options are published and freely available in the UK (e.g., Care Quality Commission or National Institute for Clinical Evidence websites), there are large ethical questions about healthcare systems that expect so much of ill patients [20]. Significant inequalities may also arise because attributes such as knowledge are strongly linked to a patient's socio-economic status.

Nutbeam [4] suggests a deficiency in the HL risk model is its tendency to measure success mostly in terms of adherence. In reality, we argue that most health literacy interventions also consider improvements in awareness, skills and motivation. It should be possible to further widen 'success' in an HL intervention to include quality of communication, patient-led outcomes and quality of care. In applied research it is common to use adherence as a desirable outcome measure for an HL intervention. This is partly because adherence measures are assumed to be simple to consistently observe and describe, and because the relationship between health literacy and adherence is not well-understood, although it has been much discussed [16], [40]. Many health literacy interventions measure success very prominently in terms of adherence to recommended advice [e.g., [23], [41], [42]. As a result, the problems of non-adherence and low HL have become tangled and seemingly endemic despite widespread intervention efforts [43]. Instead, perhaps it should be seen as normal that for a single patient, both HL levels and adherence rates vary by condition and context (an idea also discussed in Nutbeam [44]). Thus it comes as no surprise that HL needs must be assessed continuously and can be expected to fluctuate in inconsistent ways, as it is the product of a joint experience between professionals and patients, each bringing individual and inconsistent skills and investment to the process.

## Limitations and lessons learned

Our participants had a specific interest in long term chronic (particularly musculoskeletal) conditions. Longer or repeat FGD might have elicited different perspectives on the value of HL in their own lives or work. Patients barely mentioned basic reading, numeracy or memory skills, although these deficits were a significant part of HP discussions. Patients could have been more explicitly invited to discuss any difficulties they or peers might have in very basic numeracy and communication skills. A different choice of video presentation might have led to different viewpoints, too.

The focus group patients and carers presented as a relatively knowledgeable group. We did not describe or formally administer an HL instrument, partly because it did not suit our aims of soliciting unguarded opinions. It might have been intimidating or insensitive. A reasonable alternative might have been to incentivise patients (with payment) to take a HL test, and later invite them to participate in FGD. Thus we might have had more success targeting patients whose functional HL levels were more clearly diverse. However, we cannot be sure that those who opted to participate were not still the most engaged and well-informed, or whose critical HL levels might have had little relationship with tested functional skills (following the experience of Smith et al [34]). Similarly, our health professionals were reluctant to ask patients about literacy or numeracy skills for fear of causing offence. HPs might have been less resistant if we had explained assessment methods that are not reading tests. We could have described ways to detect HL deficits using just a few qualitative and non-pejorative questions (eg [45]). However, we suspect that our HPs would still have worried about drawing conclusions from subjective answers as well as insufficient time available within routine appointments (typically around ten minutes with GPs [46]). Time is pressured for those providing secondary health care, too. The British National Health Service (NHS) is publicly funded, providing care for free at the time of use (no co-payments). The NHS is over-stretched in many areas and is widely considered to be under-resourced [47]. There are nonetheless strict targets that hospitals must meet regarding waiting times for patient appointments with many suggested negative consequences for other aspects of care [48]. Hence rapid delivery of service is foremost in the mind of health professionals. Support to assess health literacy is not a target or priority in the current system.

**Recruitment Problems.** We perceive that patients and carers were very engaged with healthcare management and were relatively health literate. As with all research recruitment, we are aware that our sample may not include hard to-reach individuals, including those who do not want to think about their health more than necessary. We suspect that some people are more attracted to the focus group format, while others find it intimidating, inconvenient or uninteresting. Given that engagement is a key ingredient to good HL, we should not be surprised that our FGD patients appeared to have relatively good HL skills. The assertive and engaged atmosphere highlights an inherent shortcoming in using FGD to identify important barriers to improving HL among those most at risk. It is hard to recruit patients with minimal skills or motivation, and previous research has highlighted issues of 'shame' associated with low HL [49,50]. Some self-selection was inevitable and our findings cannot be said to be transferrable to the views of people with the most limited health literacy.

Low recruitment of carers was disappointing. It meant reduced input about HL in the context of providing for the needs of patients with cognitive or physical decline. HL skills among carers should be a particular concern in the context of ageing population profiles.

## Conclusions

It should be possible to integrate elements of both the assets and risk models of HL to produce something that better meets needs. A shift in professional and patient perspectives may be required to reemphasise quality of care rather than informed diversity of choice. The real challenge for qualitative research into HL may be to help clarify the useful purpose of the HL concept, why is it of interest and to whom. As a clinical risk factor it helps to identify communication and support needs. Beyond a fairly basic level, however, the value of the HL concept becomes less clear. It implies but yet is not the same as self-efficacy and empowerment [51], and yet success in HL promotion efforts is often measured in terms of adherence and outcomes. Patients with chronic conditions are increasingly encouraged to develop what might be called interactive or even critical HL skills, hopefully to increase patient autonomy. However, those skills may not increase confidence in recommended treatment. Perhaps not surprisingly in Smith et al. [34], patients invited to be critical of cancer screening options became less likely to choose any form of screening.

All of our participants seemed to prefer shared decision making rather than expect a norm of patient empowerment. We note that however resourceful and autonomous highly health literate patients such as ours might become, clinicians will customarily have more knowledge power due to the science-based nature of medicine [52]. Patients desire predictable interactions and search for more than knowledge, empowerment and responsibility from their engagement with healthcare. As Lupton [53] put it, we seek 'affirmation and re-enactment of cultural, psychodynamic and affective processes (to make) everyday life choices, decisions and actions'. This attendant emotional based trust and desire for, at the very least, reciprocity in healthcare, is not an idealised engagement of two independent rational 'health literate' actors but rather an intersubjective interaction influenced by a variety of human needs and qualities.

## Acknowledgments

We would like to thank Sian Smith and three anonymous reviewers, all our participants and the project Steering Group especially Caroline Ferrari, Benny Harston, Carol Crouch and Carole Williams. Also, thanks to Ina Hinz, Gill Rowlands and David Scott.

### Disclaimer

This paper outlines independent research funded by the NIHR under its Research for Patient Benefit Programme: PB-PG-1207-1524. The views expressed are those of the authors and not necessarily those of the National Health Service, the NIHR or the Department of Health. The funders had no role in study design, data collection and analysis, decision to publish, or preparation of the manuscript.

## Author Contributions

Conceived and designed the experiments: CS LM YL. Performed the experiments: CS LM. Analyzed the data: CS LM JB YL. Wrote the paper: CS JB LM YL.

## References

1. Berkman ND, Davis TC, McCormack L (2010) Health Literacy: What Is It? Journal of Health Communication 15: 9–19.
2. Sørensen K, Van Den Broucke S, Brand H, Fullam J, Doyle G, et al. (2012) Health literacy and public health: a systematic review and integration of definitions and models. BMC Public Health: 80.

3. Pearson A, Saunders M (2009) Health literacy revisited: what do we mean and why does it matter? Health Promotion International 24: 285–296.
4. Nutbeam D (2008) The evolving concept of health literacy. Social Science & Medicine 67: 2072–2078.
5. Jochelson K (2007) Health Literacy: Review Paper. London: National Social Marketing Centre. London. pp. 21.
6. Paasche-Orlow MK, Parker RM, Gazmararian JA, Nielsen-Bohlman LT, Rudd RR (2005) The Prevalence of Limited Health Literacy. JGIM: Journal of General Internal Medicine 20: 175–184.
7. HLS-EU Consortium (2012) Comparative report of health literacy in eight EU member states. The European health Literacy Survey HLS-EU.: Online Publication http://eceuropaeu/eahc/documents/news/Comparative_report_on_health_literacy_in_eight_EU_member_statespdf.
8. Australian Bureau of Statistics (2009) Australian Social Trends Canberra: ABS. cat. no. 4102.4100 p.
9. Baker, Gazmararian JA, Sudano J, Patterson M (2000) The Association Between Age and Health Literacy Among Elderly Persons. The Journals of Gerontology Series B: Psychological Sciences and Social Sciences 55: S368–S374.
10. Nielsen-Bohlman L, Panzer AM, Kindig DA (2004) Health literacy: a prescription to end confusion: National Academies Press.
11. Moser C (1999) Improving literacy and numeracy: a fresh start. Report of the working group chaired by Sir Clause Moser.
12. Nutbeam D (2000) Health literacy as a public health goal: a challenge for contemporary health education and communication strategies into the 21st century. Health promotion international 15: 259–267.
13. Chinn D (2011) Critical health literacy: a review and critical analysis. Social Science & Medicine 73: 60–67.
14. Jordan JE, Osborne RH, Buchbinder R (2011) Critical appraisal of health literacy indices revealed variable underlying constructs, narrow content and psychometric weaknesses. Journal of Clinical Epidemiology 64: 366–379.
15. Collins SA, Currie LM, Bakken S, Vawdrey DK, Stone PW (2012) Health literacy screening instruments for eHealth applications: A systematic review. Journal of biomedical informatics 45: 598–607.
16. Paasche-Orlow MK, Wolf MS (2007) The Causal Pathways Linking Health Literacy to Health Outcomes. American Journal of Health Behavior 31: S19–S26.
17. Berkman ND, Sheridan SL, Donahue KE, Halpern DJ, Crotty K (2011) Low Health Literacy and Health Outcomes: An Updated Systematic Review. Annals of Internal Medicine 155: 97–W41.
18. von Wagner C, Steptoe A, Wolf MS, Wardle J (2009) Health literacy and health actions: a review and a framework from health psychology. Health Education & Behavior 36: 860–877.
19. Baker DW (2006) The meaning and the measure of health literacy. Journal of General Internal Medicine 21: 878–883.
20. Volandes AE, Paasche-Orlow MK (2007) Health literacy, health inequality and a just healthcare system. The American Journal of Bioethics 7: 5–10.
21. Kwan B, Frankish J, Rootman I, Zumbo B, Kelly K, et al. (2006) The development and validation of measures of "health literacy" in different populations. UBC Institute of Health Promotion Research and University of Victoria Community Health Promotion Research.
22. Loke YK, Hinz I, Wang X, Rowlands G, Scott D, et al. (2012b) Impact of health literacy in patients with chronic musculoskeletal disease - systematic review PLoS One
23. Loke YK, Hinz I, Wang X, Salter C (2012) Systematic Review of Consistency Between Adherence to Cardiovascular or Diabetes Medication and Health Literacy in Older Adults. The Annals of pharmacotherapy 46: 863–872.
24. Ritchie J, Lewis J (2003) Qualitative research practice: A guide for social science students and researchers: Sage.
25. Halkier B (2010) Focus groups as social enactments: integrating interaction and content in the analysis of focus group data. Qualitative research 10: 71–89.
26. Raynor DKT (2012) Health literacy. BMJ 344.
27. Kramer G (2013) Health literacy: let's think again. http://wwwhealthorguk/blog/. Scotland: The Health Foundation.
28. Smith SG, Curtis LM, von Wagner C, Wolf MS (2013) Skill Set or Mind Set? Associations between Health Literacy, Patient Activation and Health. PLoS One.
29. Entwistle VA, Cribb A, Watt IS (2012) Shared decision-making: enhancing the clinical relevance. JRSM 105: 416–421.
30. McCaffery KJ, Smith SK, Wolf M (2010) The challenge of shared decision making among patients with lower literacy: a framework for research and development. Medical Decision Making 30: 35–44.
31. Weiss BD, Schwartzberg JG (2007) Health literacy and patient safety: Help patients understand: manual for clinicians: AMA Foundation.
32. Al Sayah F, Williams B (2012) An Integrated Model of Health Literacy Using Diabetes as an Exemplar. Canadian Journal of Diabetes 36: 27–31.
33. Smith SK, Dixon A, Trevena L, Nutbeam D, McCaffery KJ (2009) Exploring patient involvement in healthcare decision making across different education and functional health literacy groups. Social science & medicine 69: 1805–1812.
34. Smith SK, Nutbeam D, McCaffery KJ (2013) Insights into the concept and measurement of health literacy from a study of shared decision-making in a low literacy population. Journal of health psychology.
35. Joseph-Williams N, Edwards A, Elwyn G (2014) Power imbalance prevents shared decision making. BMJ: British Medical Journal 348.
36. Protheroe J, Brooks H, Chew-Graham C, Gardner C, Rogers A (2013) 'Permission to participate?'A qualitative study of participation in patients from differing socio-economic backgrounds. Journal of health psychology 18: 1046–1055.
37. Mol A (2008) The logic of care: Health and the problem of patient choice: Routledge.
38. Kmietowicz Z (2004) Doctors condemn" patient choice" initiative as no real choice at all. BMJ: British Medical Journal 329: 14.
39. Entwistle VA, Carter SM, Cribb A, McCaffery K (2010) Supporting patient autonomy: the importance of clinician-patient relationships. Journal of general internal medicine 25: 741–745.
40. Lindquist LA, Go L, Fleisher J, Jain N, Elisha Friesema BA C (2012) Relationship of health literacy to intentional and unintentional non-adherence of hospital discharge medications. Journal of general internal medicine 27: 173–178.
41. Gazmararian J, Jacobson KL, Pan Y, Schmotzer B, Kripalani S (2010) Effect of a pharmacy-based health literacy intervention and patient characteristics on medication refill adherence in an urban health system. Annals of Pharmacotherapy 44: 80–87.
42. Sheridan SL, Halpern DJ, Viera AJ, Berkman ND, Donahue KE, et al. (2011) Interventions for individuals with low health literacy: a systematic review. Journal of health communication 16: 30–54.
43. Wroe AL (2002) Intentional and unintentional nonadherence: a study of decision making. Journal of behavioral medicine 25: 355–372.
44. Nutbeam D (2009) Defining and measuring health literacy: what can we learn from literacy studies? International Journal of Public Health 54: 303–305.
45. Chew LD, Griffin JM, Partin MR, Noorbaloochi S, Grill JP, et al. (2008) Validation of screening questions for limited health literacy in a large VA outpatient population. Journal of General Internal Medicine 23: 561–566.
46. Deveugele M, Derese A, van den Brink-Muinen A, Bensing J, De Maeseneer J (2002) Consultation length in general practice: cross sectional study in six European countries. Bmj 325: 472.
47. Appleby R, Crawford R, Emmerson C (2009) How cold will it be? Prospects for NHS funding: 2011–2017.
48. McCann L, Granter E, Hassard J, Hyde P (2014) " You can't do both-something will give": limitations of the targets culture in managing UK healthcare workforces. Human resource management.
49. Wolf MS, Williams MV, Parker RM, Parikh NS, Nowlan AW, et al. (2007) Patients' shame and attitudes toward discussing the results of literacy screening. Journal of Health Communication 12: 721–732.
50. Easton P, Entwistle VA, Williams B (2013) How the stigma of low literacy can impair patient-professional spoken interactions and affect health: insights from a qualitative investigation. BMC health services research 13: 319.
51. Schulz PJ, Nakamoto K (2013) Health literacy and patient empowerment in health communication: The importance of separating conjoined twins. Patient Education and Counseling 90: 4–11.
52. Salter B (2004) The new politics of medicine: Palgrave Macmillan.
53. Lupton D (2012) Medicine as culture: illness, disease and the body: Sage.

22

# Prospects of mHealth Services in Bangladesh: Recent Evidence from Chakaria

**Fatema Khatun[1,2,3]*, SMA Hanifi[1], Mohammad Iqbal[1], Sabrina Rasheed[1], M. Shafiqur Rahman[1,4], Tanvir Ahmed[1], Shahidul Hoque[1], Tamanna Sharmin[1], Nazib Uz Zaman Khan[1], Shehrin Shaila Mahmood[1], David H. Peters[5], Abbas Bhuiya[1]**

**1** International Centre for Diarrhoeal Disease Research, Bangladesh (icddr,b), 68 Shaheed Tajuddin Ahmed Sarani, Mohakhali, Dhaka-1212, Bangladesh, **2** School of Public Health and Community Medicine, The University of New South Wales, Kensington, New South Wales 2052, Australia, **3** Asia-Pacific ubiquitous Healthcare Research Centre, School of Information Systems, Technology and Management, Australian School of Business, The University of New South Wales, Kensington, New South Wales 2052, Australia, **4** Institute of Statistical Research and Training, University of Dhaka, Dhaka-1000, Bangladesh, **5** Department of International Health, The Johns Hopkins Bloomberg School of Public Health, 615 N. Wolfe Street, Baltimore, Maryland 21205, United States of America

## Abstract

***Introduction:*** Bangladesh has a serious shortage of qualified health workforce. The limited numbers of trained service providers are based in urban areas, which limits access to quality healthcare for the rural population. mHealth provides a new opportunity to ensure access to quality services to the population. A recent review suggested that there are 19 mHealth initiatives in the country. This paper reports findings on people's knowledge, perception, use, cost and compliance with advice received from mHealth services from a study carried out during 2012–13 in Chakaria, a rural sub-district in Bangladesh.

***Methods:*** A total of 4,915 randomly-chosen respondents aged 18 years and above were interviewed.

***Results:*** Household ownership of mobile phones in the study area has increased from 2% in 2004 to 81% in 2012; 45% of the respondents reported that they had mobile phones. Thirty-one percent of the respondents were aware of the use of mobile phones for healthcare. Very few people were aware of the available mHealth services. Males, younger age group, better educated, and those from richer households were more knowledgeable about the existing mHealth services. Among the respondents who sought healthcare in the preceding two weeks of the survey, only 2% used mobile phones for healthcare. Adherence to the advice from the healthcare providers in terms of purchasing and taking the drugs was somewhat similar between the patients who used mobile phone for consultation versus making a physical visit.

***Conclusions:*** The high penetration of mobile phones into the society provides a unique opportunity to use the mHealth technology for consulting healthcare providers. Although knowledge of the existence of mHealth services was low, it was encouraging that the compliance with the prescriptions was almost similar for advice received through mobile phone and physical visits. The study revealed clear indications that society is looking forward to embracing the mHealth technology.

**Editor:** Natalie Walker, The National Institute for Health Innovation, New Zealand

**Funding:** This research study was funded by Department for International Development (DFID), grant number_ DFID/PO: 5457. The funder had no role in study design, data collection and analysis, decision to publish, or preparation of the manuscript.

**Competing Interests:** The authors have declared that no competing interests exist.

* Email: kfatema@icddrb.org

## Introduction

Bangladesh continues to be one of the 57 countries with a serious shortage of trained doctors, paramedics, nurses and midwives despite attempt for increased production in the recent years [1]. Bangladesh Health Watch reported in 2008 that there were only three physicians and two nurses per 10,000 population [2]. The presence of the limited number of qualified service providers is highly urban-centred, with 86% of the physicians; and 75% of the nurses and dentists are based in urban areas where only 20% of the population lives [2]. Rural health service delivery is dominated by informally-trained village doctors and drug-sellers practicing modern medicine. Contact rate with qualified health-care providers is low and highly inequitable in terms of socioeconomic status of the patients and place of residence [3]. The first port of call for the poor is the informally trained village doctors and drug retailers who make their living by selling drugs. They quite often use more than necessary and inappropriate drugs for treating patients [3,4]. Thus for the shortage of qualified healthcare providers and their geographic mal-distribution, access to quality healthcare by the people in general and the disadvantaged section of people in particular is constrained. Given the current level of production of trained health workforce, it is very unlikely that the situation will change drastically in the near future.

Under these circumstances, the use of Information and Communication Technology (ICT), e.g.mobile phone connectivity provides a new opportunity to increase access to quality healthcare for the population [5,6]. A recent review of the growth of mHealth services in Bangladesh documented 19 initiatives involving mHealth services from call centres sending messages from health authorities to subscribers. Details of these initiatives can be seen elsewhere [7]. Making optimum use of the ICT will depend on the development of appropriate programmes informed by research on peoples' perception about the use of ICT and mobile phone, and making use of the feedback from the user on the existing services. A continuous monitoring of the change in perception about quality and adequacy of the service, along with problems faced by the people in accessing and using the services will help further improve the existing services. Despite the potential of this technology in providing healthcare services, a systematic assessment of the people's knowledge of, attitude about, and use of mobile phone and mHealth services has been lacking in the literature. Keeping this in mind this paper presents findings from a survey on mobile phone and mHealth which was carried out in a rural area of Bangladesh. It is expected that the findings will be useful in improving the existing ones and designing new programmes.

## Methods and Materials

### Study Area

The study was carried out in eight unions of Chakaria upazilla (sub-district), under Cox's Bazar district in the south-east costal area of Bangladesh where icddr,b has been running a Health and Demographic Surveillance System (HDSS) since 1999 [8]. The surveillance covers 118,335 residents living in 20,124 households. The population density is 782 individuals/km$^2$, considerably lower than national average of 939/km$^2$. The population comprises mainly Muslims (90%), a small number of Hindus (7%), and Buddhists (3%). The Bangalees constitute 99% of the households, and others are from an ethnic minority group called *Mogh* (*Rakhain*). The main economic activities in the area have been agriculture, forestry and sea-fishing. Typographically Chakaria is similar to other coastal areas in Chittagong district but different than rest of the country. Chakaria is a relatively low-performing area in terms of health and development indicators compared to areas of the central and western part of the country [9].

The availability of health services in the area is typical of other rural areas with public and private healthcare services with a very strong presence of informal healthcare providers [10]. icddr,b has been working with a selected number of communities since 1994 mainly in the area of primary healthcare with direct involvement in running six village health posts established and managed by the community. The icddr,b healthcare providers also have been available for consultations through mobile phones for the last 10 years. The government services included an upazilla health complex as the highest level of primary care, with seven family welfare centres, one rural dispensary, 14 community clinics at the lowest level [8]. There are three private clinics with the facility of general surgery [10]. During the study period, the villagers had access to mHealth services offered by a private company at the national level, which allowed consultation from physicians in the call centres. In addition, the government physicians of the upazilla health complex were also available for consultation through mobile phones. There was also a special service from Telemedicine Referral Centre Limlited, a private call centre, for a selected group of village doctors who participated in an icddr,b programme for the improvement of quality of their services [11].

### Study design

A total of 62,459 household members aged 18 years and above living in 20,124 households in Chakaria HDSS area in November 2012 formed the sampling frame for the survey. Because of unequal distribution of the population by both age and sex [8], a stratified sampling scheme with proportional allocation was employed to determine the sample-size for the survey. Stratification was done by separating males and females based on the age groups: 18–29, 30–39, 40–49, and 50 completed years and above. In the absence of any data on the level of knowledge about mobile phone based consultation services, a value of 50% was used for calculating sample-size separately for males and females for each of the age-groups, to have a reliable estimate of proportion of respondents having knowledge, using the services, and having a positive attitude towards mHealth with 95% confidence. This gives 384 (approximately 400) samples for each group. The sample-size from each of the age groups was calculated by using the sampling fraction (400/population of the age-group with lowest population size) multiplied by number of population in the age-group. This has resulted in a sample of 400 or more number of respondents in each age-group, with a total of 5152 respondents. Finally one respondent from each household was randomly chosen from the HDSS database. This sampling design has made the total sample self-weighted, making data analysis straight forward.

Data were collected by using a questionnaire developed in Bangla language which was duly pretested before finalization. Most of the questions had the provisions of recording pre-coded and open answers. Fifteen experienced female interviewers were recruited for the survey and were given a three day training on the survey questionnaire. Two experienced supervisors looked after the data-collection process. For quality control of the data collection, the supervisors re-visited 5% of the households chosen randomly within 2 days of data collection by the field workers to recollect data on some of the key questions. The supervisors and the relevant field workers together sorted out any inconsistencies in the collected data immediately making additional field visits if required. The survey was conducted during November 2012 to April 2013.

### Ethical consideration

Ethical Review Committee of the International Centre for Diarrhoeal Disease Research, Bangladesh provided approval for the project. Informed written consent was taken from all interviewees, and confidentiality and anonymity were ensured.

### Variables

The questionnaire included background characteristics of the respondents, ownership of mobile -phones, knowledge about the use of mobile phone for health care, various mHealth services, care seeking, cost of health care, preference between physical visit and telephone consultation, attitude toward mHealth, satisfaction with health care consultation through mobile phone, and socio-economic and demographic characteristics of individuals and households.

### Data analysis

Different answers to open-ended questions for all variables were listed, and every answer was assigned a numerical code for computer entry and processing. Exploratory analysis of data including summary statistics, graphs, and cross tabulation was carried out. For each proportion, 95% confidence interval (CI) was calculated based on exact binomial distribution. In some cases, test for statistical significance (parametric or non-parametric when required) was performed.

## Results

The survey team could successfully interview 1,964 male and 2,951 female respondents through repeated visits. Males were hard to reach for interviews for their absence in the household during daytime;- three repeated visits were made to minimize the rate of non-response. Finally, 89.8% males and 99.6% females could be interviewed.

### Characteristics of the respondents

The background characteristics of the respondents are presented in Table 1. The distribution of the background characteristics of the respondents is somewhat similar to that of the population aged 18 years and above in the study area [8] with an exception for distribution of sex.

### Ownership of mobile phone

In the survey area, 45.5% of the respondents reported that they had a mobile phone (Table 2). 81% of the households had at least one phone. Data from the HDSS, independent of the present survey, recorded a steady increase in household ownership of mobile phones from 2% in 2004 to 81% in 2012 (Figure 1). The ownership of mobile phone was higher among males, younger age-groups, people from richer households, and the more-educated persons compared to females, those who were over 50 years of age, people from poorer households, and people with no education (Table 2).

### Knowledge of use of mobile phone for healthcare

In the study area, 31% (1,537) of the total respondents reported that they knew that mobile phone is being used for healthcare. Among the respondents who knew about the use of mobile phone for healthcare, knowledge about the use of mobile phone for healthcare was higher among males (39%) than females (26%) (Table 3). Only 1% knew about health helpline/call centres. Respondents perceived that the more educated and knowledgeable people tended to use mobile phone for healthcare compared to the less educated and less knowledgeable people.

### Knowledge of existing mHealth services

In terms of knowledge of the existing mHealth services very few people were aware of the services available through upazilla health complex, an initiative of the Ministry of Health or availability of special call centre numbers to call for health care (Table 4). Males, younger age- group, the better educated, and those from richer households were more knowledgeable about the existing mHealth services compared to females, those who were over 50 years of age, those who had no education and people from the poorest households (Table 4).

### Use of existing mHealth services

In terms of the actual use of mHealth services, only 11% of the respondents who knew about mHealth services actually called special numbers/call centres to seek treatment and no one actually used the mHealth services provided by upazila health complex (Table 5). Males and those from the richest households reported seeking mHealth services more than the females and those from the poorest households. Interestingly, in terms of education of the respondents, the difference was not evident (Table 5).

### Use of mobile phone and mHealth services for healthcare

Table 6 presents data on healthcare-seeking behaviour of the household members included in the survey in the case of sickness

**Table 1.** Characteristics of respondents.

| Characteristics | % of the total respondents N = 4,915 | 95%CI |
|---|---|---|
| *Age (years)* | | |
| <30 | 36.4 | (34.8–37.5) |
| 30–39 | 27.3 | (25.9–28.4) |
| 40–49 | 16.2 | (15.0–17.1) |
| 50+ | 20.1 | (18.8–21.1) |
| *Sex* | | |
| Male | 39.9 | (38.6–41.3) |
| Female | 60.0 | (58.7–61.4) |
| *Occupation* | | |
| Household | 46.8 | (45.4–48.2) |
| Formal employment and business | 9.2 | (8.4–10.1) |
| Farming | 6.2 | (5.5–6.9) |
| Menial labour | 22.1 | (20.9–23.3) |
| Unemployed | 15.7 | (14.7–16.7) |
| *Education (years of schooling)* | | |
| None | 48.1 | (46.7–49.5) |
| 1–5 | 29.3 | (28.0–30.6) |
| 6+ | 22.6 | (21.4–23.8) |

**Table 2.** Ownership of mobile phone by background characteristics.

| Characteristics | Number of respondents | % of respondents having a mobile phone | 95% CI | Statistical significance |
|---|---|---|---|---|
| *Sex* | | | | p = 0.000 |
| Male | 1964 | 61.76 | (59.6–63.9) | |
| Female | 2951 | 34.40 | (32.7–36.1) | |
| *Age (years)* | | | | p = 0.000 |
| <30 | 1791 | 49.92 | (47.6–52.3) | |
| 30–39 | 1344 | 56.10 | (53.4–58.8) | |
| 40–49 | 794 | 43.70 | (40.2–47.2) | |
| 50+ | 986 | 23.63 | (21.0–26.4) | |
| *Asset quintile* | | | | p = 0.000 |
| Poorest | 1005 | 19.20 | (16.8–21.7) | |
| 2 | 973 | 35.97 | (32.9–39.1) | |
| 3 | 1002 | 48.10 | (44.9–51.2) | |
| 4 | 954 | 53.88 | (50.7–57.1) | |
| Richest | 981 | 70.23 | (67.3–73.1) | |
| *Education (years of schooling)* | | | | p = 0.000 |
| None | 2335 | 31.31 | (29.4–33.2) | |
| 1-5 | 1462 | 51.98 | (49.4–54.6) | |
| 6+ | 1112 | 66.10 | (63.2–68.8) | |
| Total | 4915 | 45.33 | (43.9–46.7) | |

during two weeks preceding the day of data collection. Total population in the respondents' households was 26,591 at the time of the survey;. 37.7% (10,026/26,591) of the household members had a sickness during two weeks preceding the survey. For 46.83% (4,695/10,026) of those who were sick a contact with a healthcare provider was made. The most contacted healthcare provider was village doctor (57.4%) followed by village homeopath (16.5%), MBBS doctor (15.7%), trained paramedic (7.9%) and *kabiraj/ hujur* (2.4%). Based on the sample of one randomly-chosen patient per household from those who contacted a healthcare provider (2,581 patients), it was estimated that 1.9% (50 patients) contacted a provider, using a mobile phone, and 98.1% had a face-to-face consultation. Use of mobile phone was more for female (2.4%) patients than male (1.4%) in all age groups in contacting a healthcare provider for consultation. The highest use of mobile phone (2.3%) was recorded for under-five children, followed by age-group 18+ (2.1%); and the lowest use (0.9%) was observed for the 6–17 years age-group. Cold-and-fever was one of the main sicknesses for which almost half of the patients (23) contacted a doctor, using mobile phone, followed by diarrhoea (4) and indigestion (3) (Figure 2). Use of mobile phone was the highest for contacting a village doctor (58.2%), followed by an MBBS doctor (36.5%), icddr,b doctors and paramedics (4.2%), and homoeopaths (2.1%).

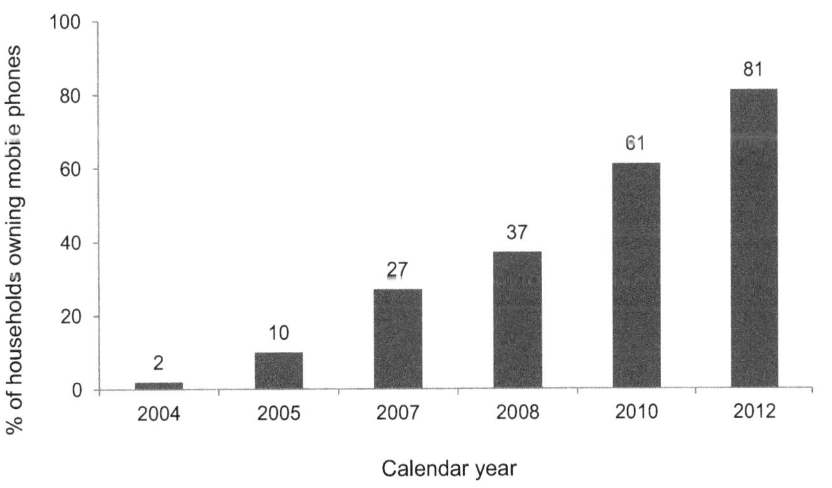


**Figure 1. Household mobile phone ownership.**

**Table 3.** Awareness about the use of mobile phone for health care services.

| Nature of awareness | % based on the respondents who knew about the service (N = 1,537) | 95% CI |
|---|---|---|
| *Possible uses of mobile phone in health care:* | | |
| Direct consultation | 79.9 | (77.8–81.9) |
| Appointment | 11.8 | (10.2–13.5) |
| Knowing availability | 4.6 | (3.6–5.8) |
| Clarification about prescription | 3.2 | (2.4–4.2) |
| Requesting home visit | 0.5 | (0.2–0.9) |
| *How people use mobile phone for health care?* | | |
| To call MBBS doctor | 69.5 | (67.1–71.8) |
| To call village doctor | 27.4 | (25.2–29.7) |
| To call helpline | 0.9 | (0.4–1.4) |
| To call hospital/clinic | 0.7 | (0.3–1.2) |
| SACMO/MA/CHCP | 0.1 | (0.01–0.4) |
| Others | 1.4 | (0.8–2.1) |
| *Perception about who uses mHealth services:* | | |
| Educated/knowledgeable | 44.2 | (41.7–46.7) |
| Upper class | 11.1 | (9.5–12.7) |
| Middle class | 5.3 | (4.2–6.5) |
| Lower class | 4.5 | (3.5–5.6) |
| Who has connection with health care providers | 24.0 | (21.9–26.2) |
| Employed/busy people | 2.3 | (1.5–3.2) |
| All types of people | 7.9 | (6.6–9.3) |
| Others | 1.8 | (1.2–2.5) |

SACMO = Sub-Assistant Community Medical Officer.
MA = Medical Assistant.
CHCP = Community Health Care Provider.

## Cost of healthcare

The median cost of treatment per patient based on all patients totaling 1886 who sought care was Taka (Tk) 150, with an interquartile range (IQR) of Tk 370 (US$ 1 = Tk 78). There was no differences in cost by sex but there was a significant difference by age ($p<0.01$), with higher cost for children under age five years, and older age groups compared to younger groups (Tk 160, Tk 100, and Tk 160 for under-five children, for those aged 6–17 years, and 18 or more years respectively). Although the difference in cost by the nature of consultation though was not statistically significant, the cost was higher in face-to-face consultations compared to consultation through mobile phone (Tk 150 versus Tk 124). Of the 2,581 patients for whom a face-to-face contact with a healthcare provider was made, 71% received advice for drugs. 87% of those who received advice for drugs bought all the drugs, 12% bought some, and 1% did not buy any. Of those who contacted a provider through a mobile phone, 68% had received advice for drugs. Of them, 88% bought all the drugs and 12% did not buy all of the drugs. Sixty-four percent of the patients who consulted using a mobile phone took all the prescribed drugs compared to 75% of those who had face-to-face consultations (Table 7).

## Intention to use mHealth services

Although the actual use of mHealth services was quite low, 29% of the respondents intended to use mHealth in the future (Table 8). Males, more educated persons, and people from richer households intended to use mHealth in the future more than females, those with no schooling and those from poorer households.

## Reasons for using mobile phone

Thirty percent of the respondents wanted to use mobile phone for seeking healthcare because of low cost, followed by time-saving (24%), instant treatment (18%), acquaintance with doctor (10%), when disease is severe (8%), no transportation cost (6%) and other causes (4%) (Table 9).

## Reasons for not using mobile phone

Forty-one percent of respondents reported that they did not want to use mobile phone for healthcare because they thought direct consultation was better, followed by not knowing which number to call (22%), not being able to explain symptoms to doctor over phone (13%), not feeling the need to use mobile phone as doctor's chamber was nearby (9%), not having ideas about availing healthcare through mobile phone (5%), and perceiving that mobile phone consultation cannot replace physical examination (3%) (Table 9).

## Discussion

The findings reflect many important aspects of mHealth services in Bangladesh including their prospects and challenges. To make the best use of the opportunity this technology offers, the potential and challenges should be well- understood to maximize the opportunity in settings similar to Bangladesh. This study focused

**Table 4.** Knowledge of existing mHealth services.

| Variable | N | Percent of respondents who knew about the existing services | | | |
|---|---|---|---|---|---|
| | | Special number % (95% CI) | Statistical significance | Upazila Health Complex % (95% CI) | Statistical significance |
| Existence of mHealth services | 4,915 | 3.9 (3.3–4.4) | | 5.0 (4.4–5.7) | |
| *Sex* | | | p = 0.00 | | p = 0.000 |
| Male | 1,964 | 7.0 (5.9–8.2) | | 7.6 (6.5–8.9) | |
| Female | 2,951 | 1.7 (1.3–2.3) | | 3.2 (2.6–3.9) | |
| *Age (years)* | | | p = 0.000 | | p = 0.000 |
| <30 | 1,791 | 6.7 (5.6–7.9) | | 6.3 (5.2–7.5) | |
| 30–39 | 1,344 | 3.4 (2.5–4.5) | | 4.3 (3.3–5.5) | |
| 40–49 | 794 | 2.1 (1.3–3.4) | | 6.3 (4.7–8.2) | |
| 50+ | 986 | 0.7 (0.3–1.5) | | 2.3 (1.5–3.5) | |
| *Education (years of schooling)* | | | p = 0.000 | | p = 0.000 |
| None | 2,335 | 1.4 (0.97–2.0) | | 2.7 (2.1–3.4) | |
| 1–5 | 1,462 | 2.1 (1.4–2.9) | | 4.7 (3.7–5.9) | |
| 6+ | 1,112 | 11.2 (9.4–13.2) | | 10.8 (9.0–12.7) | |
| *Asset quintile* | | | p = 0.000 | | p = 0.000 |
| Lowest | 1,004 | 0.1 (0.0–0.6) | | 2.5 (1.8–3.9) | |
| 2 | 973 | 1.4 (0.8–2.4) | | 2.2 (1.3–3.3) | |
| 3 | 1,002 | 1.8 (1.1–2.8) | | 3.4 (2.4–4.7) | |
| 4 | 954 | 3.1 (2.04–4.3) | | 4.3 (3.1–5.8) | |
| Highest | 981 | 12.9 (10.9–15.2) | | 12.5 (10.4–14.7) | |

on finding what may prevent people from using mobile phone services for healthcare, and to identify customers' interests in using mobile phones if the opportunity to use these for healthcare is expanded. To our knowledge this is the first study that systematically explored these aspects of mHealth in rural Bangladesh.

About 80% of the households own a phone, in this impoverished society; it is actually quite impressive and, thus mHealth has the potential to reach a larger portion of the population. The introduction of mobile phones in Bangladesh is not that old perhaps 10 years. The disturbing fact, though expected, is the high level of socioeconomic and gender inequality in the ownership. However, it should be mentioned that although ownership of

**Table 5.** Calling of the mHealth services.

| Variable | Number of respondents who knew about the special number | % of respondents called special number (95% CI) | Statistical significance |
|---|---|---|---|
| Ever called | 189 | 11.6 (7.4–17.1) | |
| *Sex* | | | p = 0.044 |
| Male | 138 | 14.5 (9.1–21.5) | |
| Female | 51 | 3.9 (0.5–13.5) | |
| *Education (years of schooling)* | | | p = 0.612 |
| None | 33 | 12.1(3.4–28.2) | |
| 1–5 | 31 | 6.5 (0.8–21.2) | |
| 6+ | 125 | 12.8 (7.5–19.9) | |
| *Asset quintile* | | | p = 0.830 |
| Poorest | 01 | 0.0(–) | |
| 2 | 14 | 7.1 (0.18–33.8) | |
| 3 | 18 | 5.6 (0.14–27.3) | |
| 4 | 29 | 10.3 (2.9–27.4) | |
| Richest | 27 | 13.4 (8.0–20.5) | |

**Table 6.** Health seeking behavior during sickness.

| Variable | Denominator | % | 95% CI |
|---|---|---|---|
| Sickness during two weeks preceding the survey | 26,591 | 37.70 | (37.1–38.3) |
| Contact with any healthcare provider | 10,026 | 46.83 | (45.8–47.8) |
| Types of healthcare provider contacted: | 4,695 | 100.0 | |
| Village doctor | | 57.44 | (56.0–58.8) |
| Homoeopath | | 16.55 | (15.5–17.6) |
| MBBS | | 15.70 | (14.7–16.8) |
| Trained paramedic | | 7.86 | (7.1–8.7) |
| Traditional (kabiraj/hujur) | | 2.45 | (2.3–2.9) |
| Use of mHealth services/mobile phone for healthcare | 2,581 | 1.93 | (1.4–2.5) |

phones ensures convenience of access to services, not owning one does not necessarily mean that members of these households are in all that disadvantageous position when there is a need to use one. Availability of shops and entrepreneurs selling mobile phone call services is abundant in Bangladesh. The 'Phone Lady' was one such initiative which comprises a woman of Grameen Bank borrower who runs a business of selling mobile phones airtime to customers in a flexible manner in terms of timing and physical availability of the services. The 'Phone Lady' has the arrangement of going to the client's households at the request of the customer, helping to ensure almost universal access to mobile phones in Bangladesh however remote or poor is the household. The gender differential in ownership may be a real hindrance in seeking healthcare for females and shows the same pattern of gender differentials against females in healthcare-seeking prevalent in this society. Globally, women are 21% less likely to own a mobile phone than men and this gender disadvantage is the highest in South Asia, followed by sub-Saharan Africa [12]. In Kenya, disparities exist in mobile phones ownership with respect to gender, age, education, literacy, urbanization and poverty [13,14]. The negative relationship between age of the respondents with the ownership should be a lesser problem in terms of restrictive access by the older members of the household because the inherent age hierarchy is in favour of seniors in this society. The higher rate of mobile phone ownership among younger members of a household also means that younger generation is more inclined to modern technology that clearly indicates the future demand of this technology and the potential it has. So is the case for education of respondents for the future generation will be more educated.

The use of mobile phones for health services is dependent on whether people are aware of this aspect of this technology. The low level of knowledge about the use of mobile phone for health services and the perception that only a small proportion of villagers use these can be one of the contributory factors in the low use of mobile phone for healthcare or mHealth services. The findings that educated and upper-class people use these services set this as an aspirational target for the others which is also indicative of a potential large future demand for the use of mobile for health and mHealth services. The higher use of mobile phones for contacting a healthcare provider in case of a female than male patient reflects the influence of the cultural factor that limits female mobility in this rural area; females are only taken out for healthcare when all other options are exhausted.

Although various mHealth services have been in place for quite some time, the level of knowledge about their existence has been low. This is also a factor contributing to the low level of use of the services from the private and public sectors. It is a prerequisite that the availability of these services be widely known for increasing the use of the services.

The high level of contacting village doctors clearly indicates the continuation of dominance of informal health care providers in delivering services to the people in this community. Thus, special mHealth services targeted to these groups of healthcare providers are likely to derive maximum benefit for the people in this community. The favorable environment for the use of mobile phone/mHealth in terms of many advantages has also been reflected in an in-depth investigation recently carried out in the study area [4].

The similar level of compliance with advice received from a face-to-face consultation versus consultation through the use of mobile phone or mHealth indicates the equal value the study population gives to both types of consultation. This is very encouraging and clearly indicates the potential the mobile phone and mHealth service has in ensuring quality services to the people. Therefore, it is evident that the respondents valuing consultation through mobile phones and mHealth has started to earn peoples' trust. It should however be mentioned that the lower cost of consultation though mobile phone compared to face-to-face consultation does not imply the absence of financial barrier because the cost of mobile telemedicine is very high for the rural

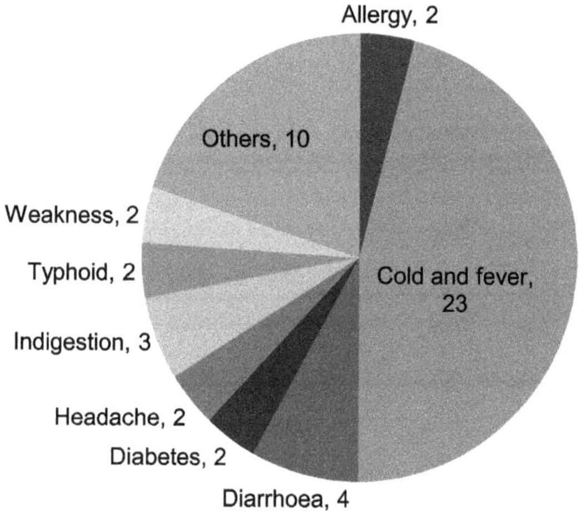


**Figure 2. Distribution of patients who contracted doctors using mobile phone by type of disease.**

**Table 7.** Cost of treatment by background characteristics.

| Variable | Median | IQR | Number of respondents who contacted doctor | Statistical significance |
|---|---|---|---|---|
| *Sex* | | | | *p = 0.40 |
| Male | 150 | 357 | 869 | |
| Female | 150 | 380 | 1017 | |
| *Age (years)* | | | | **p = 0.0001 |
| ≤5 | 160 | 244 | 397 | |
| 6–17 | 100 | 210 | 306 | |
| 18+ | 160 | 450 | 1183 | |
| *Way of contact* | | | | *p = 0.09 |
| Mobile | 124 | 248 | 41 | |
| Face-to-face | 150 | 257 | 1845 | |

*Based on Mann-Whitney non-parametric test;
**Kruskal-Wallis rank test [for compliance with prescription]; IQR = Interquartile range.

areas compared to the per-capita income in Bangladesh [15]. There is a need to find ways to reduce the cost of mHealth services in Bangladesh to ensure access for the poor and the disadvantaged population. Toll free mHealth services or free services for people who are in low socioeconomic condition would be one of the options for enhanced uptake [16,17].

The intention to use mHealth or mobile phone for health services in the future is another indication of the future demand that the use of mobile phone and mHealth has. The findings showed that nearly 70% of the respondents prefer calling a doctor by using a mobile phone for either low cost or time-saving or instant advice. These heavily weigh in favour of future large demand for this technology for healthcare. The major reasons cited by the respondents for not intending to use mHealth services for health care was their belief that direct visits were better than consulting remotely; they comprised only 40% of the respondents. The other reasons has the potential to be appropriately dealt with in favour of mobile phone or mHealth. Our findings are also in line with Akter et al. 2010 who also found that patients' perceived service quality had a strong significant impact on satisfaction and intention to continue usage [18].

The study findings have important implications for designing future mHealth programme in Bangladesh and elsewhere. It should be mentioned that despite encouraging findings from this study in favour of mHealth, the services cannot replace traditional services involving face-to-face consultation; mHealth should rather be viewed as a complimentary mechanisms where trained heath workforce is unavailable or absent. Given the weak health system and lack of awareness about mHealth services, it is now evident that strategy to dissemination of the importance and availability of mHealth is crucial. Success of mHealth will depend on the quality of the services, cost, broadening the service components, which is possible with the recent introduction of 3G in the country. It is important to have regular monitoring of the reach, quality, cost and effectiveness of mHealth services on the use of healthcare and health of the population. Policy-makers can use findings from this and other studies to institute appropriate policy measures to

**Table 8.** Intention to use mHealth in the future.

| Variable | Number of respondents | % of respondents | 95% CI | Statistical significance |
|---|---|---|---|---|
| Has intention to call in the future | 4,081 | 28.5 | (27.1–29.1) | |
| *Sex* | | | | p = 0.000 |
| Male | 1,729 | 33.6 | (31.4–35.0) | |
| Female | 2,352 | 24. 6 | (22.9–26.7) | |
| *Education (years of schooling)* | | | | p = 0.000 |
| None | 1,791 | 21.6 | (18.7–22.5) | |
| 1–5 | 1,271 | 27.1 | (24.7–29.7) | |
| 6+ | 1,013 | 42.4 | (39.3–45.5) | |
| *Asset quintile* | | | | p = 0.000 |
| Lowest | 744 | 17.6 | (14.9–20.5) | |
| 2 | 796 | 23.4 | (20.5–26.5) | |
| 3 | 832 | 26.7 | (23.7–29.8) | |
| 4 | 833 | 30.8 | (27.7–34.1) | |
| Highest | 876 | 41.7 | (38.4–45.1) | |

**Table 9.** Reasons for calling/not calling doctor for future sickness with mobile phones (First answer reported).

| Reasons for calling a doctor for future sickness with mobile phones (N = 1,161) | Percentage (95% CI) | Reasons for not calling a doctor for future sickness with mobile phones (N = 2,919) | Percentage (95% CI) |
|---|---|---|---|
| Low cost | 28.94 (26.3–31.6) | Don't know which number to call | 21.7 (20.2–23.2) |
| Saves time | 23.83 (21.4–26.4) | No idea about health care through mobile | 5.39 (4.6–6.3) |
| Instant treatment | 17.94 (15.7–20.2) | Feel shy talk to male doctor | 0.42 (0.21–0.71) |
| No transportation cost | 6.42 (5.4–7.9) | Doctor's chamber is nearby | 9.45 (8.4–10.6) |
| Doctor is known | 9.76 (8.8–11.6) | Doctor does not receive the call | 0.63 (0.36–0.97) |
| Disease is severe | 8.18 (6.7–9.9) | Direct consultation is better | 40.67 (38.3–42.5) |
| Can get treatment at home | 1.14 (0.6–1.9) | Don't have mobile phone | 2.87 (2.3–3.5) |
| To know the presence of doctor in chamber | 2.20 (1.5–3.3) | Can't explain the medical condition | 13.27 (12.1–14.5) |
| Others | 1.58 (0.9–2.4) | Can't take physical examination | 3.29 (2.7–4.0) |
| | | Can get treatment, not medicine | 0.74 (0.47–1.2) |
| | | Others | 1.62 (1.2–2.1) |

enhance access, utilization and effectiveness of mHealth in a country like Bangladesh.

In conclusion, the environment is quite favorable to the use of mobile phone for healthcare and or mHealth. It is indicative of the potential this technology-based platform has in providing quality healthcare services to the mass people, especially in settings where there is shortage and/or unavailability of trained health workforce. However, it is important to have regulatory framework and monitoring system in place to ensure accountability and quality of services.

## Acknowledgments

icddr,b gratefully acknowledges the following donors which provide unrestricted support to its research efforts: Australian Agency for International Development (AusAID), Government of the People's Republic of Bangladesh, Canadian International Development Agency(-CIDA), Swedish International Development Cooperation Agency (Sida), and Department for International Development, UK (DFID). We acknowledge Dr. Md. Mahabubur Rahman, Mohammad Nahid Mia, Amena Sultana and Ashish Paul for field implementation and data management.

## Author Contributions

Conceived and designed the experiments: AB MI SMAH FK SR TA SSM MSR SH TS NZK. Performed the experiments: MI TA SH. Analyzed the data: AB SMAH MSR. Contributed reagents/materials/analysis tools: AB SMAH MSR. Wrote the paper: AB SMAH MSR FK. Critical review, input and revision of the manuscript: AB FK SMAH MSR DHP. Critical review and final approval of the manuscript: AB SMAH MSR FK TA MI SR SH TS NZK SSM DHP.

## References

1. World Health Organization (2007) WHO Bangladesh Country Cooperation Strategy 2008–2013. Dhaka, Bangladesh World Health Organization.Country office for Bangladesh.
2. Bangladesh Health Watch (2008) The state of health in Bangladesh 2007: Health workforce in Bangladesh; Who constitutes the healthcare system?. Dhaka, Bangladesh.
3. Mahmood SS, Iqbal M, Hanifi SM, Wahed T, Bhuiya A (2010) Are 'Village doctors' in Bangladesh a curse or a blessing? BMC International Health Human Rights 3: 10–18.
4. Bhuiya A, Iqbal M (2013) Use of mHealth to improve the quality of services of the village doctors Recent learning from Chakaria, Bangladesh. Dhaka, Bangladesh International Centre for Diarrhoeal Disease Research, Bangladesh.
5. United Nations foundation & Vodafone foundation (2009) mHealth for Development: The opportunity of mobile technology for healthcare in developing world.
6. The Earth Institute at Columbia University, Promise. M, (UNDP). TUDP (2010) Millennium villages project The impact of mobile connectivity on the Millennium Development Goals in Africa.
7. Ahmed T, Bloom G, Iqbal M, Lucas H, Rasheed S, et al. (2014) E-health and M-Health in Bangladesh: Opportunities and Challenges. Brighton, UK: Institute of Development Studies.
8. Hanifi SMA, Rasheed S, Mamun AA, Urni F, Hoque S, et al. (2011) Chakaria Health and Demographic Surveillance System Focusing on the Poor and Vulnerable. Mohakhali, Dhaka 1212, Bangladesh. ICDDR, B.
9. National Institute of Population Research and Training (NIPORT), MEASURE Evaluation (2011) Bangladesh Demographic and Health Survey.
10. Bhuiya A, editor (2009) Health for the rural masses: insights from Chakaria: International Centre for Diarrhoeal Disease Research, Bangladesh.
11. Wahed T, Rasheed S, Bhuiya A (2012) Doctoring the Village Docotrs. Dhaka, Bangladesh: Iternational Centre for Diarrhoeal Disease Research, Bangladesh.
12. GSMA Development Fund, Cherie Blair Foundation for Women&Vital Wave Consulting (2010) Women & Mobile: A Global Opportunity. A Study on the Mobile Phone Gender Gap in Low and Middle-Income Countries. London: GSMA, London.
13. Wesolowski A, Eagle N, Noor AM, Snow RW, Buckee CO (2012) Heterogeneous mobile phone ownership and usage patterns in Kenya. PLoS One 7: e35319.
14. Zurovac D, Otieno G, Kigen S, Mbithi AM, Muturi A, et al. (2013) Ownership and use of mobile phones among health workers, caregivers of sick children and adult patients in Kenya: cross-sectional national survey. Global Health 9: 20.
15. Ivatury G, Moore J, Bloch A (2009) A doctor in your pocket: Health hotlines in developing countries,Innovations: Technology, Governance & Globalization. MIT Press Journal (online) 4: 119–153.
16. Huq NL, Koehlmoos TP, Azmi AJ, Quaiyum MA, Mahmud A, et al. (2012) Use of mobile phone: Communication barriers in maternal and neonatal emergencies in rural Bangladesh. International Journal of Sociology and Anthropology 4.
17. Mobile Alliance for Maternal Action (MAMA) Reaches Moms and Babies in 22 Countries with Critical Health Information.
18. Akter S, D'Ambara J, Ray P. User Perceived Service Quality of mHealth Services in Developing Countries; 2010 6–9 June; Pretoria, South Africa.

# Permissions

All chapters in this book were first published in PLOS ONE, by The Public Library of Science; hereby published with permission under the Creative Commons Attribution License or equivalent. Every chapter published in this book has been scrutinized by our experts. Their significance has been extensively debated. The topics covered herein carry significant findings which will fuel the growth of the discipline. They may even be implemented as practical applications or may be referred to as a beginning point for another development.

The contributors of this book come from diverse backgrounds, making this book a truly international effort. This book will bring forth new frontiers with its revolutionizing research information and detailed analysis of the nascent developments around the world.

We would like to thank all the contributing authors for lending their expertise to make the book truly unique. They have played a crucial role in the development of this book. Without their invaluable contributions this book wouldn't have been possible. They have made vital efforts to compile up to date information on the varied aspects of this subject to make this book a valuable addition to the collection of many professionals and students.

This book was conceptualized with the vision of imparting up-to-date information and advanced data in this field. To ensure the same, a matchless editorial board was set up. Every individual on the board went through rigorous rounds of assessment to prove their worth. After which they invested a large part of their time researching and compiling the most relevant data for our readers.

The editorial board has been involved in producing this book since its inception. They have spent rigorous hours researching and exploring the diverse topics which have resulted in the successful publishing of this book. They have passed on their knowledge of decades through this book. To expedite this challenging task, the publisher supported the team at every step. A small team of assistant editors was also appointed to further simplify the editing procedure and attain best results for the readers.

Apart from the editorial board, the designing team has also invested a significant amount of their time in understanding the subject and creating the most relevant covers. They scrutinized every image to scout for the most suitable representation of the subject and create an appropriate cover for the book.

The publishing team has been an ardent support to the editorial, designing and production team. Their endless efforts to recruit the best for this project, has resulted in the accomplishment of this book. They are a veteran in the field of academics and their pool of knowledge is as vast as their experience in printing. Their expertise and guidance has proved useful at every step. Their uncompromising quality standards have made this book an exceptional effort. Their encouragement from time to time has been an inspiration for everyone.

The publisher and the editorial board hope that this book will prove to be a valuable piece of knowledge for researchers, students, practitioners and scholars across the globe.

# List of Contributors

**Jocelyn R. Wilder, Michael Z. David, Robert Daum and Diane S. Lauderdale**
The Department of Health Studies, The University of Chicago, Chicago, Illinois, United States of America

**Duane T. Wegener,**
The Department of Psychology, The Ohio State University, Columbus, Ohio, United States of America

**Charles Macal**
The Department of Health Studies, The University of Chicago, Chicago, Illinois, United States of America
Decision and Information Sciences Division, Argonne National Laboratory, Argonne, Illinois, United States of America

**Teresa Leonardo Alves, Auramarina F. Martins de Freitas and Aukje K. Mantel-Teeuwisse**
World Health Organization Collaborating Centre for Pharmaceutical Policy and Regulation, Utrecht Institute for Pharmaceutical Sciences (UIPS), Utrecht University, Utrecht, The Netherlands

**Martine E. C. van Eijk**
Independent Consultant, Utrecht, The Netherlands

**Bart Victor**
Owen Graduate School of Management, Vanderbilt University, Nashville, Tennessee, United States of America
Vanderbilt Institute for Global Health, Vanderbilt University, Nashville, Tennessee, United States of America

**Meridith Blevins**
Vanderbilt Institute for Global Health, Vanderbilt University, Nashville, Tennessee, United States of America
Department of Biostatistics, Vanderbilt University School of Medicine, Nashville, Tennessee, United States of America

**Ann F. Green**
Vanderbilt Institute for Global Health, Vanderbilt University, Nashville, Tennessee, United States of America

**Elisée Ndatimana and Lázaro Gonzá lez-Calvo**
Friends in Global Health, Maputo, Mozambique

**Edward F. Fischer**
Vanderbilt Center for Latin American Studies and Department of Anthropology, Vanderbilt University, Nashville, Tennessee, United States of America

**Alfredo E. Vergara,**
Department of Preventive Medicine, Vanderbilt University School of Medicine, Nashville, Tennessee, United States of America
Vanderbilt Institute for Global Health, Vanderbilt University, Nashville, Tennessee, United States of America
US Centers for Disease Control and Prevention, Maputo, Mozambique

**Sten H. Vermund and Troy D. Moon**
Vanderbilt Institute for Global Health, Vanderbilt University, Nashville, Tennessee, United States of America
Department of Pediatrics, Vanderbilt University School of Medicine, Nashville, Tennessee, United States of America
Friends in Global Health, Maputo, Mozambique

**Omo Olupona**
World Vision International, Maputo, Mozambique

**Sherwin I. DeSouza, Agalya P. Vasanthi, Suchitha Maria Joseph and Rashmi Rodrigues**
St. John's National Academy of Health Sciences, Bangalore, India

**M. R. Rashmi**
St. John's National Academy of Health Sciences, Bangalore, India
Department of Community Medicine, Saveetha Medical College, Thandalam, Chennai, Tamil Nadu, India

**Jessica Y. Lee**
Department of Pediatric Dentistry, School of Dentistry, University of North Carolina at Chapel Hill, Chapel Hill, NC, United States of America
Department of Health Policy and Management, UNC Gillings School of Global Public Health, University of North Carolina at Chapel Hill, Chapel Hill, NC, United States of America

**Kimon Divaris**
Department of Pediatric Dentistry, School of Dentistry, University of North Carolina at Chapel Hill, Chapel Hill, NC, United States of America
Department of Epidemiology, UNC Gillings School of Global Public Health, University of North Carolina at Chapel Hill, Chapel Hill, NC, United States of America

**Darren A. DeWalt**
School of Medicine and Cecil G. Sheps Center for Health Services Research, University of North Carolina at Chapel Hill, Chapel Hill, NC, United States of America

**A. Diane Baker and William F. Vann, Jr.**
Department of Pediatric Dentistry, School of Dentistry, University of North Carolina at Chapel Hill, Chapel Hill, NC, United States of America

**Ziya Gizlice**
Center for Health Promotion and Disease Prevention, University of North Carolina at Chapel Hill, Chapel Hill, NC, United States of America

**R. Gary Rozier**
Department of Health Policy and Management, UNC Gillings School of Global Public Health, University of North Carolina at Chapel Hill, Chapel Hill, NC, United States of America

**Meskerem Abate**
Sabian Health Centre, Dire Dawa Health Office, Dire Dawa, Ethiopia

**Nega Assefa and Tadesse Alemayehu**
College of Health and Medical Sciences, Haramaya University, East Harerge, Ethiopia

**Abdul Rashid**
Department of Public Health Medicine, Penang Medical College, Georgetown, Penang, Malaysia

**Azizah Ab Manan, Noorlia Yahya and Lailanor Ibrahim**
Penang State Health Department, Georgetown, Penang, Malaysia

**Kyoko Miura**
School of Public Health and Social Work, Faculty of Health, Queensland University of Technology, Kelvin Grove, Queensland, Australia
Cancer and Population Studies Group, QIMR Berghofer Medical Research Institute, Herston, Queensland, Australia

**Gavin Turrell**
School of Public Health and Social Work, Faculty of Health, Queensland University of Technology, Kelvin Grove, Queensland, Australia

**Ji-Yeon Shin**
Department of Preventive Medicine, School of Medicine, Eulji University, Daejeon, Republic of Korea

**Hye Young Shim and Jae Kwan Jun**
National Cancer Control Institute, National Cancer Center, Goyang, Republic of Korea

**Qiuli Zhao, Li Yang, Xiao Zhang, Xuemei Zhu, Qingqing Zuo, Liu Yang, Wei Gao, Minghui Li and Shanshan Cheng**
School of Nursing, The 2nd Affiliated Hospital of Harbin Medical University, Harbin Medical University, Harbin, China

**Yanni Wu**
Department of Nursing department, The 2nd Affiliated Hospital of Harbin Medical University, Harbin Medical University, Harbin, China

**Tommy Tsz Man Hung, Vico Chung Lim Chiang and Regina Lai Tong Lee**
School of Nursing, The Hong Kong Polytechnic University, Hung Hom, Kowloon, HKSAR

**Angela Dawson**
Health Services and Practice, Faculty of Health, University of Technology, Sydney, Australia

**Showket Hussain, Vilas Nasare and Mausumi Bharadwaj**
Division of Molecular Genetics & Biochemistry, Institute of Cytology & Preventive Oncology (ICMR), Noida, Uttar Pradesh, India

**Malasha Kumari**
Division of Clinical Oncology, Institute of Cytology & Preventive Oncology (ICMR), Noida, Uttar Pradesh, India

**Shashi Sharma**
Division of Biostatistics & Epidemiology, Institute of Cytology & Preventive Oncology (ICMR), Noida, Uttar Pradesh, India

**Mohammad Aijaz Khan**
Division of Behaviour Oncology, Institute of Cytology & Preventive Oncology (ICMR), Noida, Uttar Pradesh, India

**Bhudev C. Das**
Division of Molecular Oncology, Institute of Cytology & Preventive Oncology (ICMR), Noida, Uttar Pradesh, India

**Christiane Montag, Laura Haase, Martin Bayerl and Jürgen Gallinat**
Charité University Medicine Berlin (Charité Universitätsmedizin Berlin), Department of Psychiatry and Psychotherapy, Campus Mitte, Berlin, Germany

**Dorothea Seidel**
Charité University Medicine Berlin (Charité Universitätsmedizin Berlin), Department of Psychiatry and Psychotherapy, Campus Mitte, Berlin, Germany
Weissensee School of Art (Kunsthochschule Berlin-Weißensee), Art Therapy Department, Berlin, Germany

**Uwe Herrmann and Karin Dannecker**
Weissensee School of Art (Kunsthochschule Berlin-Weißensee), Art Therapy Department, Berlin, Germany

**Dong-Hee Kim**
Department of Nursing, College of Nursing, Pusan National University, Yangsan, Gyeongsangnamdo, South Korea

**Hak Sun Yu**
Department of Parasitology, School of Medicine, Pusan National University, Yangsan, Gyeongsangnamdo, South Korea
Immunoregulatory therapeutics group in Brain Busan 21 project, Busan, South Korea

**Muhammad Ashraf Majrooh, Seema Hasnain, Javaid Akram and Arif Siddiqui**
Allama Iqbal Medical College, Lahore, Pakistan

**Zahid Ali Memon**
Population Survives International - Greenstar, Karachi, Pakistan

**Darren Flynn, Nick Steen and Richard G. Thomson**
Institute of Health and Society, Newcastle University, Newcastle upon Tyne, United Kingdom

**Gary A. Ford and Helen Rodgers**
Institute for Ageing and Health (Stroke Research Group), Faculty of Medical Sciences, Newcastle University, Newcastle upon Tyne, United Kingdom

**Christopher Price**
Wansbeck General Hospital, Northumbria Healthcare NHS Foundation Trust, Ashington, United Kingdom

**Uhana Seifert Guimarães Suga, Raquel Sano Suga Terada, Adriana Lemos Mori Ubaldini, Mitsue Fujimaki, Renata Corrêa Pascotto**
Department of Dentistry, State University of Maringá, Maringá, Brazil

**Adelia Portero Batilana and Ricardo Pietrobon**
Department of Surgery, Duke University Medical Center, Durham, North Carolina, United States of America

**João Ricardo N. Vissoci**
Department of Surgery, Duke University Medical Center, Durham, North Carolina, United States of America
Department of Medicine, Faculdade Ingá, Maringá, Brazil

**Clarissa G. Rodrigues**
Department of Surgery, Duke University Medical Center, Durham, North Carolina, United States of America
Instituto de Cardiologia do Rio Grande do Sul - Fundação Universitária de Cardiologia (IC-FUC), Porto Alegre, Brazil

**Farah Seedat, Sally Hargreaves and Jonathan S. Friedland**
International Health Unit, Section of Infectious Diseases and Immunity, Commonwealth Building, Hammersmith Campus, Imperial College London, London, United Kingdom

**Wendy T. M. Pots**
University of Twente, Department of Psychology, Health & Technology, Enschede, the Netherlands
Dimence, Community Mental Health Center, Almelo, the Netherlands

**Peter A. M. Meulenbeek**
University of Twente, Department of Psychology, Health & Technology, Enschede, the Netherlands
GGNET, Community Mental Health Center, Warnsveld, the Netherlands

**Martine M. Veehof and Ernst T. Bohlmeijer**
University of Twente, Department of Psychology, Health & Technology, Enschede, the Netherlands

**Jorinde Klungers**
GGNET, Community Mental Health Center, Warnsveld, the Netherlands

**Ernestina Coast, Eleri Jones and Samantha R. Lattof**
Department of Social Policy, London School of Economics and Political Science, London, United Kingdom

**Anayda Portela**
Department of Maternal, Newborn, Child and Adolescent Health, World Health Organization, Geneva, Switzerland

**Charlotte Salter, Julii Brainard, Lisa McDaid and Yoon Loke**
Norwich Medical School, Faculty of Medicine & Health Sciences, University of East Anglia, Norwich, NR4 7TJ, United Kingdom

**Fatema Khatun**
International Centre for Diarrhoeal Disease Research, Bangladesh (icddr,b), 68 Shaheed Tajuddin Ahmed Sarani, Mohakhali, Dhaka-1212, Bangladesh
School of Public Health and Community Medicine, The University of New South Wales, Kensington, New South Wales 2052, Australia
Asia-Pacific ubiquitous Healthcare Research Centre, School of Information Systems, Technology and Management, Australian School of Business, The University of New South Wales, Kensington, New South Wales 2052, Australia

**SMA Hanifi, Mohammad Iqbal, Sabrina Rasheed, Tanvir Ahmed, Shahidul Hoque, Tamanna Sharmin, Nazib Uz Zaman Khan, Shehrin Shaila Mahmood and Abbas Bhuiya**
International Centre for Diarrhoeal Disease Research, Bangladesh (icddr,b), 68 Shaheed Tajuddin Ahmed Sarani, Mohakhali, Dhaka-1212, Bangladesh

**M. Shafiqur Rahman**
International Centre for Diarrhoeal Disease Research, Bangladesh (icddr,b), 68 Shaheed Tajuddin Ahmed Sarani, Mohakhali, Dhaka-1212, Bangladesh
Institute of Statistical Research and Training, University of Dhaka, Dhaka-1000, Bangladesh

**David H. Peters**
Department of International Health, The Johns Hopkins Bloomberg School of Public Health, 615 N. Wolfe Street, Baltimore, Maryland 21205, United States of America

# Index